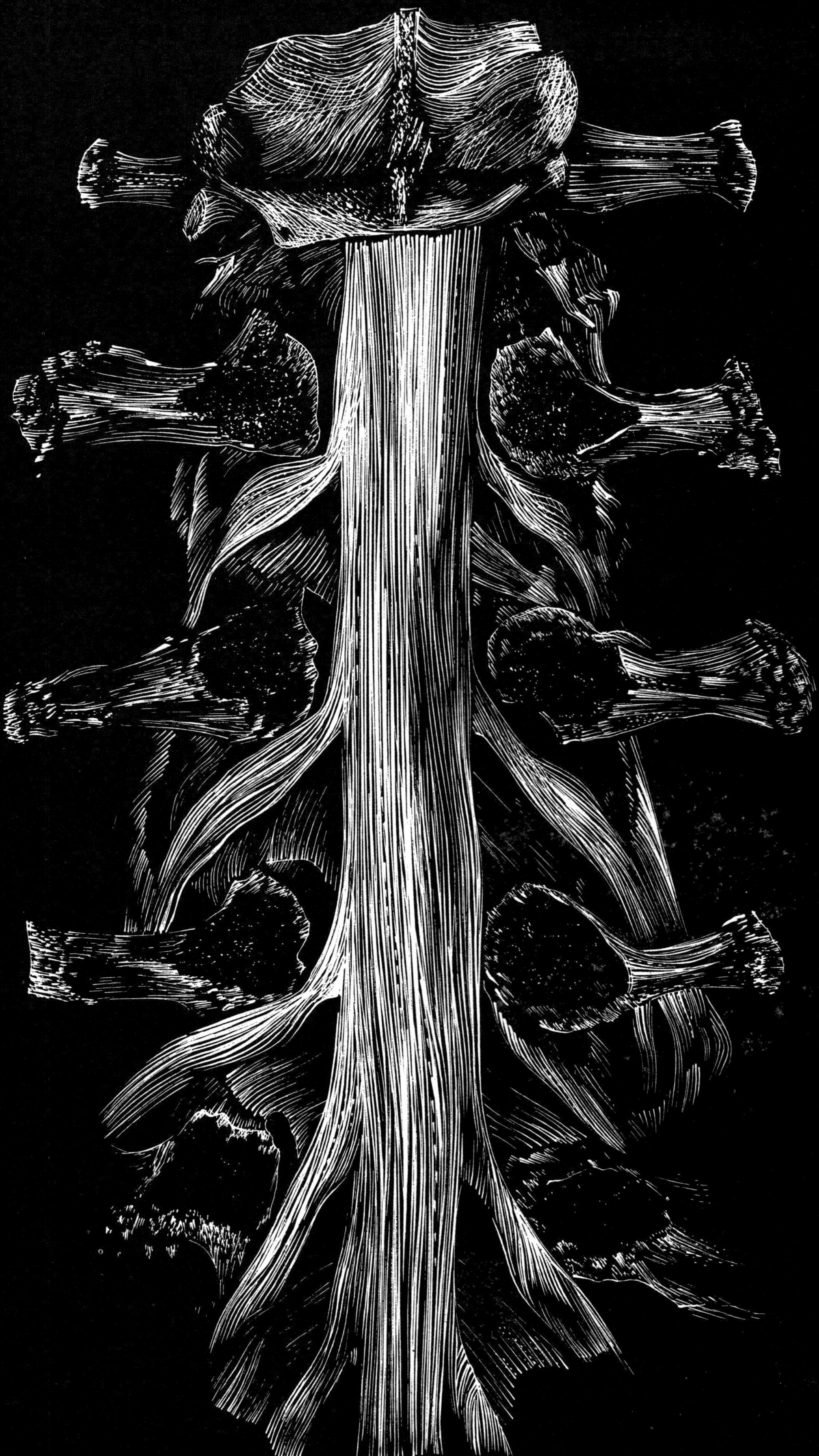

Henry V. Crock

Practice of Spinal Surgery

With a Contribution on
The Management of Spinal Injuries
by Sir George Bedbrook

Springer-Verlag
Wien New York

Henry Vernon Crock, M.D., M.S., F.R.C.S., F.R.A.C.S.
Senior Orthopaedic Surgeon, St. Vincent's Hospital, University of Melbourne, Australia

Sir George Bedbrook, Hon.M.D. (Perth), M.S. (Melbourne), F.R.C.S., F.R.A.C.S.
Senior Orthopaedic Surgeon, Royal Perth Hospital, Western Australia

Printed in Austria by Manzsche Buchdruckerei, A-1090 Wien

With 234 partly coloured Figures

Frontispiece: From a wood-block by the artist Tate Adams, based on a dissection of the lumbar spine prepared by Dr. Carmel Crock.

Library of Congress Cataloging in Publication Data. Crock, Henry Vernon. Practice of Spinal Surgery. Bibliography: p. Includes index. 1. Spine–Surgery. 2. Spine–Wounds and injuries. I. Bedbrook, Sir George. II. Title. [DNLM: 1. Spine–Surgery. 2. Intervertebral disk–Surgery. WE 725 C938p.] RD533.C76. 1983. 617'.375. 83-465

ISBN 3-211-81738-7 Springer-Verlag Wien-New York
ISBN 0-387-81738-7 Springer-Verlag New York-Wien

Foreword

It is not long since surgery of the spine dealt with fracture-dislocation and tuberculosis, little else. With the advent of contrast X-ray and anatomical study a wide range of disease entities has been categorized and become the subject of corrective and ameliorative treatment.

The principal author of the present book has played a distinguished part in widening knowledge of the anatomy of the bones, ligaments, blood vessels, neural features and the natural history of diseases relevant to hard structure disorder. He has done this in relation to the development of highly refined surgical techniques based strictly upon structural requirements in relation to the disease processes under treatment. The result is a comprehensive account of his integrative conceptualisation and the relevant principles of the methods used. His component, the major part of the book, is in the tradition of John Hunter, Bland Sutton, Kanavel and others who improved their understanding and treatment by the discipline enforced by the discipline of basic investigation. In the era of proliferation of specialties and books of single author chapters it is refreshing to meet one man's mind extended.

By Sir George Bedbrook adding the fruits of his years of experience and thought about the treatment of spinal injury the book is enriched. As the best of two investigative practitioners, it reflects the best features of the surgical calling and should be studied not only for its material but especially for its reflection of high professional endeavour.

Melbourne, June 1983

Professor Emeritus Sir Douglas Wright
Chancellor, University of Melbourne

Preface

In writing this book I have attempted to prepare a document which may prove of practical use to surgeons in what I see as a phase of transition in spinal surgery.

This book will be published nearly fifty years after Mixter and Barr's historic description of intervertebral disc prolapse–an entity now in eclipse.

Since the mid 1950s emphasis has moved to the more common problems of spinal canal and nerve root canal stenosis–the latter being caused in some cases by quite a different form of disc disease–isolated disc resorption.

Let us not forget that there are two laboratories from which progress in medicine may emanate: the laboratory of the field–clinical practice, the chief investigator being the busy practitioner; and the other–laboratories of our great medical scientific institutions.

In this book I have attempted to focus attention on a particular clinical problem described in Chapters 2 and 7 as Internal Disc Disruption. I believe that the study of the histochemistry and immunology of internal disc disruption presents a formidable challenge for science in the 1980s. This is a challenge which will only be met effectively by the joint efforts of clinicians who recognize this disabling entity and who can provide fresh disc tissues from their patients for analysis and study by those qualified to identify biochemical abnormalities in living tissues.

Perhaps that will be the direction of the next leap forward.

Melbourne, June 1983 *Henry V. Crock*

Acknowledgements

This book is based on experience gained in the past twenty years in busy practice and in orthopaedic research carried out at St. Vincent's Hospital, in the University of Melbourne. I am deeply grateful to the Sisters of Charity for their help in supporting my work.

During that time it has been my pleasure to have many visiting international fellows work with me, to all of whom I express my thanks. Among this group I single out for special thanks:

Dr. S. Sihombing (Indonesia), Professor P. R. Chari (India), Dr. S. K. Kame (India), Dr. A. Fujimaki (Japan), Mr. Robert Venner (Scotland).

Dr. H. Yoshizawa (Japan), co-author of one of my books, has continued to inspire me.

I wish to thank my orthopaedic colleagues throughout Australia, especially from Tasmania, who have referred many difficult cases on which my clinical experience has been built. Many of my ideas on the nature of intervertebral disc disorders evolved during my association with a remarkable physician, the late Dr. Joseph Silver Collings, to whose memory I wish to pay homage.

The following surgeons have kindly given me illustrations for use in this book; Messrs. B. J. Dooley, J. Cloke, B. Davie, C. Haw, J. K. Henderson, and K. Mills.

Experience with the use of special surgical techniques such as those required for anterior interbody fusion operations, can only be acquired slowly, with help from anaesthetists, general and thoracic surgeons. I thank my anaesthetic colleagues for their patience, Drs. E. Kenny, J. Forster, W. Stanisich, I. Sutherland, and D. Taylor who, from his vantage point at the head of the operating table, has designed an excellent retractor for use during these operations.

I am deeply indebted to the following general surgeons; Messrs. P. K. Steedman, I. Vellar, B. Collopy, J. L. Connell, and the late E. Ryan. I wish to thank Messrs. J. K. Clarebrough and A. Wilson for teaching me the principles of thoracic surgery applied to spinal operations.

 Acknowledgements

For permission to reproduce material from my earlier publications, I am indebted to:

1. The Medical Journal of Australia, Sydney.
2. Journal of Bone and Joint Surgery, London.
3. Clinical Orthopaedics and Related Research, Philadelphia.
4. Revue de Chirurgie Orthopédique, Paris.
5. North Holland Publishing Co., Amsterdam.
6. Butterworths, London.

The Frontispiece was prepared by Tate Adams of Melbourne, one of the greatest living woodblock artists. The author's portrait on the jacket was drawn by Louis Kahan, an old family friend.

Most of the drawings in this book have been prepared by Dayle Howat. I thank him sincerely for his splendid work.

A number of drawings have been prepared by one of my international Fellows, Dr. Hideki Matsuda from Osaka, Japan. He has inherited an artistic talent from his father, a talent which he put to good use on my behalf. I thank him sincerely for his contributions.

Mr. Bob Morton, of LaTrobe Studios, Pty. Ltd., Melbourne, has helped with colour printing.

For help in the maintenance of my laboratory at St. Vincent's Hospital, I thank particularly Mr. Laurie McMahon and Mr. Fred Green.

Mr. Dennis Cahill, chief technician in the Pathology Department at the University of Melbourne, has prepared many excellent histological slides for me, and for Mr. Miron Goldwasser, one of my co-research workers.

Financial support for this work has come from many sources. I thank, in particular, Mr. R. A. Chappell, Mr. Peter Norris, and Mr. H. D. T. Williamson. I thank also the Trustees of the William Angliss Charitable Trust, the William Buckland Foundation, the Hecht Trust, the National Trustees and Executors Agency, and the Rowden White Trust.

To my colleagues in Paris, Professor Jean Cauchoix and Dr. J. Zucman, I express particular thanks for their help in translating and facilitating the publication of my work on nucleus pulposus calcification.

Professor R. C. Bennett, Professor of Surgery, St. Vincent's Hospital, Melbourne, has continued to support my work over many years.

The tedious process of criticism on which the final quality of a manuscript depends so heavily has been undertaken once again by my friend, Dr. W. McCubbery. The manuscript has also been checked carefully by my wife, Dr. M. C. Crock, and by Dr. Paul DiMartino from New York.

My wife has performed some of the anatomical dissections, photographs of which are reproduced in this book. For fifteen years she has assisted at surgery during all my private operations. Without her help and the forbearance of my children, this book may never have been published.

My children, Elizabeth and Damian, have helped with secretarial work, Vernon with photographic work and Catherine and Carmel with constant encouragement.

I owe a special debt of thanks to my identical twin brother, Professor G. W. Crock of Melbourne.

The preliminary typing of the manuscript was done by my secretary, Mrs. Sandra Koukouras. However, the real burden of preparation of this manuscript has fallen on Mrs. Beverley Vaudrey.

I am grateful to Professor Emeritus Sir Douglas Wright, Chancellor of the University of Melbourne, my former teacher, mentor and friend, who has kindly agreed to write the Foreword.

Finally, I wish to thank my Publishers, Springer-Verlag in Vienna, particularly Mr. Frank Chr. May for his untiring help and careful attention to details, and especially Dr. W. Schwabl for his constant encouragement.

Henry V. Crock

Contents

6. The Surgical Management of Spinal Canal Stenosis 157

7. Surgery of the Cervical Spine 179

Introduction

Nineteen hundred and thirty four marked a turning point in the history of the understanding of sciatica when Mixter and Barr's paper on rupture of the intervertebral disc was published in the New England Journal of Medicine. In 1927 Putti had drawn attention to the importance of facet osteoarthritis as a cause of sciatica. His work was overshadowed by the impact of the description of prolapse of the intervertebral disc. Indeed the entity of prolapsed disc soon emerged as the only intervertebral disc lesion which was considered in dealing with the clinical problems of sciatica.

Dandy (1941) hinted at the need for a wider understanding of intervertebral disc pathology in his short paper on "Concealed Ruptured Intervertebral Discs", but once again the profound influence of the concept of disc prolapse held sway and his work also was overshadowed. In 1957 Morgan and King drew attention to the derangement of movement which may occur between adjacent vertebrae due to circumferential and incomplete radial annular tears within the discs, as a cause of backache. This paper presented an important new concept in the understanding of disc pathology applied to clinical practice, yet it failed to receive wide acclaim. The biophysical basis of their observations has since been expounded by Farfan *et al.* (1970) in their paper "The Effects of Torsion on the Lumbar Intervertebral Joints: The Role of Torsion in the Production of Disc Degeneration."

Without doubt, Mixter and Barr's work, viewed in historical perspective over the past 48 years, has exerted a profound effect on the practice of medicine relating to the diagnosis and treatment of sciatica. They presented for the first time a simple concept to explain the basis of this age-old scourge.

The impact of this work has been such, that, since its publication, every medical graduate in the world has had some familiarity with prolapse of the intervertebral disc.

Paradoxically the powerful psychological impact of this work on medical practitioners has had a number of adverse reactions. Their acceptance of the concept has tended to be blind, so that clinically, they recognize no other disc pathology apart perhaps from the vague entity of disc degeneration, widely held to be a cause of back pain. By adopting this exclusive view of disc pathology some are apt to develop aggressive attitudes and behaviour towards patients whose problems they have diagnosed as being due to disc prolapse. This is particularly so if the patient continues to complain of pain after surgery for suspected disc herniation, when none was actually found.

Even among radiologists attitudes have been strongly conditioned, so that many think of intervertebral disc pathology exclusively in terms of its capacity to produce space-occupying lesions within the vertebral column. Many are not aware of the existence of non-prolapsing disc disorders. Likewise, many neurologists have adopted a purely mechanical view of disc pathology; as a result, their concept of sciatica due to disc disease relates strictly to nerve-root impingement, pain without "signs" being beyond their imagined view of the pathology.

In the 1950s the view prevailed that prolapse of the intervertebral disc was the most common cause of low back pain and sciatica, a view which became tradition to the detriment of many thousands of patients. *Disc prolapses may be the cause of back pain and sciatica in only a small percentage of all the patients who complain of those symptoms.* Sciatica from this cause is usually unilateral and if surgery is indicated, the result of excision of the disc fragments is usually excellent. What deserves to be recognized is the fact that the results of operations for suspected but non-existent disc prolapses are often disastrous.

The recognition in recent years of a range of disorders of the intervertebral discs has made a significant difference to the results of their surgical treatment. Lesions such as prolapsed intervertebral disc and isolated disc resorption produce their adverse clinical effects mechanically, while others, such as post-traumatic internal disc disruption and nucleus pulposus calcification have complex biochemical abnormalities which probably cause pain at histochemical levels.

The four principal disorders of intervertebral discs discussed in the following chapters will be presented in order of their frequency in clinical practice.

1

Nerve Root Canal Stenosis

1.1. Isolated Lumbar Disc Resorption

This condition is characterized by gross narrowing of one affected disc space, with sclerosis of the adjacent vertebral bodies. Occurring commonly as an isolated affection in an otherwise normal lumbar spine, even late in life, it is seen most commonly at L5/S1, occasionally at L4/5 and rarely at L3/4.

Attention was drawn first to the importance of "reduced lumbo-sacral joint space: its relation to sciatic irritation", by Williams in 1932. The term *isolated disc resorption* was coined by Crock in 1970, though he was unaware of the existence of Williams' paper at that time.

Isolated disc resorption causes back and leg pain more commonly than does prolapse of an intervertebral disc. This condition therefore assumes great clinical importance and warrants identification as a specific form of disc disease. By combining observations on the pathological findings in isolated disc resorption with a sound knowledge of surgical anatomy, different forms of surgical treatment can be planned to suit individual cases. When these cases are treated by the standard operation of "laminectomy" used in the management of disc prolapse, the results are often poor, whereas excellent results may be obtained by performing *bilateral nerve root canal decompressions* or more rarely by performing some form of local spinal fusion.

a) Natural History

This condition of narrowing of a single lumbar intervertebral disc space usually progresses slowly over a number of years, the clinical course being punctuated by repeated bouts of acute low back pain lasting for three to four days and then resolving completely. Following trauma, particularly a fall on to the buttocks, the symptoms may extend to include severe bilateral buttock and leg pains. In some cases buttock and leg pain may be aggravated by physical exercise or walking. The description *nerve root claudication* may then be used to describe this particular symptom pattern.

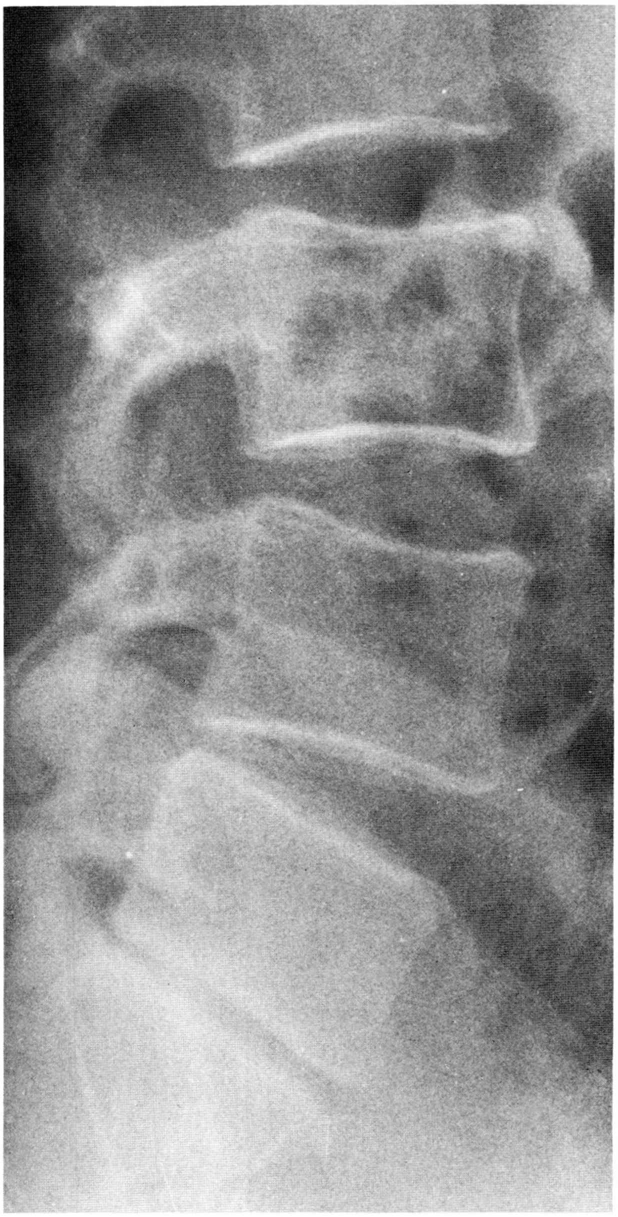

Figure 1.1. A lateral radiograph of the lumbar spine of a 48 year-old man showing the classical features of isolated disc resorption at the lumbo-sacral junction

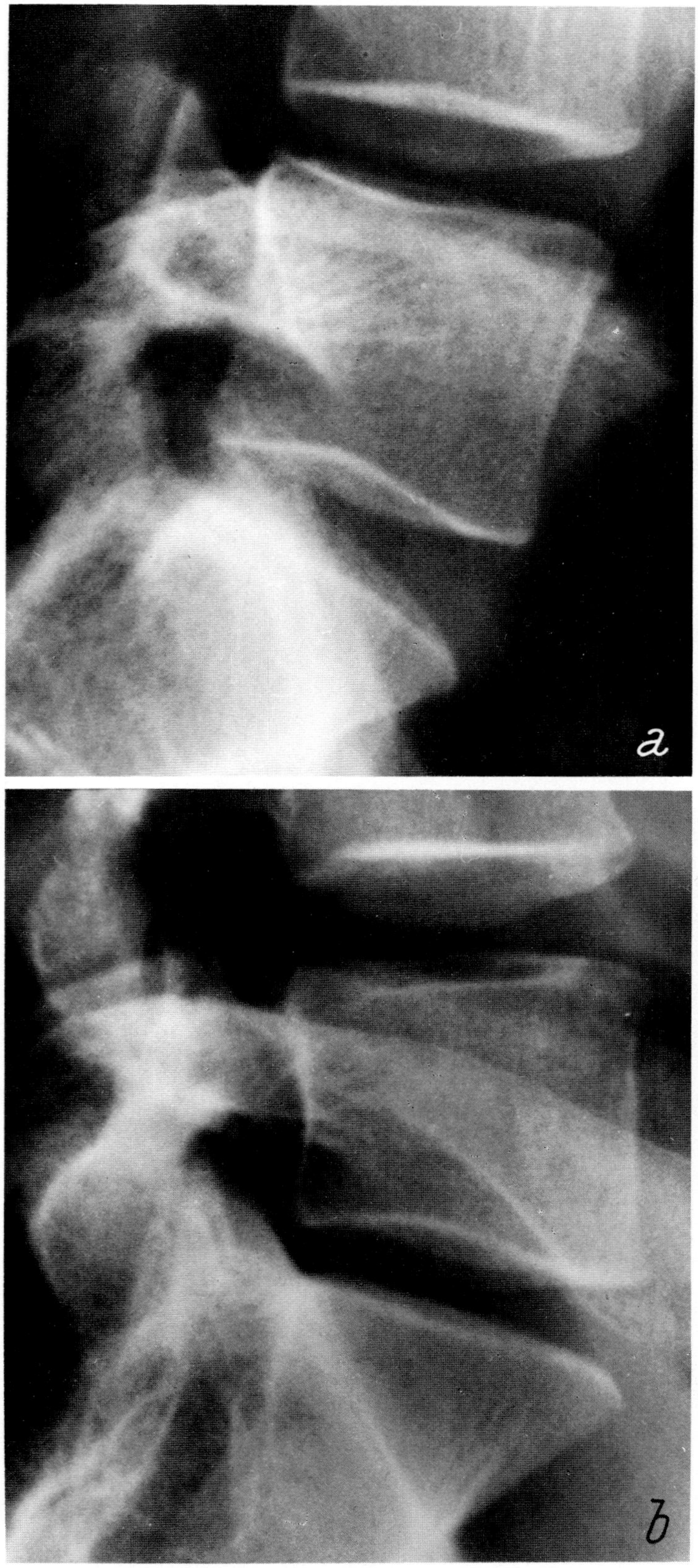

Figures 1.2 a–c. Lateral radiographs of the lower lumbar spine in a 39 year-old woman who had intractable bilateral buttock pain and unilateral leg pain. Films taken in 1970 **a,** 1972 **b** and 1974 **c** illustrate the progressive narrowing of the lumbo-sacral disc in a case of isolated lumbar disc resorption

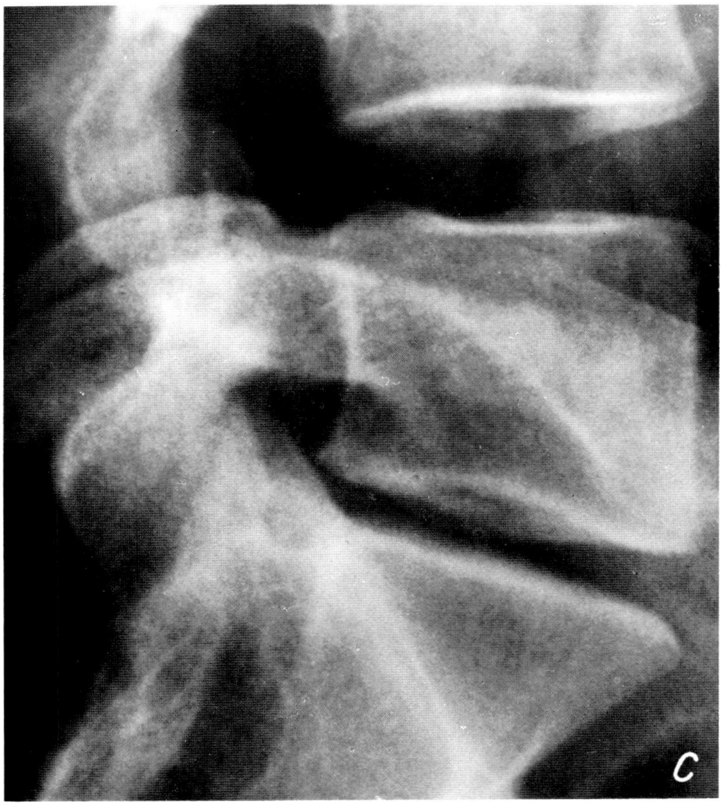

Figure 1.2 c

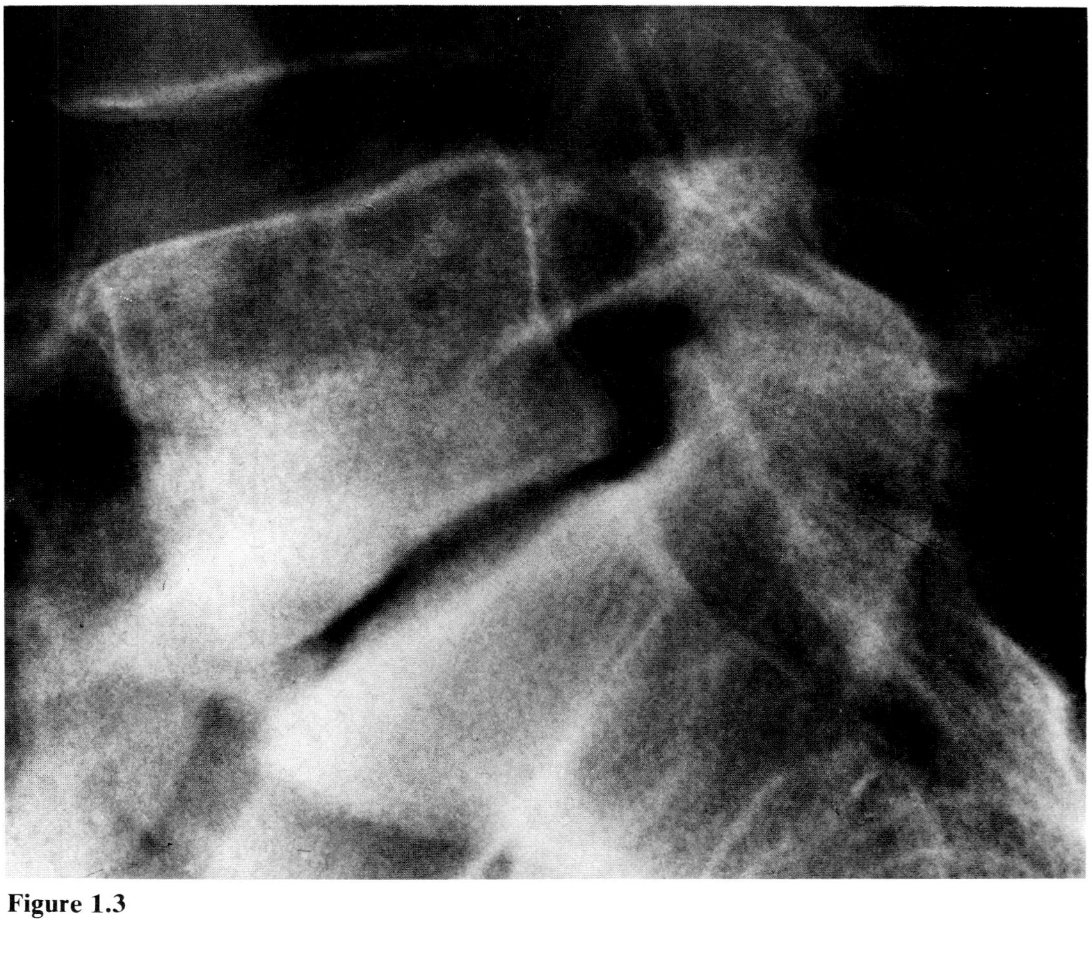

Figure 1.3

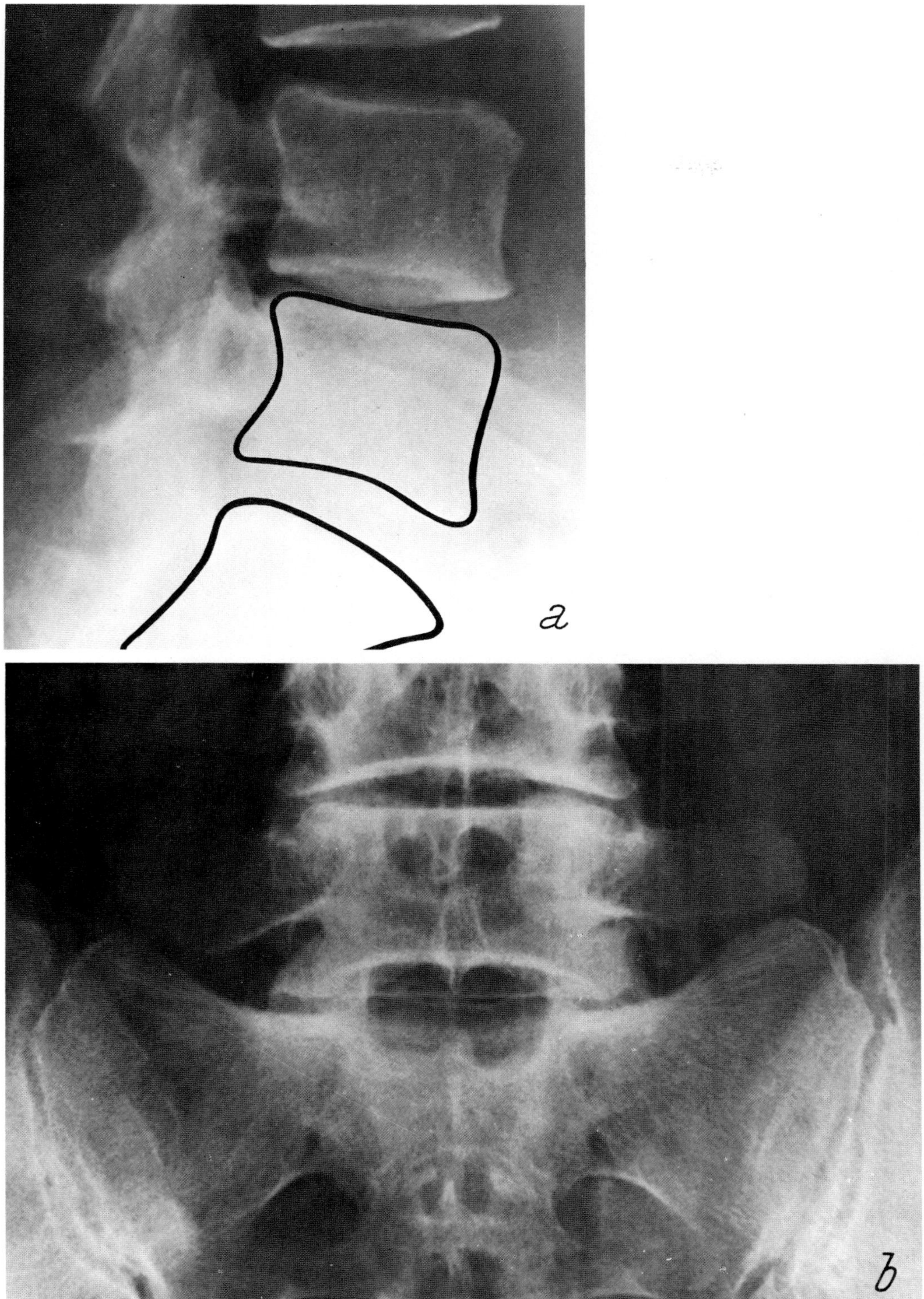

Figures 1.4 a and **b.** Isolated disc resorption at L4/5. A 48 year-old woman had longstanding back pain, with bilateral leg pain. She was treated by bilateral nerve root canal decompression laminectomy. The L4/5 disc was not disturbed at operation. **a** Lateral radiograph, and **b** antero-posterior radiograph of the spine showing features of isolated disc resorption at the L4/5 level, the vertebral end-plates remaining parallel to each other in (b)

Figure 1.3. A lateral radiograph of the lumbar spine of a woman aged 52 years showing a normal L4/5 disc space and isolated disc resorption at the L5/S1 level. The familiar vacuum sign described by Knuttson is seen

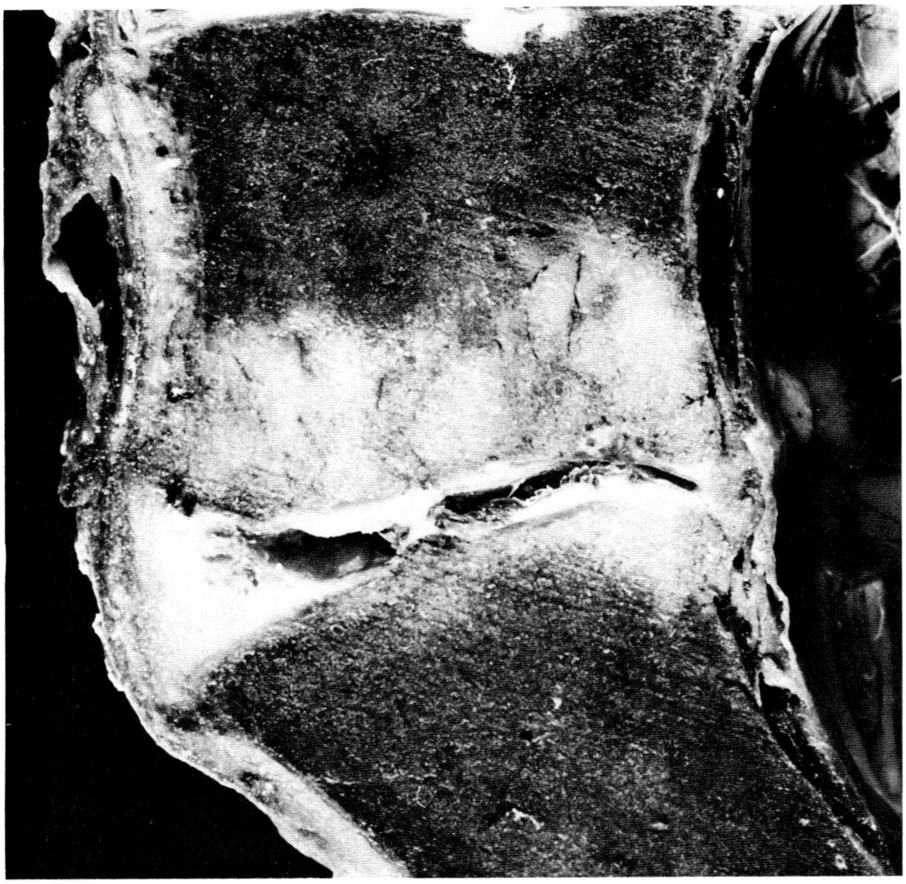

Figure 1.5. A photograph of a mid-line sagittal section of the lumbar spine of a man aged 69 years. The pathological features of isolated disc resorption are well shown, with vertebral end-plate remnants in the posterior two-thirds of the disc space visible on either side of an otherwise empty disc space. Note the marked sclerosis of the vertebral bodies on either side of the disc space

In parallel with the natural history of the symptoms, repeated radiological examination will reveal a progressive loss of disc height at the affected level (Figs. 1.2 a–c). In the lower lumbar region in adults, the disc height between adjacent vertebral end-plates ranges from 10–15 mm. In established cases of isolated lumbar disc resorption the height of the intervertebral disc space may be reduced to 3 mm. The vacuum phenomenon of Knuttson is another prominent radiological feature which may become evident if the X-ray is taken with the patient standing with the lumbar spine hyperextended. A black gas shadow will then appear in the disc space. Sclerosis of the adjacent vertebral bodies is found, while marginal osteophyte formation is minimal. Occasionally a ridge of bone covered with a thin layer of annular fibre remnants may be found projecting into the spinal canal (Figs. 1.3–1.5). For example at L5/S1 subluxation of the facet joints with intrusion of the superior facets of S1 into the intervertebral foramina and lumbar nerve root canals will also be seen (Figs. 1.6 a, b).

The disc space narrowing which accompanies sacralization anomalies is not to be confused with that occurring in isolated lumbar disc resorption.

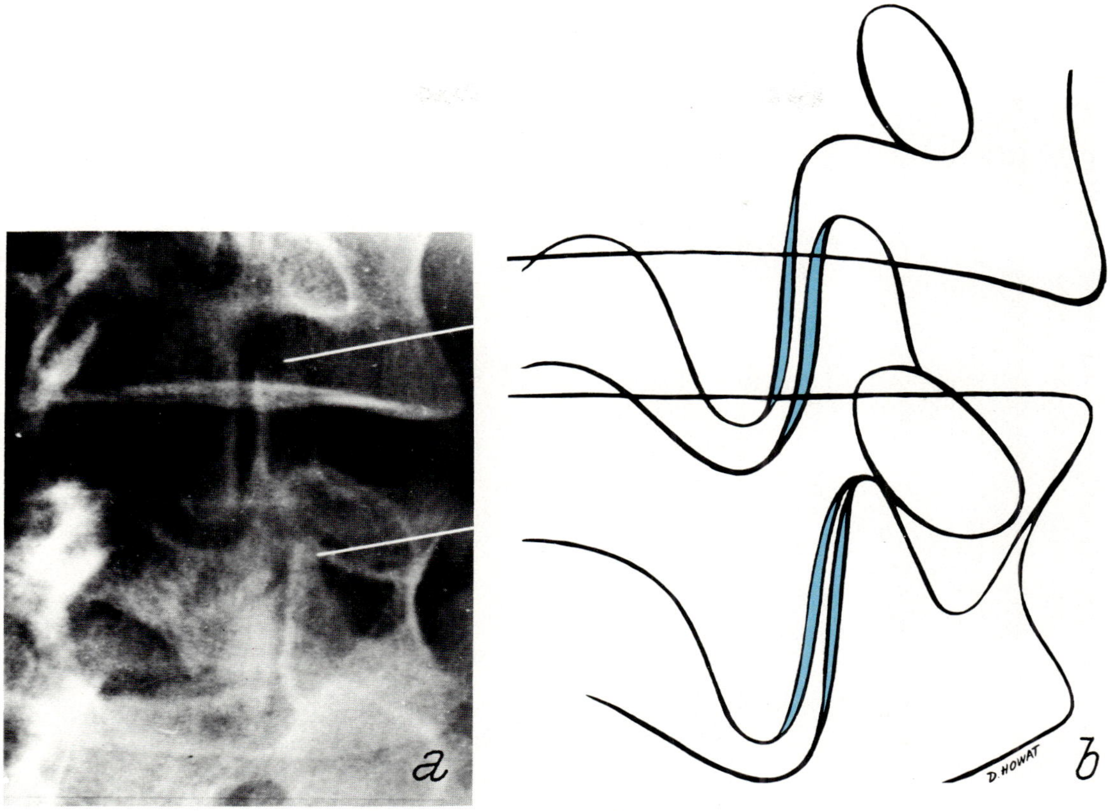

Figures 1.6 a and **b.** An oblique view of the lower lumbar spine showing normal relationships of the facets of the L 4/5 level, top marker, and subluxation of S1 up against the pedicle of L 5 on the bottom marker, with an explanatory line drawing alongside

In established cases where the disc space has become very narrow, with parallel vertebral end-plate settling, the symptoms of buttock and leg pain, if intractable, are usually bilateral.

Earlier in the course of this disease, a small number of patients may present with unilateral sciatica. These patients may exhibit the classic features of neurological defects in either L 5 or S1 nerve roots. Usually they will be found to have a sequestrated fragment of vertebral end-plate cartilage impinging on the affected nerve root. This finding is one of the striking features of this disease process. At operation in such cases, the disc space is virtually empty and clearly recognizable necrotic vertebral end-plate cartilage will be found causing the nerve root compression.

b) Anatomy of Nerve Root Canals

i) Normal

The anatomy of the lumbar nerve root canals and intervertebral foramina will be described to assist with the understanding of the genesis of the symptoms and signs which may occur in cases of isolated disc resorption.

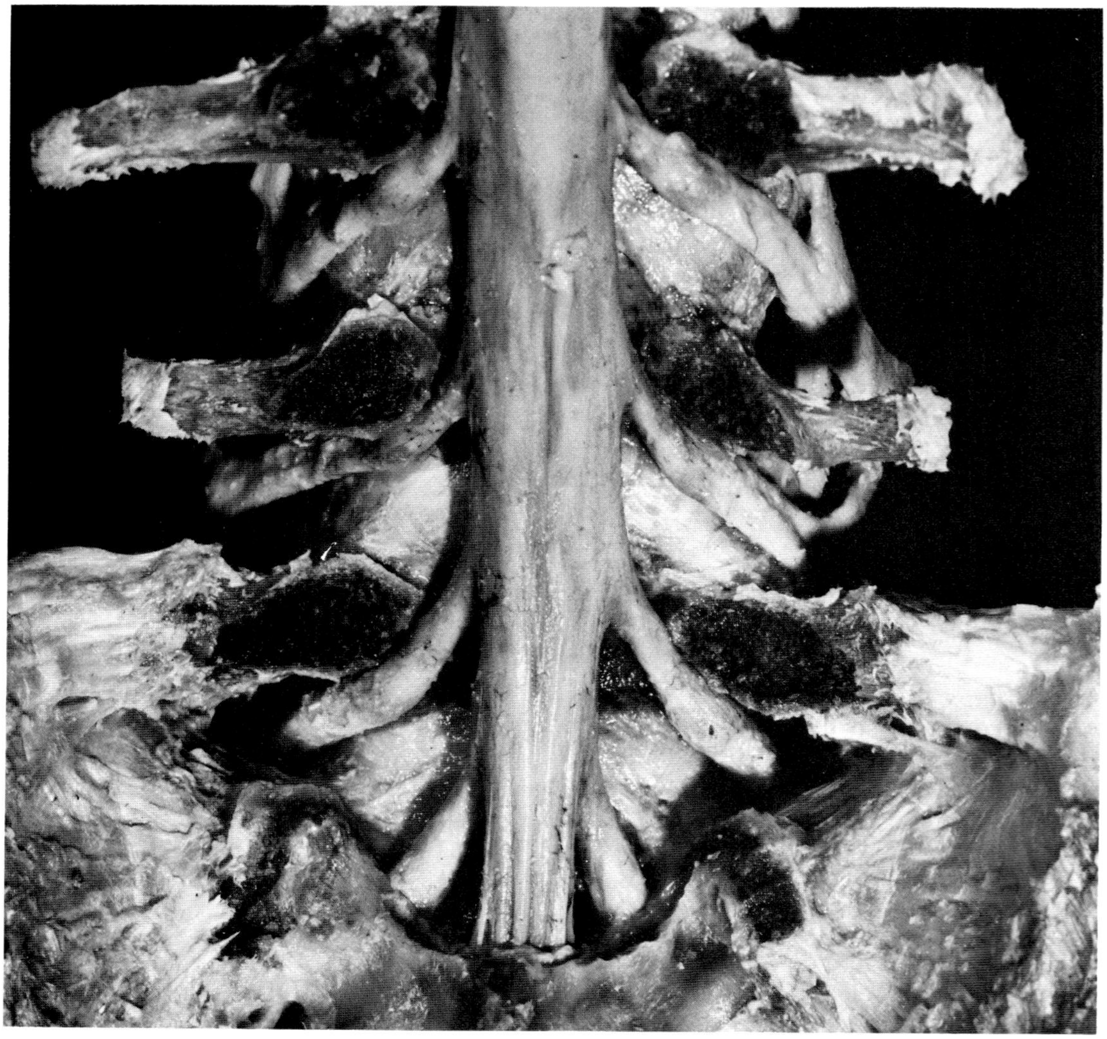

Figure 1.7. A photograph of a dissection of the lower lumbar spine in an adult to show some of the relations of the lumbar nerve roots. Note especially the origins of the nerve root sleeves from the dural sac and the courses of the nerve roots in relation to the pedicles. (Dissected by Dr. M. C. Crock)

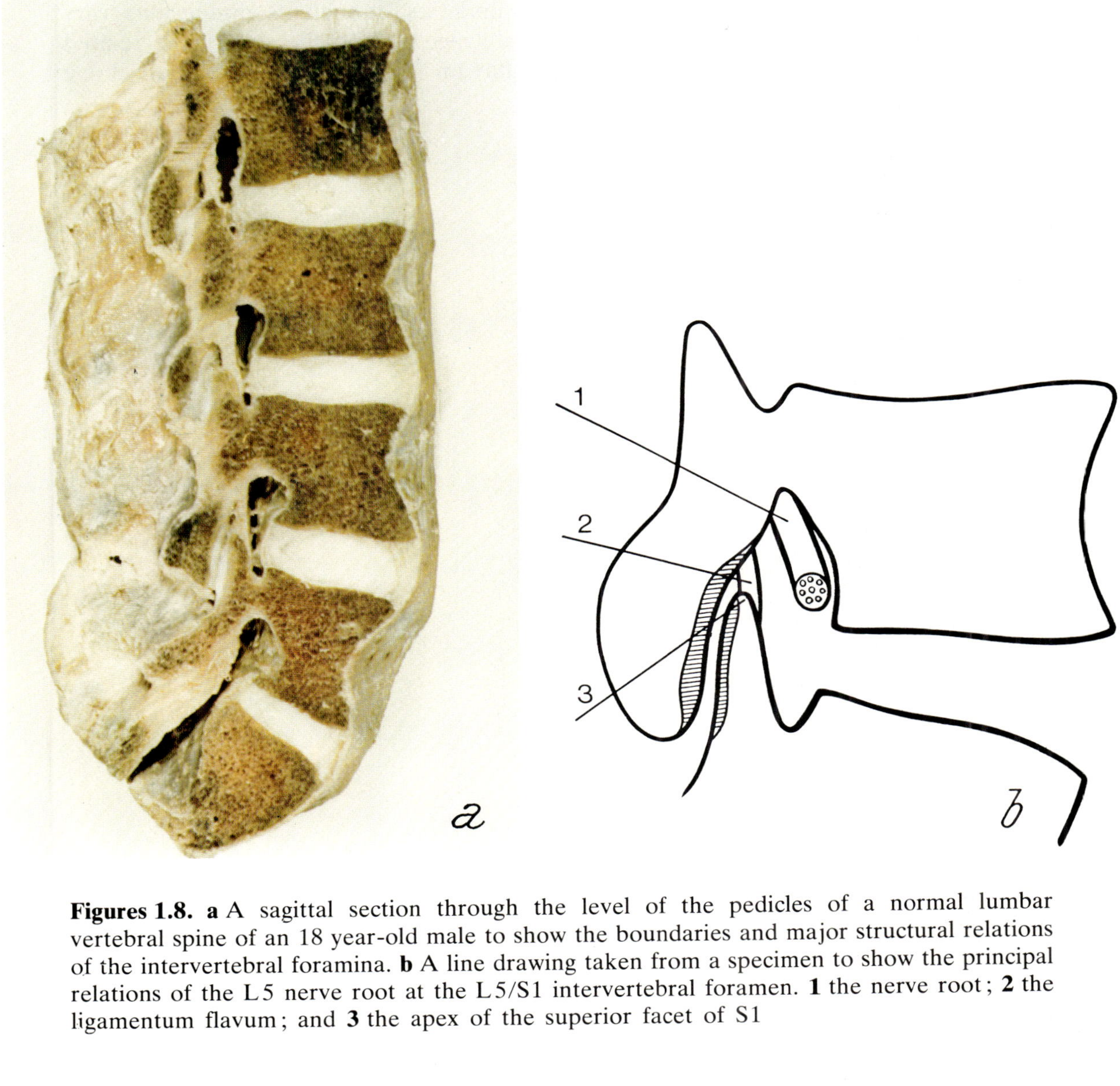

Figures 1.8. a A sagittal section through the level of the pedicles of a normal lumbar vertebral spine of an 18 year-old male to show the boundaries and major structural relations of the intervertebral foramina. **b** A line drawing taken from a specimen to show the principal relations of the L5 nerve root at the L5/S1 intervertebral foramen. **1** the nerve root; **2** the ligamentum flavum; and **3** the apex of the superior facet of S1

The lumbar nerves run obliquely downwards and laterally from the lateral aspects of the dural sac, emerging at their respective intervertebral foramina and lying inferior to the lumbar pedicle in the upper part of each foramen (Fig. 1.7). Anomalies excluded, each nerve root is intimately related to the medial and inferior aspects of the adjacent vertebral pedicle.

The intervertebral foramen has fixed boundaries, though its dimensions vary depending on the height of the individual disc space and on the size of the related facet joints and thickness of the ligamentum flavum (Figs. 1.8a, b). Bounded above and below by the vertebral pedicles, the floor from above downwards is formed by the postero-inferior margin of the superior vertebral body, the intervertebral disc and the postero-superior margin of the inferior vertebral body (Fig. 1.9). The roof is formed by the ligamentum flavum, terminating at its outer free edge, and posterior to this structure lies the pars interarticularis and the apophyseal joint formed between the adjacent inferior and superior vertebral facets (Fig. 1.10). The intervertebral foramen is analogous to the doorway at the end of a passage, its vertical height being determined by the vertical height of the corresponding intervertebral disc space.

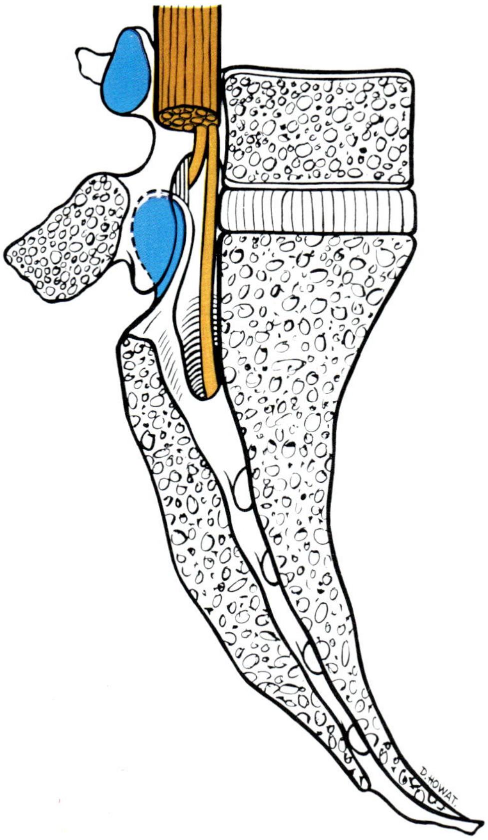

Figure 1.9. A drawing showing the relations of the S1 spinal nerve root canal viewed from within the spinal canal

A nerve root canal, by contrast, is a tubular canal of variable length, arising from the lateral aspect of the dural sac. Viewed from within the sac, the hiatus through which the component motor and sensory nerve roots pass to the spinal nerve has the

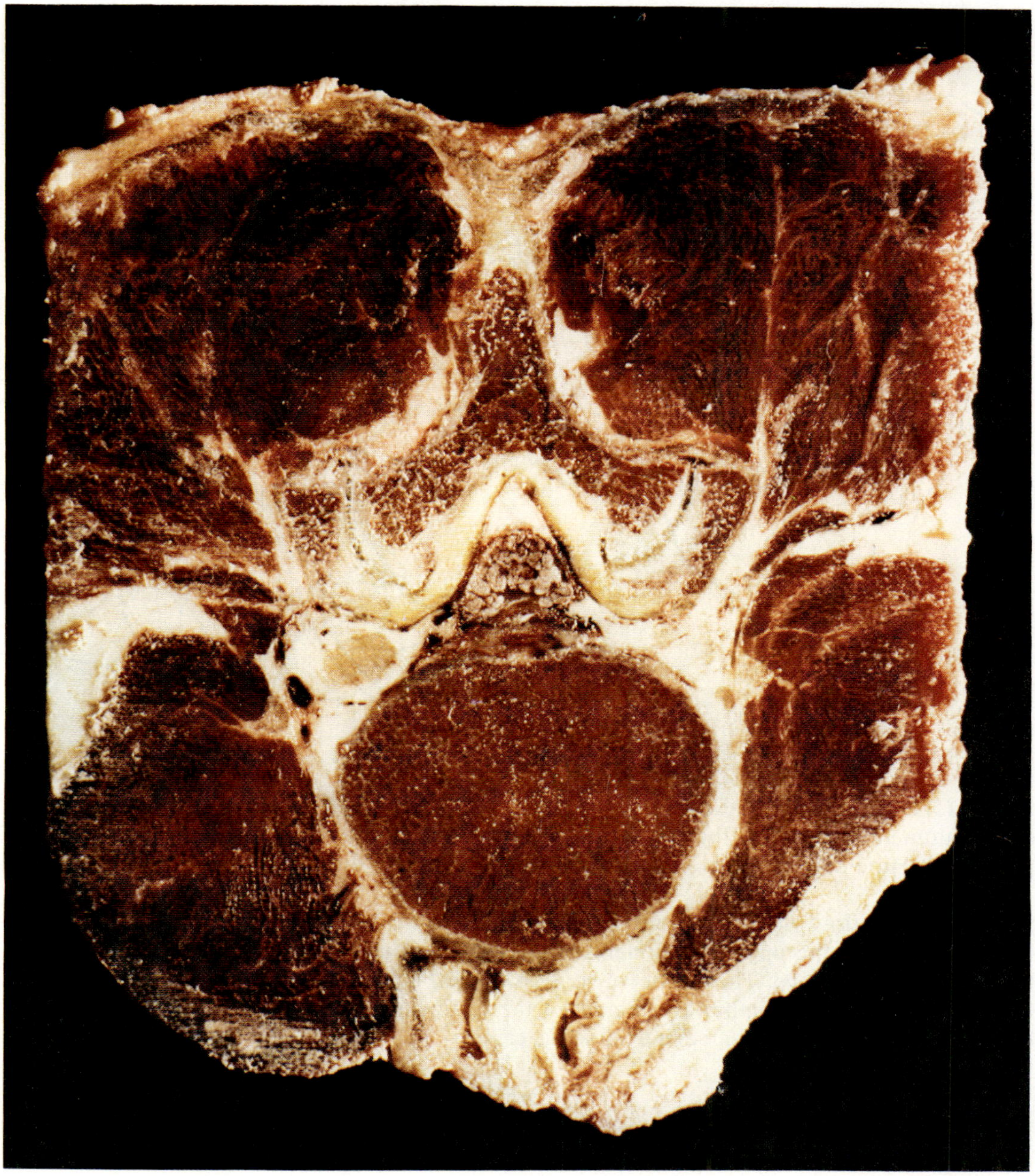

Figure 1.10. A transverse section through the lower lumbar spine at the level of the intervertebral foramen, the section passing through the vertebral body. On the left of the specimen note the posterior relations of the nerve root. In the mid-line, the cauda equina can be clearly seen, easily distinguished from the epidural fat

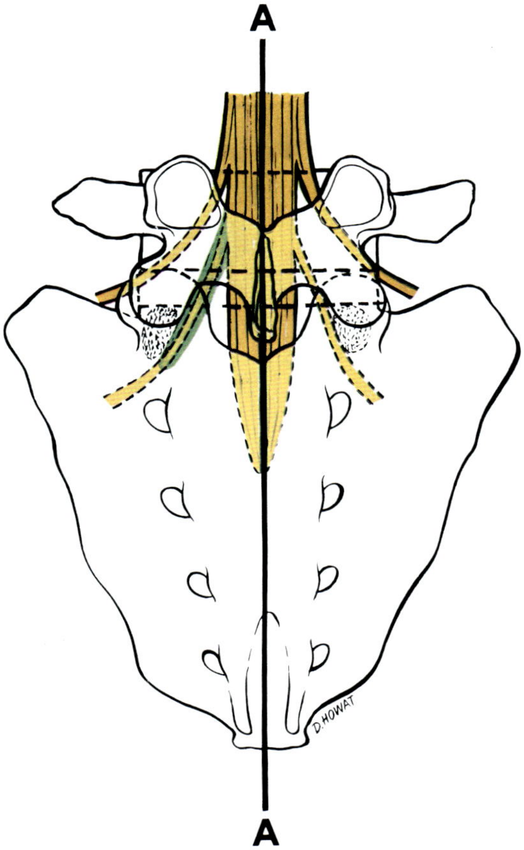

Figure 1.11

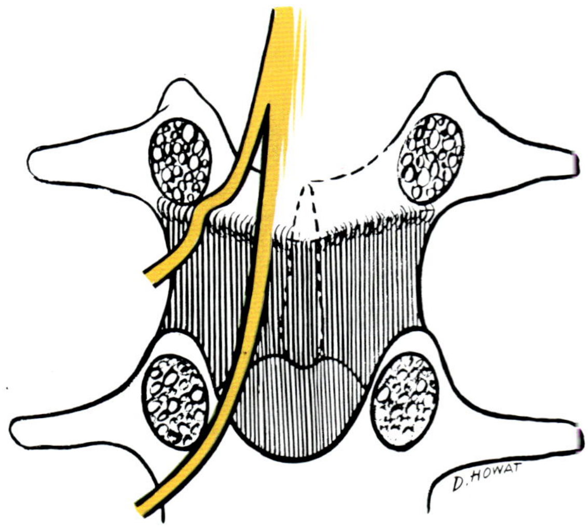

Figure 1.12

Figure 1.11. A drawing of the normal lumbo-sacral junction. Note the spinal nerve root canal of S1 outlined in green on the left side of the diagram. The line marked AA represents the plane of section for drawings illustrated in Figs. 1.9, 1.16, and 1.20

Figure 1.12. A drawing of two lumbar laminae viewed from within the spinal canal, showing the bony ridge of the upper attachment of the ligamentum flavum to the superior lamina at the intervertebral space. The L5 nerve root on the left side is shown kinked forwards by this ridge at the level of the upper attachment of the ligamentum flavum. The S1 nerve root may be similarly deformed from behind in some cases

shape of a funnel. Viewed from without, the dural sheath clothes the spinal nerve on all sides as it courses obliquely downwards and laterally towards the intervertebral foramen (Fig. 1.11). The upper lumbar nerve roots are often orientated almost at right angles to the dural sac and their intraspinal portions are, therefore, very short. The nerve root canal in such cases becomes, in effect, a useless concept, as the dural sac lies against the medial wall of the upper lumbar pedicle. The emerging lumbar spinal nerve passes at once into the intervertebral foramen at its upper boundary immediately below the pedicle.

The shape of the dural sac changes from a rounded tubular outline, tapering progressively from the level of L3 downwards. Contrasting with the upper two lumbar spinal nerves, the lower lumbar nerves are longer and come off at more acute

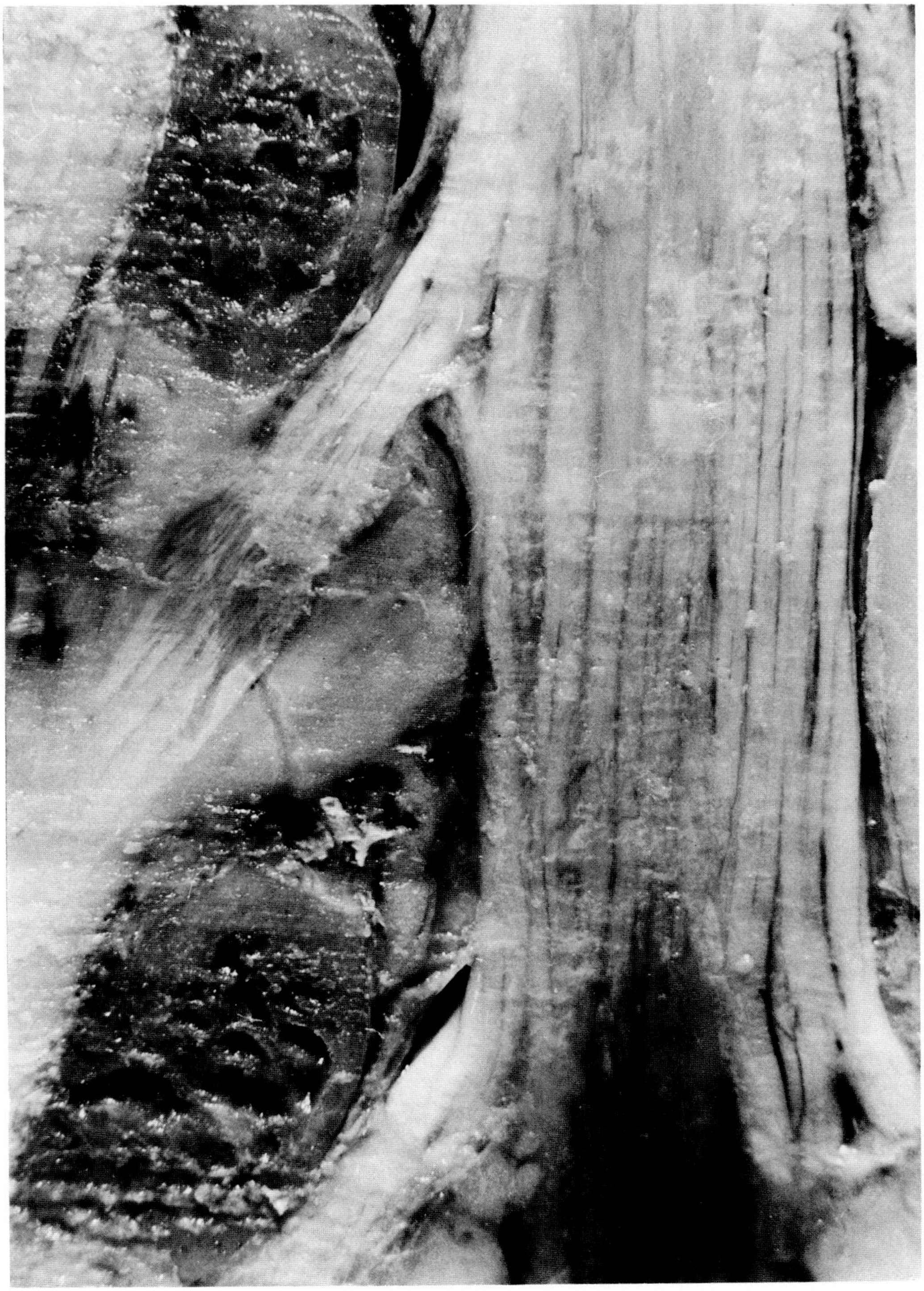

Figure 1.13. A coronal section of the mid-lumbar region of an adult, showing the cauda equina and two lumbar nerve roots on the left, each related to a vertebral pedicle. Note the extra-dural fat pads around the upper of the two nerve roots

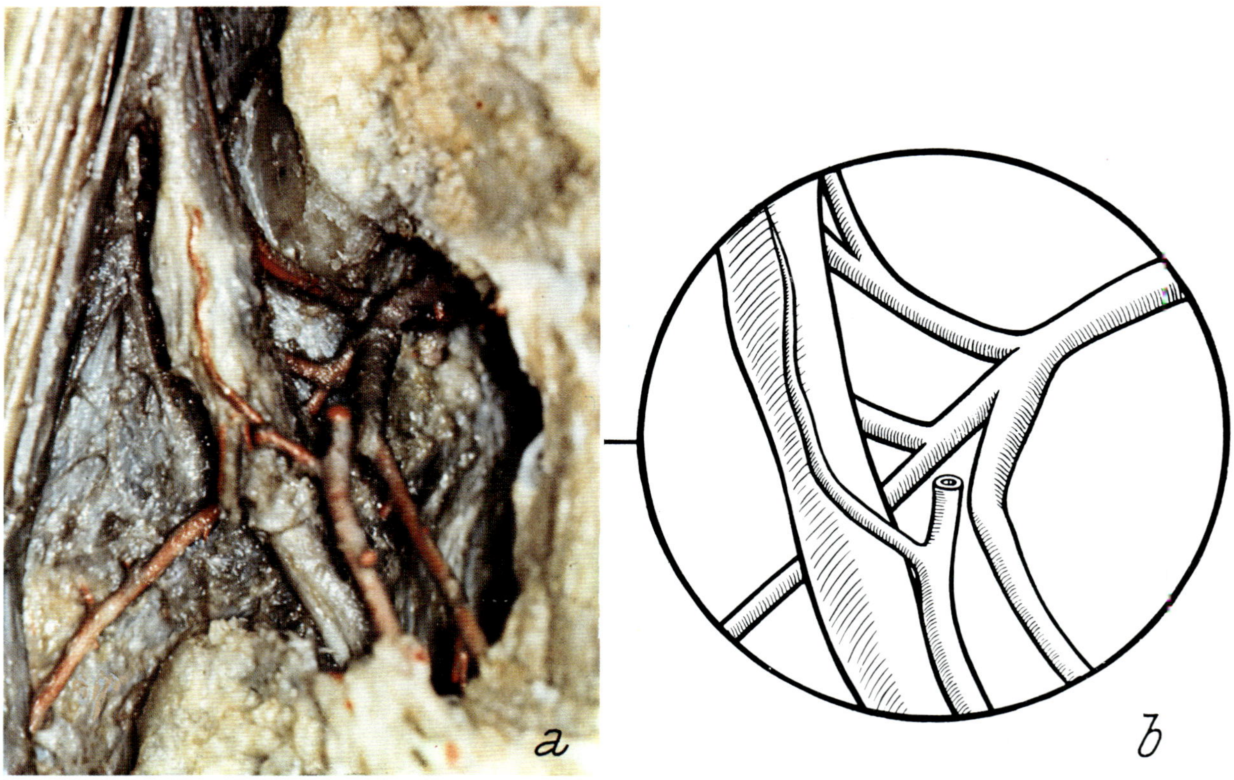

Figures 1.14 a and **b.** A detailed photograph to show the anterior spinal canal branches of the lumbar artery lying anterior to the emerging lumbar nerve root at the intervertebral foramen, together with the ascending anterior and posterior nerve root branches of the lumbar artery, from a female aged 18 years

angles from the sides of the dural sac. *The concept of a nerve root canal is of greatest significance in relation to the two lower-most lumbar and first sacral nerves.*

In Fig. 1.11, the origin of the S1 nerve from the dural sac is shown just below the level of the inferior margin of the fifth lumbar pedicle. Medially at its origin it is related to the lateral aspect of the dural sac. The nerve courses downwards and obliquely as it passes laterally, lying first medial to the fifth lumbar nerve root and below that, medial to the L5/S1 intervertebral foramen; it then lies adjacent to the medial aspect of the pedicle of S1. At the lower border of this pedicle it enters the first sacral intervertebral foramen (Figs. 1.9, 1.11).

The anterior relations of the S1 nerve root canal from above downwards are: the posterior aspect of the body of L5, the intervertebral disc, the posterior aspect of the body of S1. These constitute the floor of the canal when viewed from behind (Figs. 1.9, 1.11).

The posterior relations vary considerably depending on the length of the individual nerve root and on the orientation of the lamina of L5, which will vary with the lumbo-sacral angle. From above downwards, the uppermost posterior relation of the root canal at its origin is the bony ridge raised on the anterior aspect of the lamina of L5 by the superior attachment of the ligamentum flavum (Fig. 1.12). The nerve root is then covered by the antero-medial aspect of the S1 facet (Fig. 1.11).

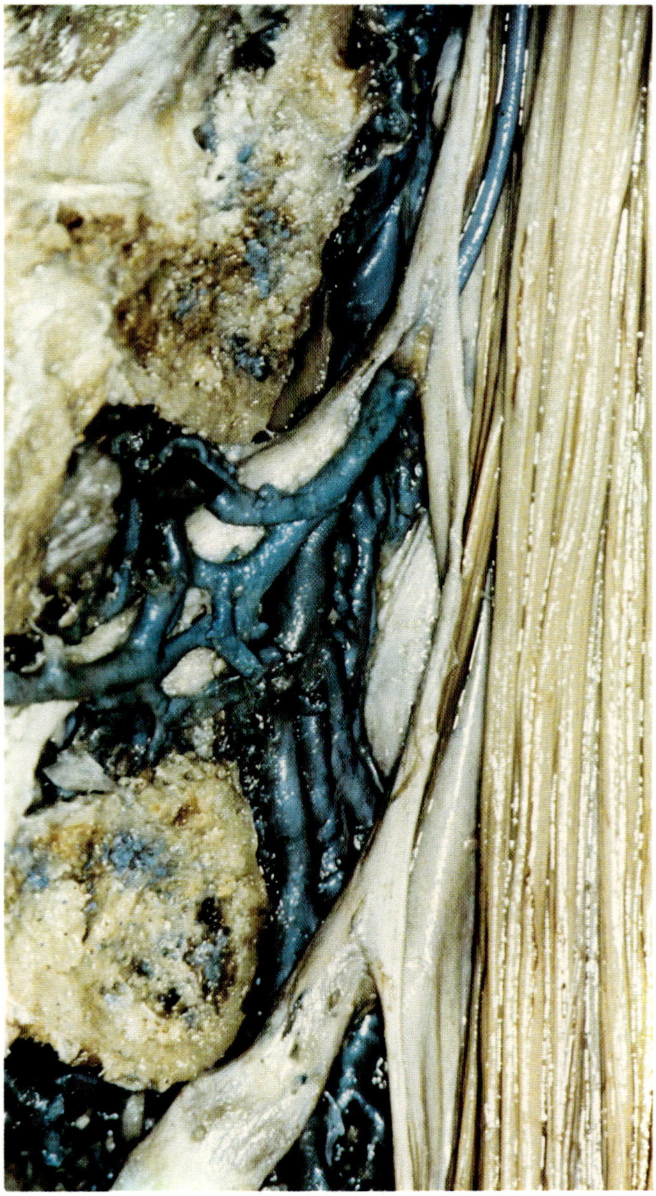

Figure 1.15. A photograph of a dissection to show details of the anterior internal vertebral venous plexus from a male aged 71 years. The plexus was injected with latex rubber. Note the large radicular vein joining the plexus

Epidural fat surrounds the spinal nerve root throughout its course to the intervertebral foramen (Fig. 1.13).

The arterial and venous relations of the spinal nerve roots are of great importance.

Knowledge of the anatomy of these veins helps the surgeon to conserve them during spinal exploration, avoiding venous haemorrhage which may lead to faulty technique in root canal decompression, simply because the fine structures cannot be identified in the pool of blood in the depth of the dissection. *Venous obstruction is a cause of symptoms in nerve root canal stenosis* and the task of relieving it is made easy by a knowledge of this local vascular anatomy.

Relations of the nerve root arteries assume practical significance during difficult spinal canal operations. These vessels should be protected when spinal nerves are being manipulated. Diathermy of their branches should be kept to a minimum, thereby minimizing the risk of iatrogenic nerve root injury which may be permanent.

Detailed descriptions of these vessels have been given by Crock and Yoshizawa (1977). The salient features of this anatomy are seen in the accompanying illustrations on pp. 16 and 17 (Figs. 1.14a, b, 1.15).

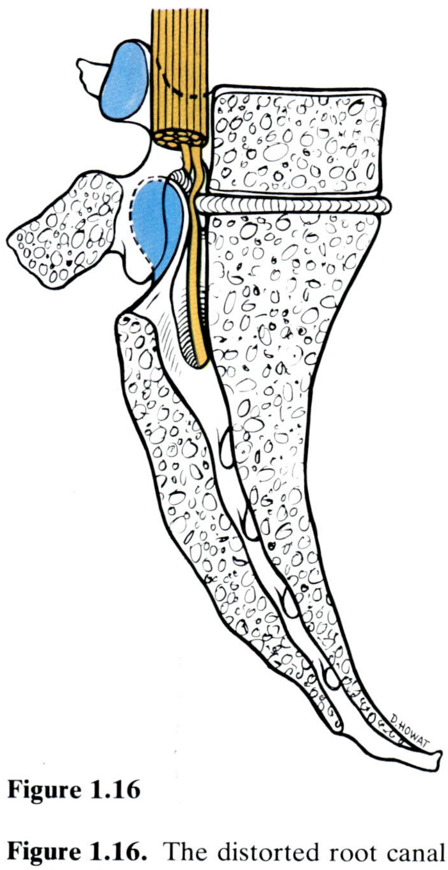

Figure 1.16

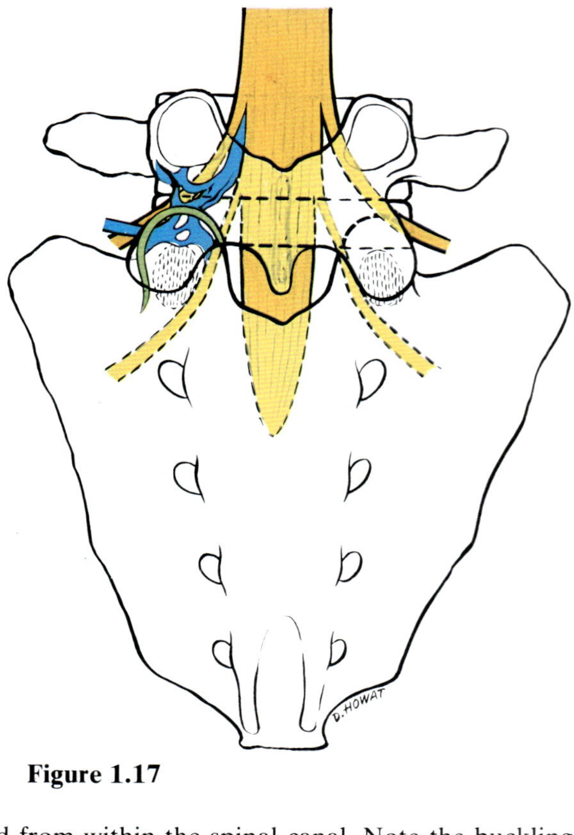

Figure 1.17

Figure 1.16. The distorted root canal viewed from within the spinal canal. Note the buckling of the ligamentum flavum into the intervertebral foramen, compressing the L5 nerve root

Figure 1.17. A drawing showing the normal neural and venous vascular relations at the L5/S1 level. The outline of the upper border of the S1 facet is shown in green

ii) Pathological

When the vertical height of the lumbo-sacral disc space is greatly reduced, changes occur in the floor and roof of the S1 nerve root canal and also in the L5/S1 intervertebral foramen (Fig. 1.5). A narrow transverse bulging ridge formed by posterior fibres of the remaining annulus fibrosus and posterior longitudinal ligament protrudes into the floor of the S1 nerve root canal. Coupled with the movement upwards of the S1 facet towards the pedicle of L5, the anterior and medial edges of the S1 facet come to lie very close to this ridge and occasionally even to the postero-inferior surface of the fifth lumbar vertebral body. In consequence, mechanical obstruction to the S1 nerve root develops (Fig. 1.16).

In some cases, in addition to the infolding of ligamentum flavum, hypertrophy of the bony ridge for its upper attachment may occur, further contributing to stenosis of both the S1 nerve root canal at its origin and, immediately lateral to it, to stenosis of the L5 nerve root canal just medial to the L5 pedicle (Fig. 1.12).

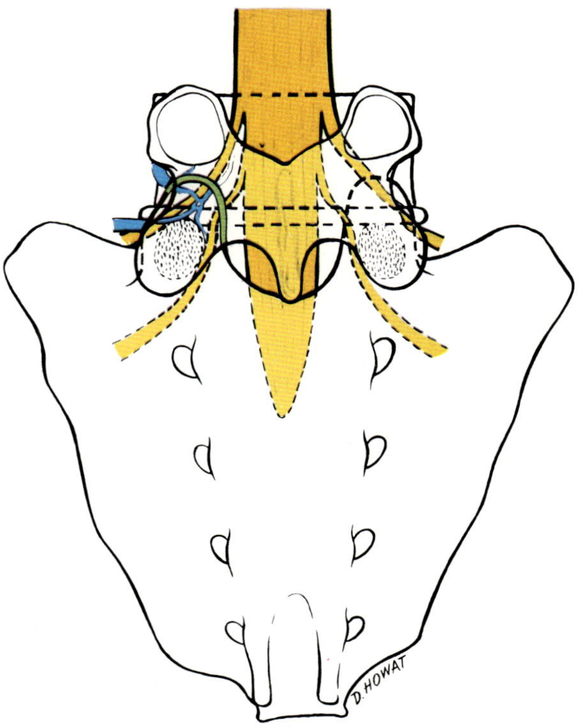

Figure 1.18

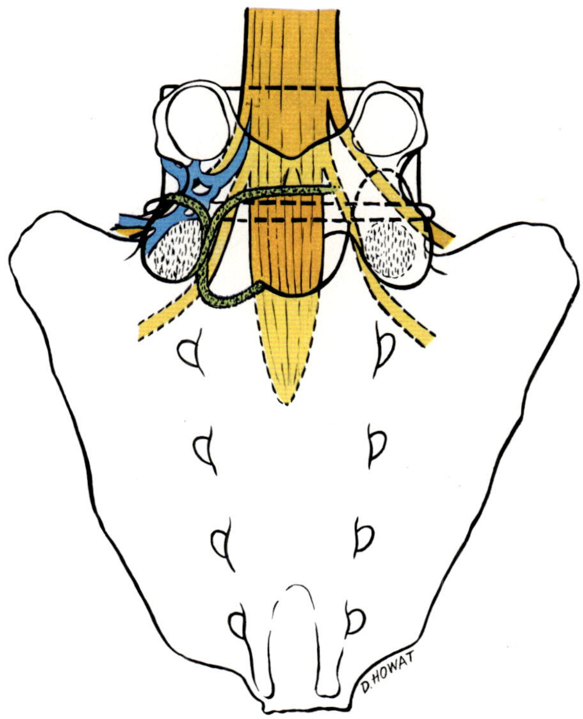

Figure 1.19

Figure 1.18. A drawing showing distortion of the S1 nerve root canal and of the L5/S1 intervertebral foramen due to subluxation upward of the S1 facet in isolated disc resorption of the L5/S1 disc. Note particularly the obstructed veins around the nerve roots. The outline of the medial and apical portions of the S1 facet are shown in green

Figure 1.19. A drawing showing the restoration of normal neuro-vascular relations after decompression of the S1 nerve root canal and L5/S1 intervertebral foramen on the left side at the L5/S1 level. The central portion of the neural arch of L5 has not been removed. The outline of the cut surfaces of bone are shown in stippled green and black

Appreciating these various contributing factors in the stenosis which may affect the S1 nerve root canal and the L5 nerve root at the L5/S1 intervertebral foramen, the planning of an effective surgical decompression can be logically organized (Figs. 1.17–1.20).

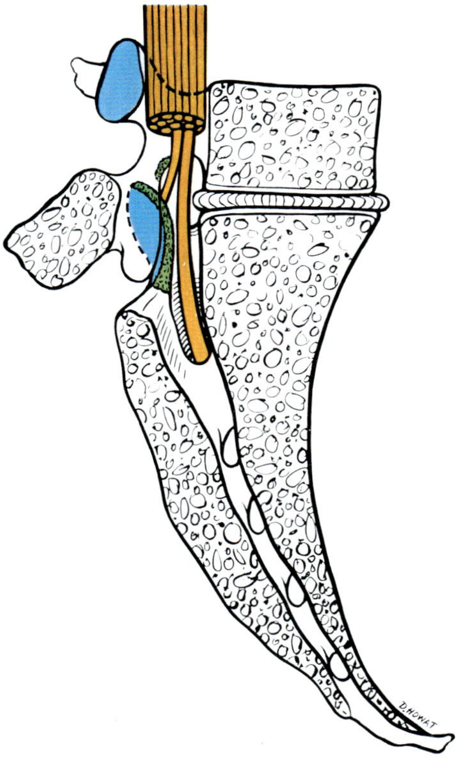

Figure 1.20. A view from within the canal after decompression. The ligamentum flavum has been totally excised. A stippled green and black outline indicates the extent of bony excision of the superior facet of S1 and of the bony ridge on the anterior aspect of the lamina of L5 at the level of the upper attachment of the ligamentum flavum. The L5 spinal nerve is shown emerging unimpeded through the intervertebral foramen

c) Venous Obstruction

While the mechanical obstruction to the S1 nerve root in its canal can be readily appreciated in the condition of isolated disc resorption, the finding of venous obstruction is less widely known. The occlusion of veins that is found in advanced cases of isolated disc resorption is demonstrated in Fig. 1.18. These veins are shown refilled after the operative procedure which is designed to relieve symptoms in this condition (Figs. 1.19, 1.20).

d) Clinical Studies

In recent work published by Venner and Crock in 1981 an analysis was made of the symptoms and signs in a group of 50 patients suffering from isolated disc resorption at the L5/S1 level. 94% of these patients complained of low lumbar pain, and 48%

noted radiation of pain to one or both buttocks: 76% had pain in one or both legs, and 50% complained of paraesthesia. Only 8% reported exacerbation of their pain on coughing, but 18% gave a history of increasing leg pain or paraesthesia on walking distances up to 500 yards (root claudication). Some patients had weakness and occasional dragging of the feet or difficulty in standing, but these symptoms settled on resting, usually by sitting. 94% had lumbar tenderness, but only 8 patients had reduced lumbar movement as defined by Moll and Wright (1976).

Signs of root irritation, evidenced by limited straight leg raising, painful bowstring test or sciatic nerve tenderness were detected in only 6%; and reduced nerve conduction indicated by wasting, motor weakness, sensory abnormality or reflex depression in 16%. One or both ankle jerks were absent in 10%.

In Table 1.1, measurements of the height of the L5/S1 intervertebral disc space in these 50 patients are recorded.

Table 1.1. Height of the L5/S1 intervertebral disc (50 patients)

	Anterior Height			Posterior Height	
	>10 mm*	10–5 mm	< 5 mm	> 5 mm	< 5 mm
Male	7	20	3	5	25
Female	3	14	3	4	16
Totals	10	34	6	9	41

* In only one patient was the height more than 15 millimetres.

e) Investigations

i) Plain X-Rays

Radiological findings are the key to the diagnosis of this condition; plain X-ray examination alone usually suffices to confirm it. Typical findings are: gross disc space narrowing, vertebral body sclerosis especially close to the vertebral end plates, the Knuttson vacuum sign on the lateral extension film, minimal evidence of osteophyte formation and evidence of facet joint subluxation–best seen on oblique views, with intrusion of one facet into the intervertebral foramen seen in the lateral view.

ii) Lumbar Myelography

Disc prolapse is not seen in the established case, so that lumbar myelography is unnecessary except in special circumstances; for example, when the patient has severe unilateral leg pain. Disc prolapse at another level may be found, or vertebral end-plate sequestration at the level of the disc resorption may be confirmed.

The myelogram in a typical case may be normal in appearance and this could influence a surgeon who is not fully aware of the nature of this condition to advise against the surgery that is indicated.

iii) Lumbar Discography

Isolated disc resorption rarely occurs with pathological changes in adjacent intervertebral discs so that lumbar discography is not routinely indicated. An example of a normal discogram at L4–5 above an isolated disc resorption at L5/S1 is shown where the dye injected at L5/S1 has leaked extra-durally into the spinal canal (Fig. 1.21).

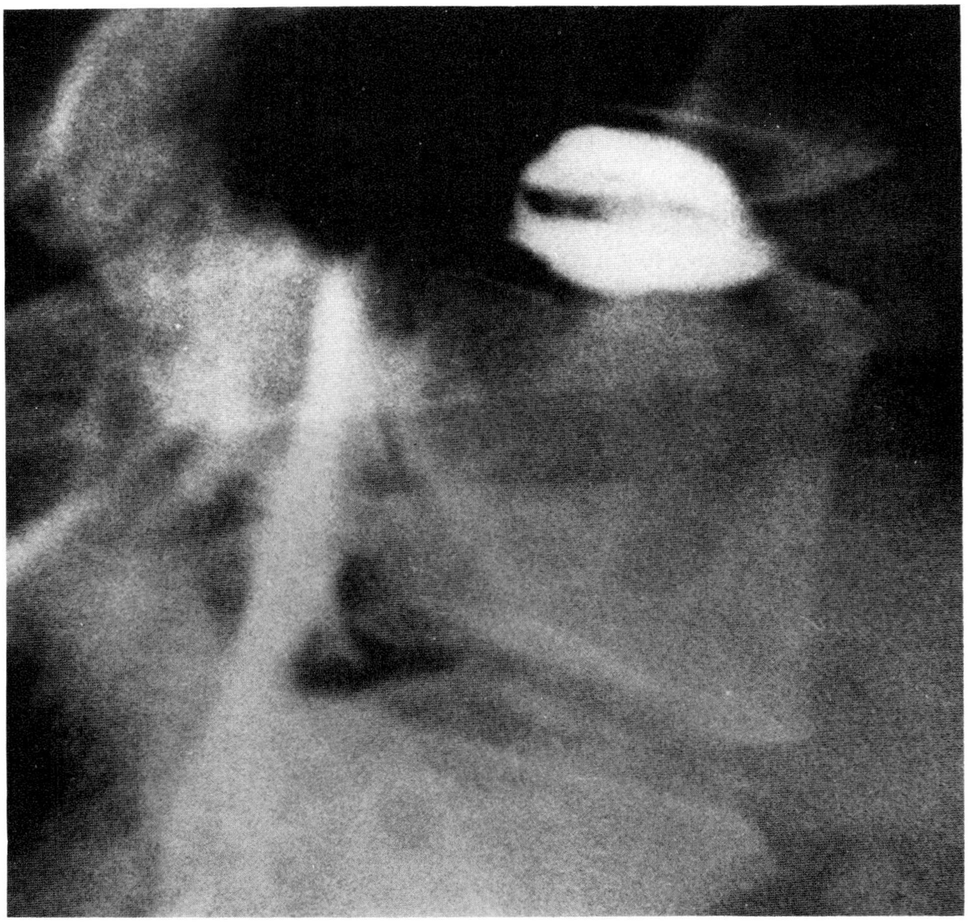

Figure 1.21. A radiograph showing a normal discogram at L4/5 with gross extravasation of dye into the extra-dural space at L5/S1 at the level of an isolated disc resorption

iv) Computerized Axial Tomography

Reconstructed C.T. Scanning is useful in confirming the foraminal and nerve root canal stenosis that occurs in this condition. However, transverse scanning at the lumbo-sacral junction is difficult to interpret in relation to the demonstration of root canal stenosis.

v) Epidural Venography

Obstruction of the intervertebral veins can be demonstrated satisfactorily with this special investigation. However, its demonstration is of theoretical interest as the venous obstruction is a concomitant pathological finding in established cases of isolated disc resorption with facet joint subluxation, facet intrusion into the intervertebral foramen and ligamentum flavum buckling.

f) Operations

i) Types

The treatment of choice in cases with bilateral buttock and leg pain is bilateral nerve root canal decompression. The technique of this operation will be outlined below and described in detail on pp. 23–27.

In cases where there is an associated unilateral sciatica, a sequestrum of necrotic vertebral end-plate cartilage will usually be present. The protruding fragment should be removed and the vertebral end-plate cartilage remnants curetted and extracted from the disc space. At the same time bilateral nerve root canal decompression should be performed.

If, at the time of nerve root canal decompression, marked vertebral instability is noted at the site and the patient's symptoms have included the complaint of intractable back pain, then spinal fusion should be carried out. Inter-transverse-alar sacral fusion is recommended. Theoretically, in this circumstance, the ideal procedure is posterior interbody fusion using either the Cloward or Wiltberger techniques, because the grafts fit accurately between the vertebral bodies, producing a strictly localized spinal fusion.

When low back pain is the dominant symptom, primary anterior interbody fusion at the affected level may be indicated.

The cause of the back pain in these cases is not related to nerve root canal and foraminal stenosis, but emanates from either the vertebral bodies, or the arthritic subluxed facet joints.

ii) Technique of Lumbar Nerve Root Canal Decompression at L5/S1 Level

The approach to the L5/S1 interspace is described on pp. 110–117. Details of the technique of nerve root canal decompression are set out below:

The whole of the ligamentum flavum is removed, laterally at the intervertebral foramen and superiorly from its uppermost laminal attachment. The soft tissues are now separated carefully from the anterior surfaces of the lamina and from the superior and inferior facets at the interspace. This is best done with a probe of the Watson-Cheyne type. Forward-angled laminal punches of varying sizes may be used then, under direct vision, minimizing the risks of venous haemorrhage or of dural or nerve root injury (Figs. 1.22–1.24). The upper edge of the inferior lamina is excised together with the overhanging border of its superior articular process, flush with the medial margin of the pedicle. The tip of the superior articular process is then removed and the inner edge of the overhanging inferior articular process of the

Figure 1.22. A photograph of a Watson-Cheyne dissector. The curved tip on the right hand side is sharp and the left-handed end is a blunt probe

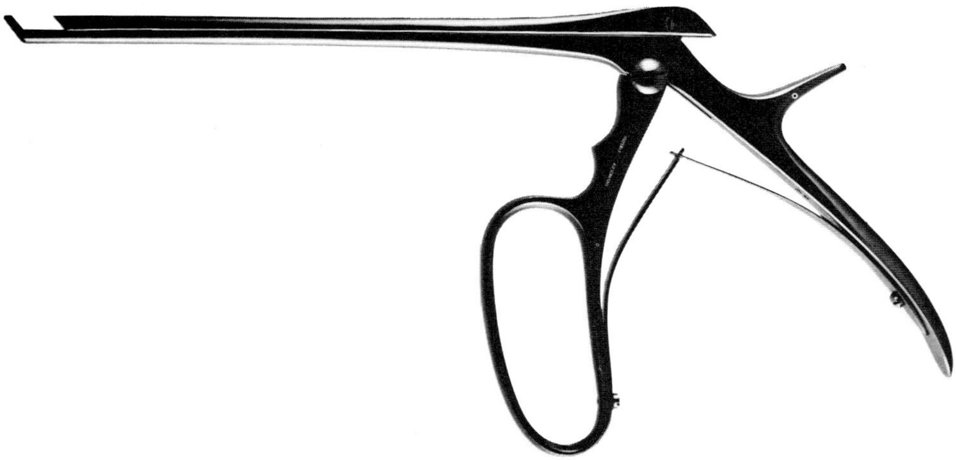

Figure 1.23. A photograph of a 45° forward-angled pituitary punch

superior lamina is trimmed flush with the medial edge of the superior facet, using a right-angled forward cutting laminal rongeur.

In cases where nerve root canal stenosis is severe–as may occur in isolated disc resorption, or facet osteoarthrosis–the anterior surface of the superior facet on the inferior side of a particular vertebral interspace may be closely applied to the posterior surface of the intervertebral disc. Insertion of a forward-angled rongeur between the roof and floor of the nerve root canal may be difficult. The risk of injuring the entrapped nerve root is high in such circumstances so that use of an assortment of different instruments may become necessary to decompress it and to relieve the concomitant venous obstruction in the nerve root canal and intervertebral foramen. Use of a fine sucker, its tip covered with a patty, held as a dural retractor in one hand is recommended. Meanwhile, with a Watson-Cheyne probe in the other hand, the medial edge of the superior facet is defined, soft tissues separated from its anterior surface and the site of maximal obstruction of the nerve root canal determined. Only then, in a bloodless field, can the tactics be planned and the most suitable instruments chosen for the task of nerve root canal decompression. Fine, straight and curved chisels, a variety of forward-cutting laminal rongeurs and fine straight pituitary rongeurs should be available. Some powered tools such as the Quintron oscillating gouge and curette system or air drills may be useful for this delicate work. Powered instruments are potentially dangerous unless they are used with caution (Figs. 1.25, 1.26).

Assuming that one is dealing with a very tight nerve root canal and foraminal stenosis at L5/S1, the site of maximal compression of the S1 nerve root is usually related to the upper, inner and middle thirds of the superior articular facet of S1. The foraminal stenosis is due largely to the apex of the S1 facet together with the ligamentum flavum which has buckled into the foramen. The accompanying diagrams

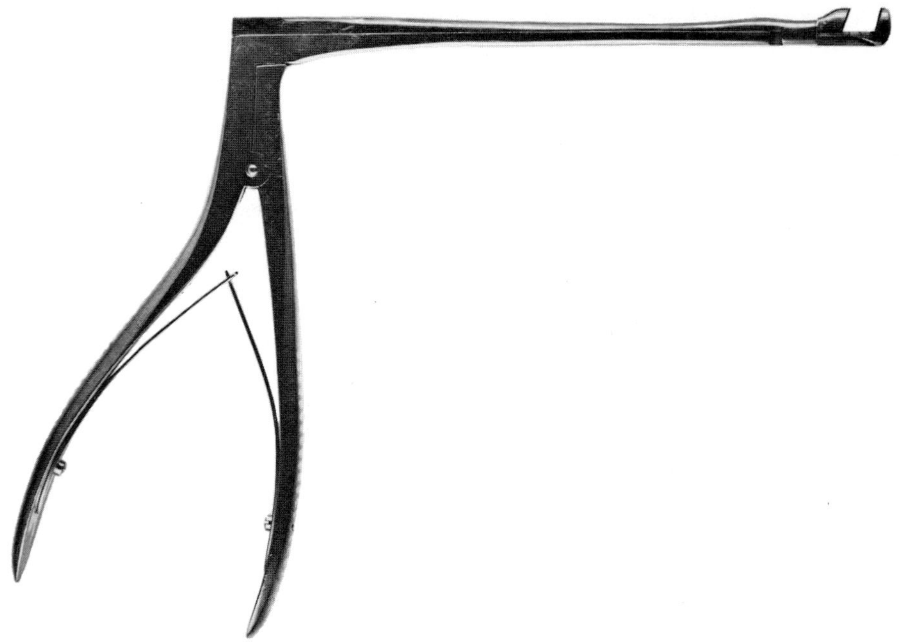

Figure 1.24. A photograph of a 90° forward-angled punch

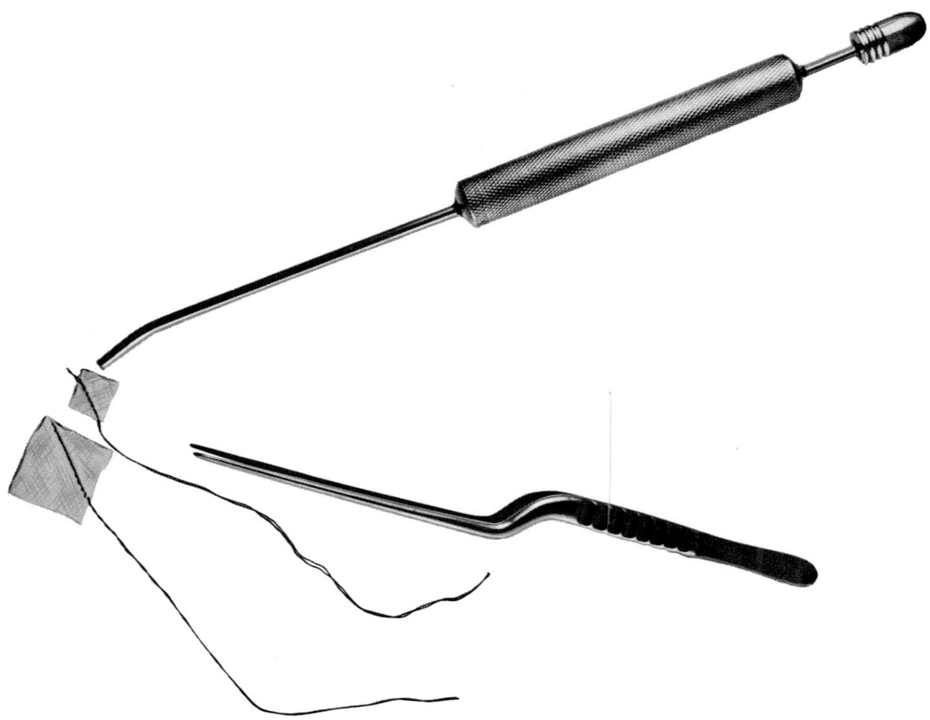

Figure 1.25. A photograph showing a sucker and bayonet forceps with patties of different sizes, all vital for use in spinal canal explorations

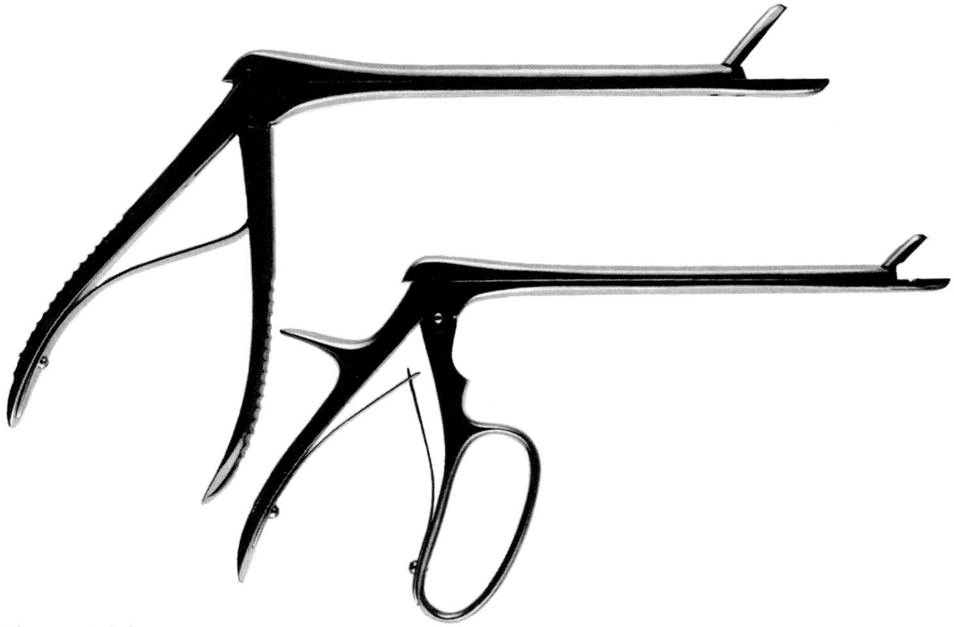

Figure 1.26

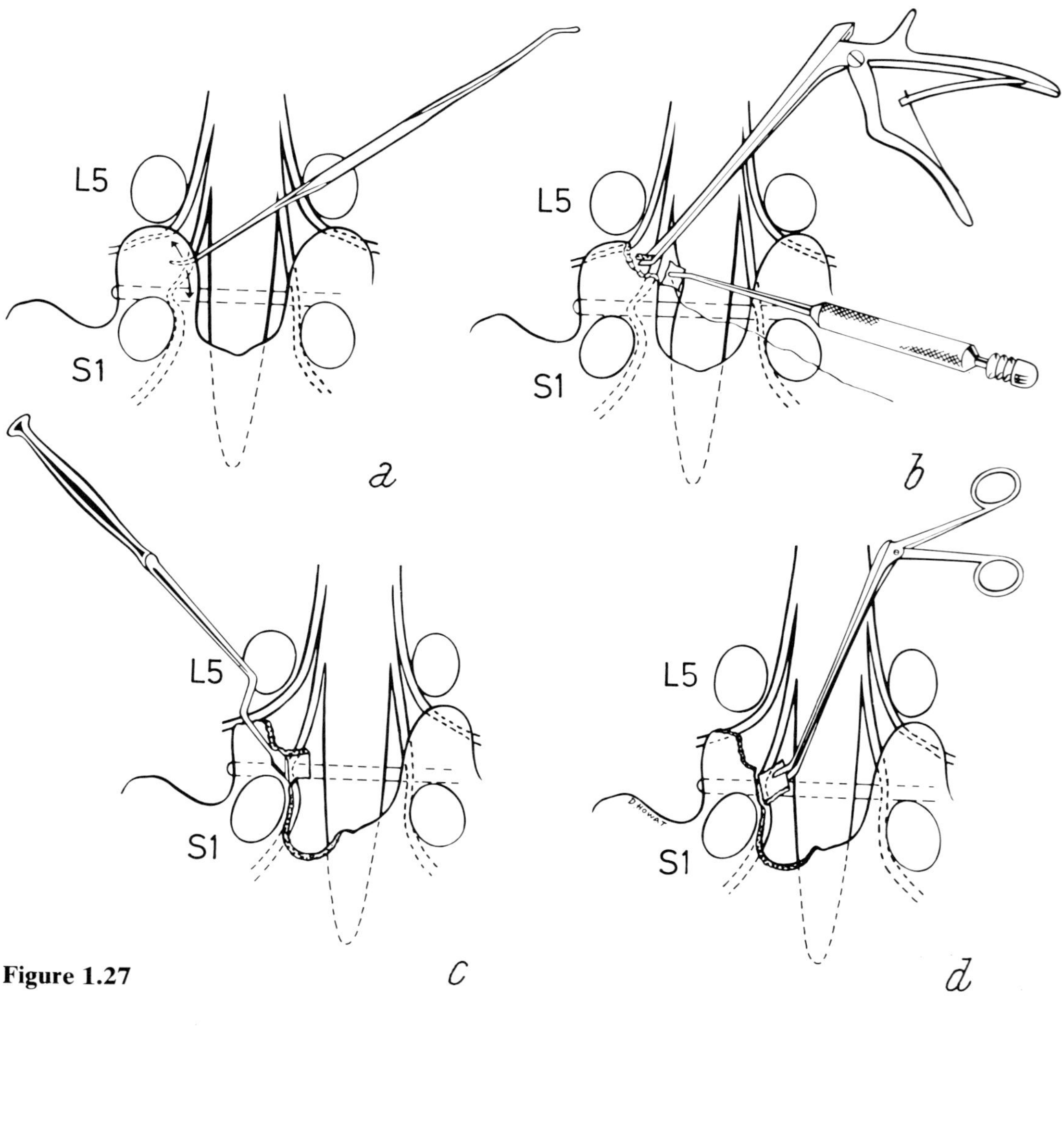

Figure 1.27

depict alternative methods of relieving these stenotic lesions, minimizing risks of nerve root, dural or vascular damage (Figs. 1.27a–d).

During the excision of the medial margin and apex of the S1 facet, obstruction of the intervertebral veins and internal vertebral venous plexus will be noted. When this surgical dissection has been completed the refilling of these veins is dramatic (Figs. 1.28a, b).

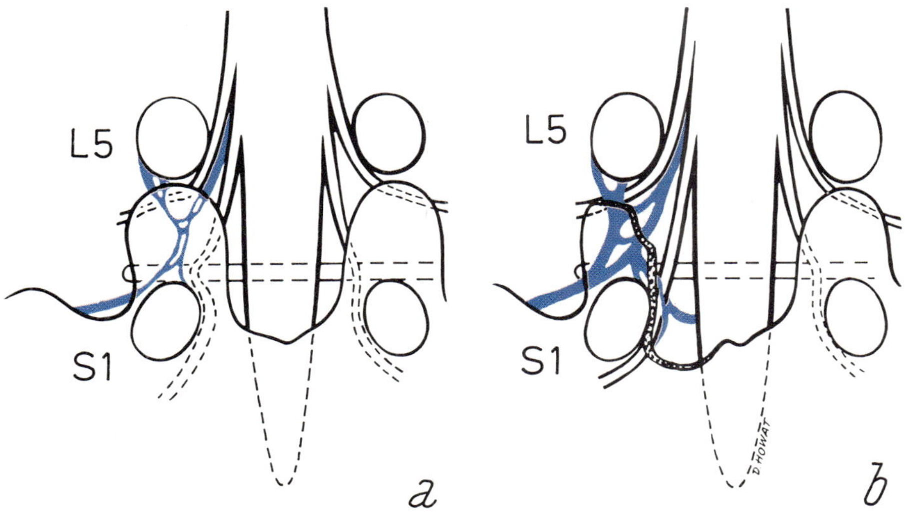

Figures 1.28. **a** A drawing to highlight the feature of venous obstruction which is a concomitant of foraminal and nerve root canal stenosis at L5/S1 in a case of isolated disc resorption. **b** On the right, following decompression by excising the apical and medial portions of the S1 facet and the ligamentum flavum, *note that the mechanical obstruction of the nerve roots is relieved and the venous drainage re-established*

In some instances excision of the bony ridge and upper attachment of the ligamentum flavum can be achieved only after excision of the central arch of the lamina of L5. When this becomes necessary, care is taken to preserve the partes interarticulares of this lamina on both sides, leaving the cut bony surfaces smooth and coating them with bone wax; excision of the apex of the S1 facet, together with the lateral edge of the ligamentum flavum is then facilitated.

Rarely is it necessary to interfere with the floor of the S1 spinal nerve root canal in cases of isolated lumbar disc resorption. Occasionally a sub-rhisal vertebral end-plate sequestrum will be found and this obstruction should be removed from beneath the S1 nerve root.

Figure 1.26. A photograph showing straight pituitary rongeurs of varying sizes. A range of these must be available for use during spinal canal decompressions

Figures 1.27. **a** A diagramatic representation of the findings of S1 nerve root canal stenosis at the L5/S1 level in isolated disc resorption. Note the use of the curved pointed end of the Watson-Cheyne dissector being used to free the soft tissues anterior to the medial edge of the S1 facet. **b** Note the disposition of the sucker and patty and the use of a forward-angled 45° fine cup pituitary punch to excise the apical portion of the facet of S1. **c** A drawing depicting the use of a fine chisel to split off the remnants of the medial aspect of the S1 facet where the S1 nerve root canal is most tightly constricted. **d** A drawing depicting the removal of the segment of the S1 facet to complete the decompression of the S1 nerve root canal. A fine-pointed forward-angled pituitary rongeur is used for this purpose

Results

Symptoms arising from isolated lumbar disc resorption have been shown to be severely disabling. The study published by Venner and Crock in 1981 suggests that nerve root canal decompression in isolated disc resorption is a useful addition to the surgical armamentarium for the treatment of pain in the back and leg. In a series of 45 patients with isolated disc resorption independently reviewed on an average of 45 months after surgical decompression of the S1 or lower lumbar nerve roots, complete success was achieved in 62% of the patients and partial success in 24%.

Table 1.2. Success rate of the operation for isolated disc resorption based on six criteria (45 patients)

Criteria	Success rate for each individual criterion (per cent)	Overall success rate of operation (per cent)	
Operation considered by the patient to be "worthwhile"	84	Complete success (6 criteria)	62
Functional disability reduced	71		
Return to work	78	Partial success (3–5 criteria)	24
Relief of backache	84		
Relief of pain in the legs	91	Failure (< 3 criteria)	14
Independent Observer's Assessment: Dr. R. M. Venner	71	Good	71

1.2. Miscellaneous Causes of Nerve Root Canal Stenosis

a) Congenital Abnormalities

Some congenital abnormalities of the lumbar spine may easily go unnoticed. Congenital hypertrophy of facets is an important cause of nerve root canal stenosis which may be overlooked, particularly if the intervertebral disc spaces are of normal height (Figs. 1.29a–c).

Congenital deficiencies of facets are less common and the defects are sometimes unilateral (Figs. 1.30a–c).

b) Space Occupying Lesions

Occasionally, in an otherwise normal spinal canal, space-occupying lesions related to abnormalities in the dura or arachnoid may occur. Extra-dural arachnoid cysts, of the Schreiber type or peri-neurial cysts of the Tarlov type, may produce symptoms of nerve root canal stenosis (Figs. 1.31a, b) (Gimeno, 1978).

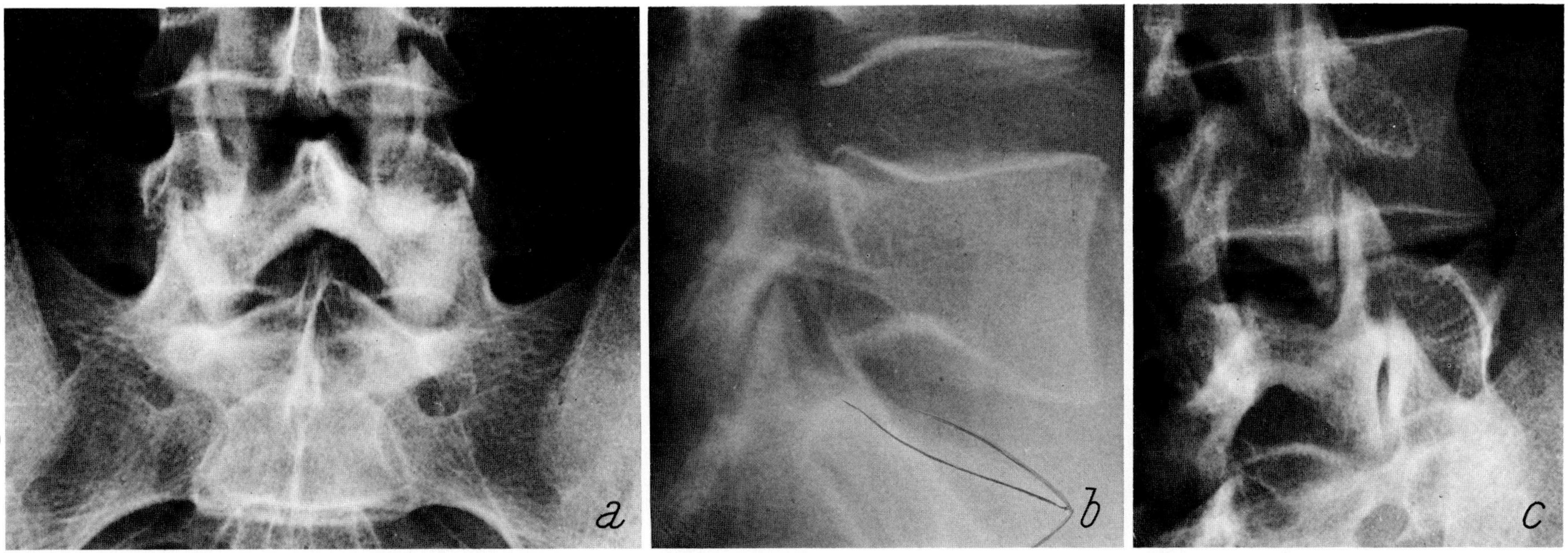

Figures 1.29. **a** An antero-posterior radiograph of the lower lumbar spine in a man aged 38 years presenting with symptoms of bilateral buttock and thigh pain extending to the back of the knee, aggravated by standing, sitting or walking. Note the orientation of the facets at L5/S1 with the apices of the S1 facets visible on the A-P view in close proximity to the inferior borders of the pedicles of L5. **b** A lateral radiograph of the spine in the same patient showing normal discs at L4/5 and L5/S1. Note the *congenital large S1 facets* projecting upwards into the intervertebral foramen at L5/S1, the apex of the facet being visible close to the inferior surface of the pedicle of L5. **c** An oblique view of the same spine showing the hypertrophic S1 facet, the apex of which lies close to the inferior border of the pedicle of L5. The relationships of the apex of the superior facet of L5 and the pedicle of L4 provide a marked contrast to the findings at the lower level

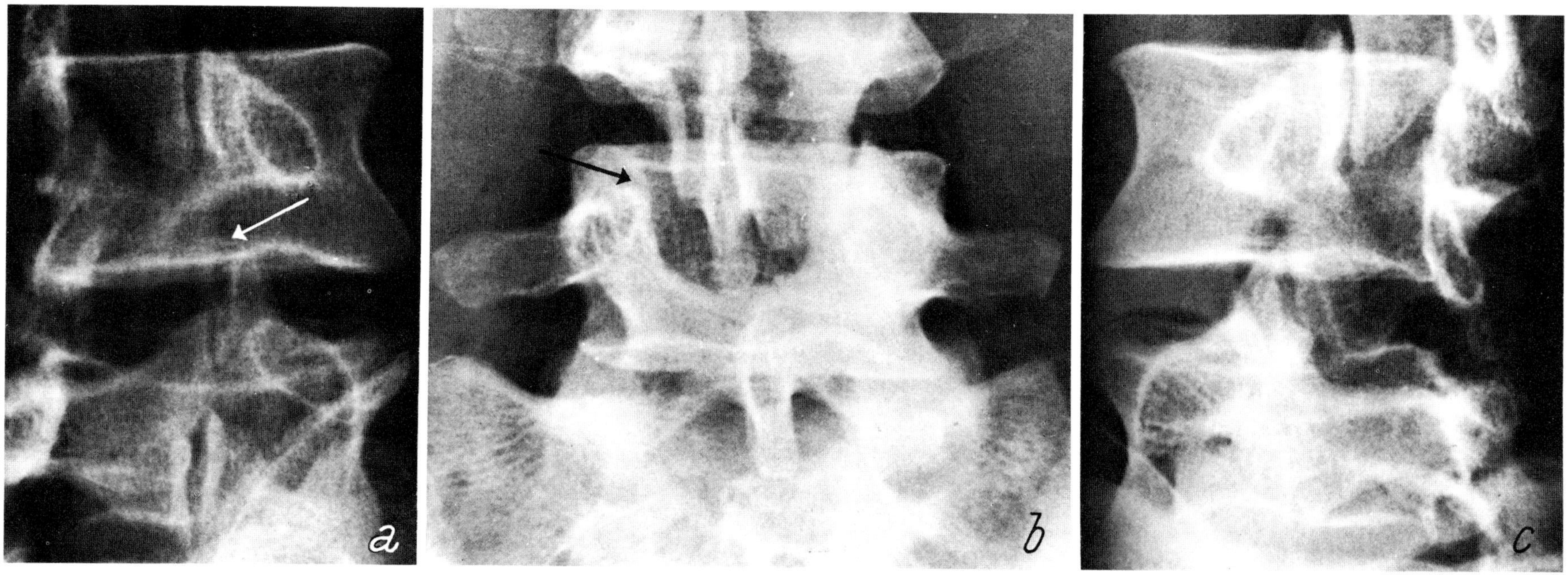

Figures 1.30. **a** An oblique view of the lower lumbar spine of a woman aged 34 who presented with unilateral buttock and leg pain aggravated by standing and walking. The arrow points to the congenital abnormality at the pars interarticularis with absence of the inferior facet of L 4. **b** An antero-posterior radiograph of the same spine showing the unilateral congenital abnormality with absence of the facet of L 4 on one side. In the area indicated at the tip of the arrow, there was a bulky mass of soft tissue found at operation; semicartilagenous in consistency, it was causing root canal stenosis. **c** An oblique view of the opposite side of the spine showing the normal laminal arrangement and intact inferior facet

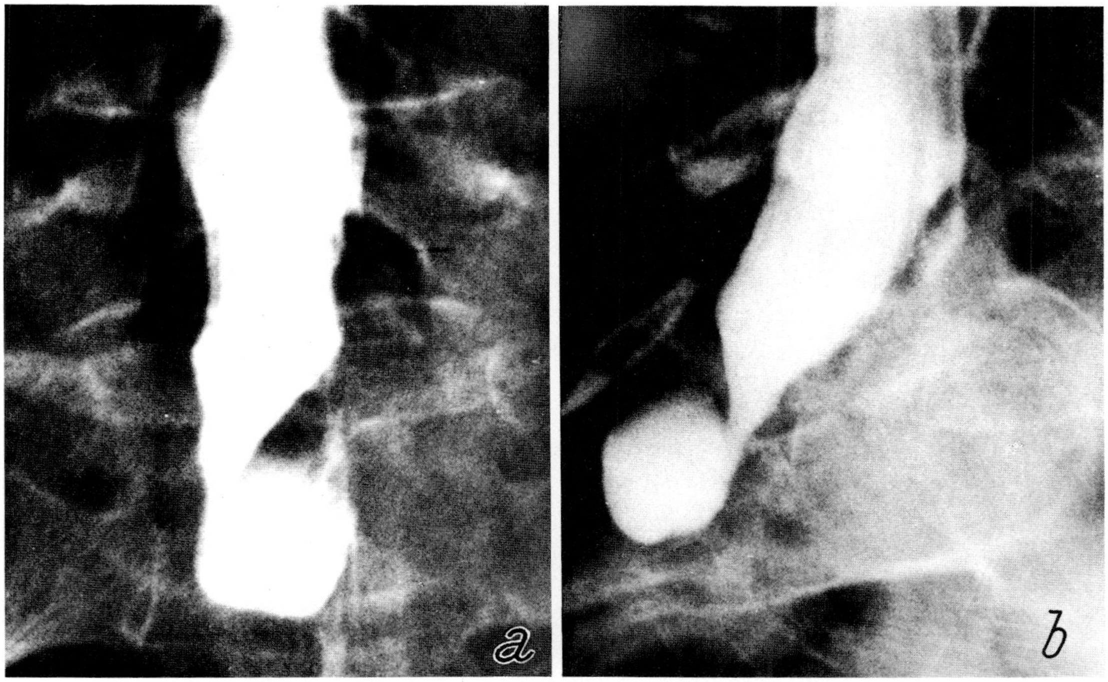

Figures 1.31. a An antero-posterior radiograph of the lower lumbar and upper sacral area showing a myelographic defect produced by an *extra-dural arachnoid cyst of the Tarlov type.* **b** A lateral radiograph of the myelogram in the same spine, showing the deformation of the lower end of the lumbo-sacral dural sac produced by a large extra-dural arachnoid cyst, acting as a space-occupying lesion in the nerve root canal in this area, there being no associated abnormality of the disc or vertebral column

c) Localized Degeneration

More common causes of nerve root canal stenosis are seen in localized degenerative disorders.

i) For example, in isolated disc resorption, retrolisthesis of L5 on S1 may occur, aggravating the tendency for the development of spinal nerve root canal stenosis which occurs commonly in this condition (Fig. 1.32).

ii) Retrolisthesis of one lumbar vertebra on another often occurs in association with disc resorptive changes in the first mobile segment above sacralization anomalies in the lower lumbar spine.

iii) Unilateral facet osteoarthritis may occur at a single level, most commonly at the lumbo-sacral junction, where it can produce unilateral sciatica (Figs. 1.33a, b).

The use of myelography in the diagnosis of these problems is recommended and typical changes, with gross local deformity, can be seen in a number of the miscellaneous causes referred to in this text (Figs. 1.34a, b). However, it is very important to recall that the myelogram may be reported as normal in many of these cases. The surgeon must then fall back on his clinical assessment of the patient, aided by plain X-ray findings, while deciding whether or not to recommend surgical treatment in a particular case.

Accuracy of diagnosis has been enhanced since the advent of C.T. scanning, though it must be remembered that these expensive instruments are not yet universally available. In addition, unless the computer facility allows for reconstructions in three planes, its value in the diagnosis of these particular problems is seriously restricted. *Problems in the nerve root canal are not readily appreciated throughout its length by studies of transverse sections alone.* Unless this is appreciated, together with the fact that myelography may not define the anatomy of the nerve root canals completely in particular cases, the surgeon presented with apparently normal myelography and normal C.T. scanning in the transverse plane alone, may be disinclined to believe that the patient is seriously disabled and so deny him or her the surgical treatment which would relieve the symptoms.

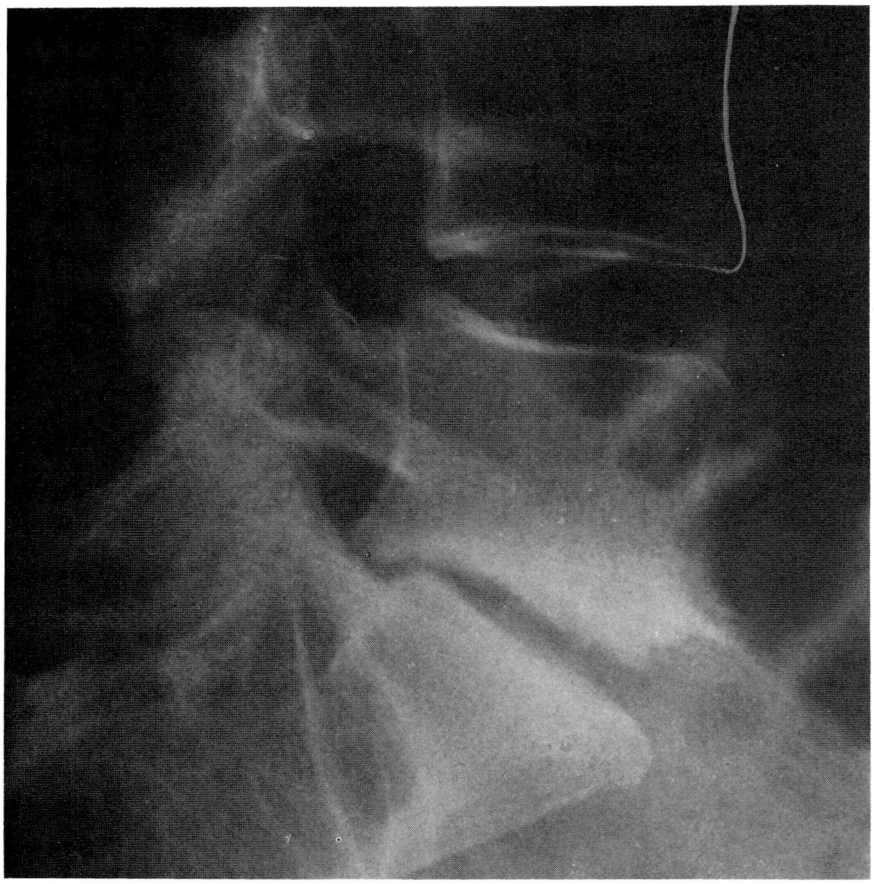

Figure 1.32. A lateral radiograph of the lower lumbar spine showing an example of *retro-spondylolisthesis complicating isolated disc resorption at the lumb-sacral junction,* one of the rarer causes of root canal stenosis complicating this localized degenerative disc disease in the lower lumbar spine

Figures 1.33. **a** A radiograph of the lower lumbar spine in a woman aged 49 years showing unilateral facet hypertrophy due to osteoarthritis, leading to unilateral nerve root canal stenosis. **b** An antero-posterior radiograph of the lower lumbar spine of a man aged 30 with unilateral osteoarthritis of a facet at L5/S1 producing root canal stenosis

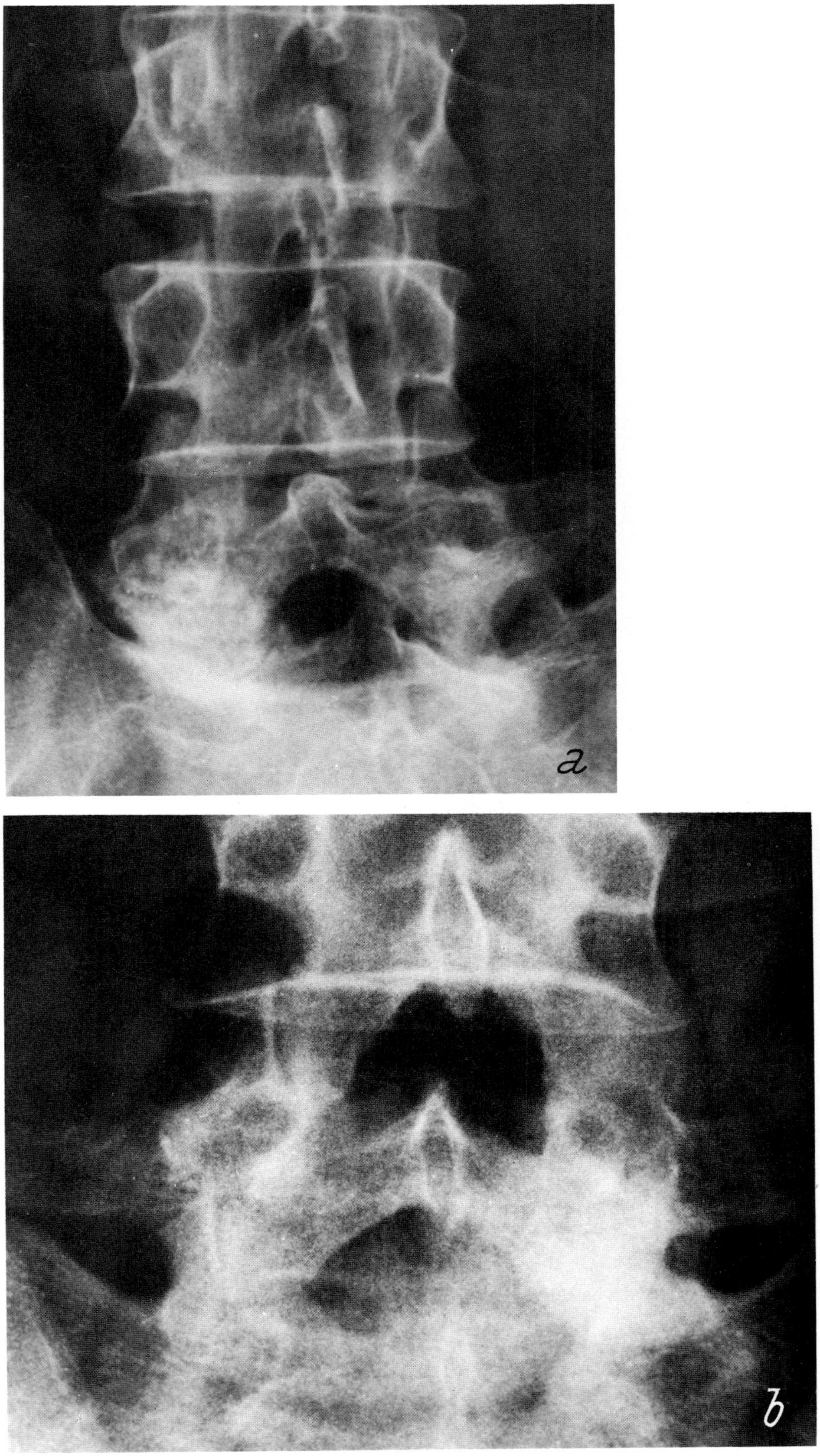

Figures 1.33

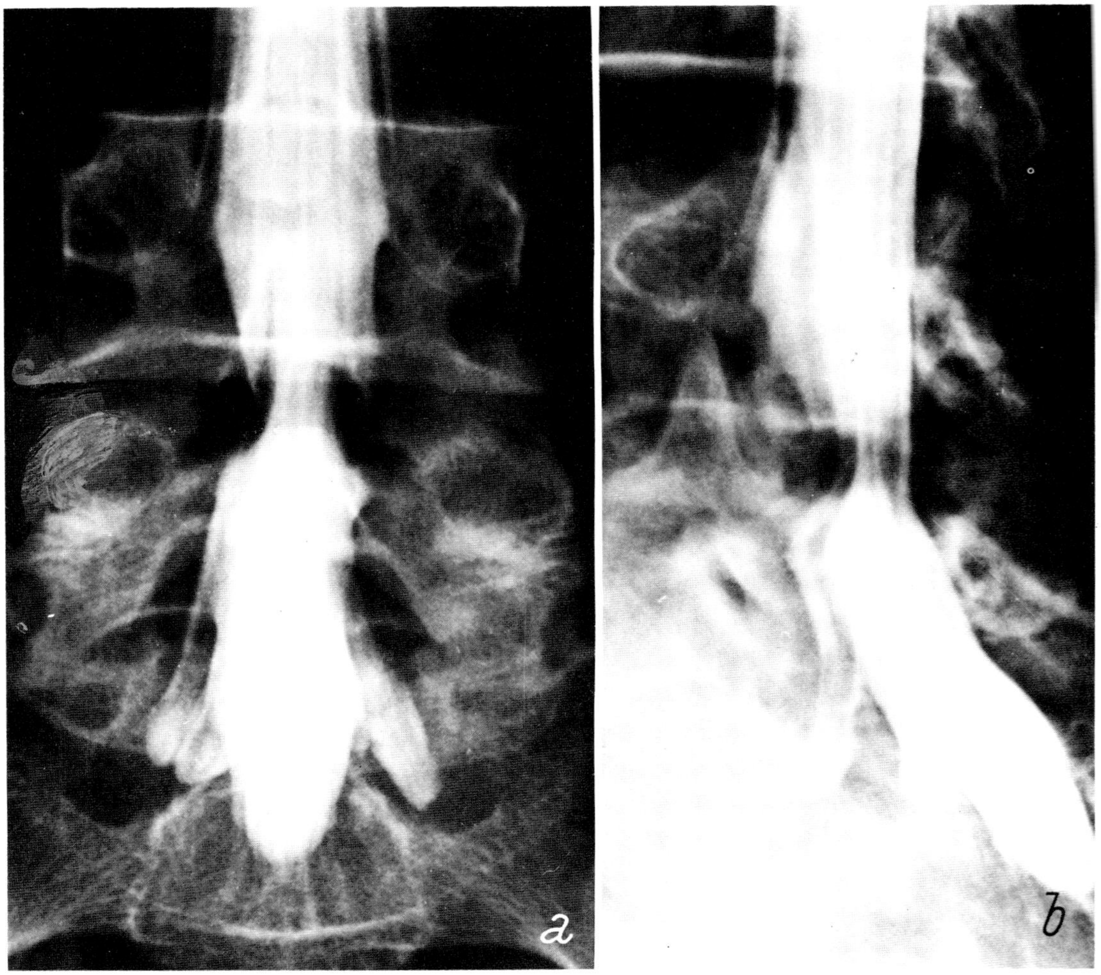

Figures 1.34. **a** An antero-posterior radiograph of the lower lumbar spine to show a myelographic defect (metrizamide) with partial spindling of the main column produced by bilateral facet hypertrophy of the inferior facets of L4. **b** An oblique radiograph of the metrizamide myelogram highlighting the relationship of the deformity in the column of dye to the medial border of the inferior facet of L4. Although there is an element of spinal canal stenosis present in such a case, the principal effect is seen in stenosis of the nerve root canal

2

Internal Disc Disruption

This term was introduced in a paper titled: "A reappraisal of intervertebral disc lesions", published in the Medical Journal of Australia in 1970.

The condition is common and should be readily identified clinically, though discography is essential for its confirmation.

The clinical syndrome which may be associated with this type of disc disorder usually follows severe trauma inflicted on the disc, for example, by sudden unexpected weight lifting, or by forces transmitted through the disc or discs during high speed accidents.

2.1. Clinical Features

a) Symptoms

Patients affected by severe grades of internal disc disruption present with an array of symptoms which should arouse the clinician's suspicion early in the course of management, especially if the history of the mechanism of injury is placed in its proper perspective. Back pain is prominent, having the character of a deep-seated dull ache. Their description of referred limb pain differs remarkably from that given by those with disc prolapses. The patient with limb pain due to internal disc disruption always finds difficulty in describing this type of pain. Usually it seems to be widespread in the limb, or deep inside it, having an intolerable aching character. Except for short remissions the symptoms are rarely alleviated by conservative physical therapy and may be aggravated by spinal manipulation or traction.

When these patients first present for treatment, one may be unimpressed with their description of symptoms and struck by the complete absence of abnormal physical signs in many of them. Observation over two or three months will reveal their low tolerance for physical activity. Their symptoms may become widespread with severe occipital headache, intractable spinal pain, nausea and weight loss.

There has been a tendency to label as "functional" or "psychological" many of the symptoms described by patients with lumbar disc disruption including those of headache and temperature dysaesthesia in the legs (Hakelius *et al.,* 1969).

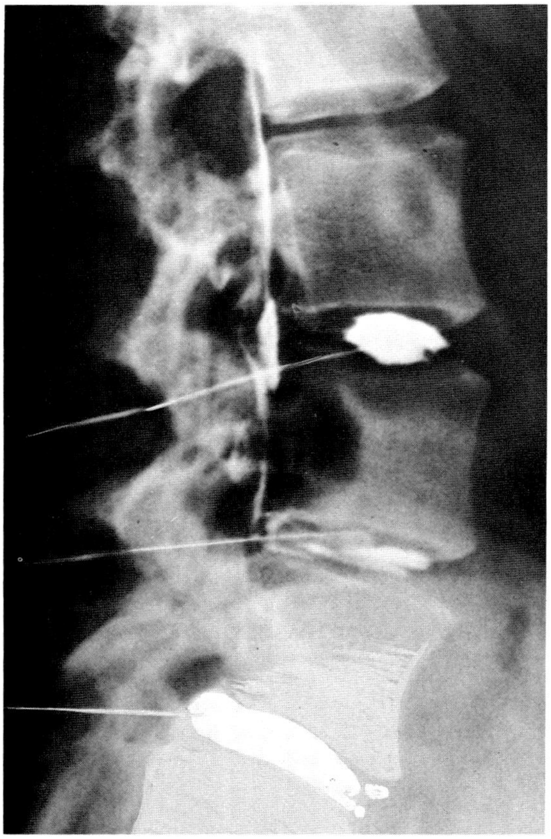

Figure 2.1. A lateral radiograph of the lower lumbar spine from a girl aged 18 showing a normal discogram at L3/4. At L4/5, gross disc disruption is evident with extra-thecal leakage of dye into the spinal canal extending to the level of L2/3. The L5/S1 discogram shows gross disc disruption with dye extending back to the level of the spinal canal but not leaking into it. This is an example of post-traumatic internal disc disruption sustained following a fall from a horse three years previously

b) Spinal Movements

When standing, many have great difficulty in rising from a flexed position. They usually assist themselves by placing the palms of their hands on the anterior aspects of their thighs, literally climbing up from the stooped position using the hands as props. Similarly, when attempting to sit up from a lying position, they may find it impossible without placing both hands flat on the bed behind them and exerting pressure on the upper limbs to raise themselves to a sitting position. At other times they may turn on to one side and get up into a sitting position by rolling their legs over the side of the bed and then levering themselves up slowly and awkwardly, obviously in pain. Spasm of the paraspinal muscles, as seen in cases with disc prolapse, is very uncommon in this condition.

c) Body Weight Loss

In patients who are clearly constitutionally ill as a result of internal disc disruption, weight loss may be profound over the course of a few months, ranging from 6–18 kg.

Conversely, some patients actually gain weight, due to their enforced physical inactivity.

d) Neurological Signs

Abnormal neurological signs in the limbs are uncommon, though complaints of weakness, clumsiness, and sympathetic nervous system disturbances as described above, are often made.

e) Psychiatric Disturbances

The psychological responses to this form of disc injury are partly predictable. These patients are usually incapacitated for many months before the diagnosis is established. They soon realize that their symptoms are a mystery not only to themselves but often to their doctors also. They feel that their problems are being taken too lightly. Financial worries soon begin to plague them and shortly the whole fabric of their lives begins to disintegrate, leading to an acute anxiety state. The view is often expressed that these problems and others, glibly described as litigation neurosis, will not loom as major obstructions to recovery if treatment is undertaken quickly (Macnab, 1969). Iatrogenically induced neurosis is often seen in these patients, especially if they have been under treatment for more than nine months without relief of symptoms.

There is a range of psychiatric disturbances seen in this group which is distinct from the simpler psychological disturbances seen in patients with disc prolapse requiring surgery.

Following total disc excision and interbody fusion for internal disc disruption, a significant, but small percentage of these patients, develop an acute psychiatric illness within a few days. They often become disorientated and violent. This phenomenon is rarely seen following any other orthopaedic operation. One is tempted to relate such disturbances to some biochemical abnormality in the damaged disc tissue, postulating that the psychiatric upset is caused by the sudden release of a sensitizing substance into the general circulation at the time of operation.

In managing patients with this type of disc disorder, it is desirable to work closely with a psychiatrist who has a special interest in these matters. The following comments come from the pen of such a consultant psychiatrist, H.G. Stevenson, writing in 1970:

"Psychiatric problems following disc disease appear to be labelled functional by the surgeon whose treatment has failed to relieve symptoms, and iatrogenic by his colleagues in the profession who have been fortunate not to be involved in the actual surgical onslaught. Neither of these labels appears to be justifiable in the vast majority of cases.

i) Acute Psychotic Reaction

"Two major patterns of disturbance are seen. Firstly, an acute psychotic reaction occurring shortly after operation on either the cervical or lumbar spine varying from a manic type of reaction to one which appears to be schizophrenic in type. The nearest parallel to these are the puerperal psychoses which are accepted as being due to a sudden alteration in biochemical function of the individual following the major physiological alterations of birth, and considered to occur only in patients with a covert psychosis.

"In those who react in this way to spinal surgery, there is probably an underlying covert psychotic make-up which may otherwise never have become apparent without the operation. The acute reaction is usually short-lived, responds to conservative anti-psychotic treatment readily and seldom needs intensive psychiatric or physical treatment.

"Given that patients, suffering from this syndrome, are probably prone individuals of whom there is no dearth in the normal community, it could be fairly said that even with a mild whiplash injury to the neck, a state of depression follows.

ii) Reaction to Prolonged Disease

"With more serious disc disease–particularly of the cervical spine–one finds the second typical syndrome, characterized by irritability, intolerance to noise, periods of severe depression, headaches starting at the back of the head, going over the front of the head and often causing blurring of the vision, a gross degree of introspection which is again probably a factor of a true depressive illness, reduced sexual function in both male and female and extending particularly in the male to the state of complete impotence, dizziness often postural in type and frequently directly related to the intensity of the headache; pain in the limbs not corresponding to the anatomical areas of sensory supply but notably consistent over a great number of patients, a poor memory and reduced concentration. The overall syndrome responds poorly to anti-depressive medication and the added anxiety of litigation increases the failure of therapy. However, even without litigation this typical syndrome is seen and the 'cure' appears to be more an adjustment to an altered way and principle of living than a return to 'normal'. Whether the cause is biochemical, or due to alteration in the blood supply to the base of the brain, or affection of the sympathetic nervous system is questionable, but this in turn appears to be in parallel with the disc injury rather than a result of the prolonged symptoms or the failure of orthopaedic treatment. Physical strain patterns following damage to the head and neck suggest that the centre of stress is in the region of the hypothalamus, which area has been the focus of attention in most research on depressive states, and this in itself could bring about an alteration in the biochemical balance, particularly in relation to the 5-hydroxytryptamine and plasma cortisol levels.

"Follow-up studies on these patients, suggest that the depressive state persists for a considerable time, that it tends to recur, perhaps in that the patient has learned a depressive form of reaction to stress and this then becomes his normal pattern to stress in the future. The alteration in the personality adjustment in at least some cases, appears to be permanent. The relationship of strain from lower back disease affecting the upper regions of the spine and a typical depressive state occurring in parallel is also seen. Most attention has been centred on the medico-legal aspects, and efforts by Cole (1970), Stevenson (1970) and Parker (1972) have thrown some doubt on Miller's (1961) article on accident neuroses, so that more accurate psychiatric diagnosis in these post-traumatic spinal conditions is gaining acceptance.

"The role of physical psychiatric treatment including electroconvulsive therapy and intravenous amobarbital (Amytal) is doubtful. These methods of treatment are used only when the extent of the psychiatric disability warrants their use, irrespective of the physical condition in the spine."

When internal disc disruption goes unrecognized on the clinical features described above, the patients drift from doctor to doctor, often seeing as many as ten, including family doctors, general surgeons, neurologists, neurosurgeons, orthopaedic surgeons and psychiatrists. Many seek relief in fringe medicine.

2.2. *Pathology*

a) Macroscopic Changes

The primary defects appear to lie in the field of histochemical pathology and probably also in alterations to the mechanism of disc nutrition.

Macroscopically, disrupted disc tissue is soft, often slightly yellow in colour but otherwise indistinguishable from disc tissue in the early phases of degeneration.

Circumferential tears between adjacent rings of the annulus fibrosus or radial tears in these fibres, short of complete extension to the outer annular layers, can be demonstrated radiographically by discography. After many years of clinical observation, the conclusion is inescapable that in certain individuals these changes in the discs are associated with biological dynamics which lead to a disabling syndrome, precipitated by trauma and further aggravated by repeated minor trauma.

That some dynamic pathological process is active gains support in observations made during vertebral interbody fusion operations for this condition. For example, the lumbar sympathetic trunk may be found matted to such an affected disc and the adjacent paravertebral lymph nodes seen to be enlarged. In addition, the vascularity of the vertebral bodies adjacent to such a disc appears to be increased and their bony densities are reduced.

The significance of these findings relates to observations made during experiments on auto-immunity in the intervertebral discs of rabbits, reported by Bobechko and Hirsch (1965). Credit for first drawing attention to the possible auto-immune basis to the development of biochemical changes in disc prolapse should be given to Naylor (1962). With added knowledge of the anatomy of the circulation in the region of the vertebral end plates, Crock and Yoshizawa (1977), Crock and Goldwasser (1983), and with further evidence on the movement of radio-opaque dyes from disc tissues into the veins of the vertebral bodies (Figs. 2.2.–2.6), it seems likely that *auto-immunity* may play an important role in the development of the severe disabilities that afflict patients with the syndrome of *internal disc disruption*.

Site of Lesions

The lower lumbar discs are most commonly affected (Figs. 2.7a, b, 2.8).

b) Genesis of Symptoms

In these cases there appear to be three probable causes for the symptoms described: (i) irritation of adjacent nerve roots resulting from abnormal vertebral movements with or without some diffuse disc bulging, (ii) irritation of structures adjacent to the affected disc, the spinal nerves and sympathetic system, due to catabolites diffusing

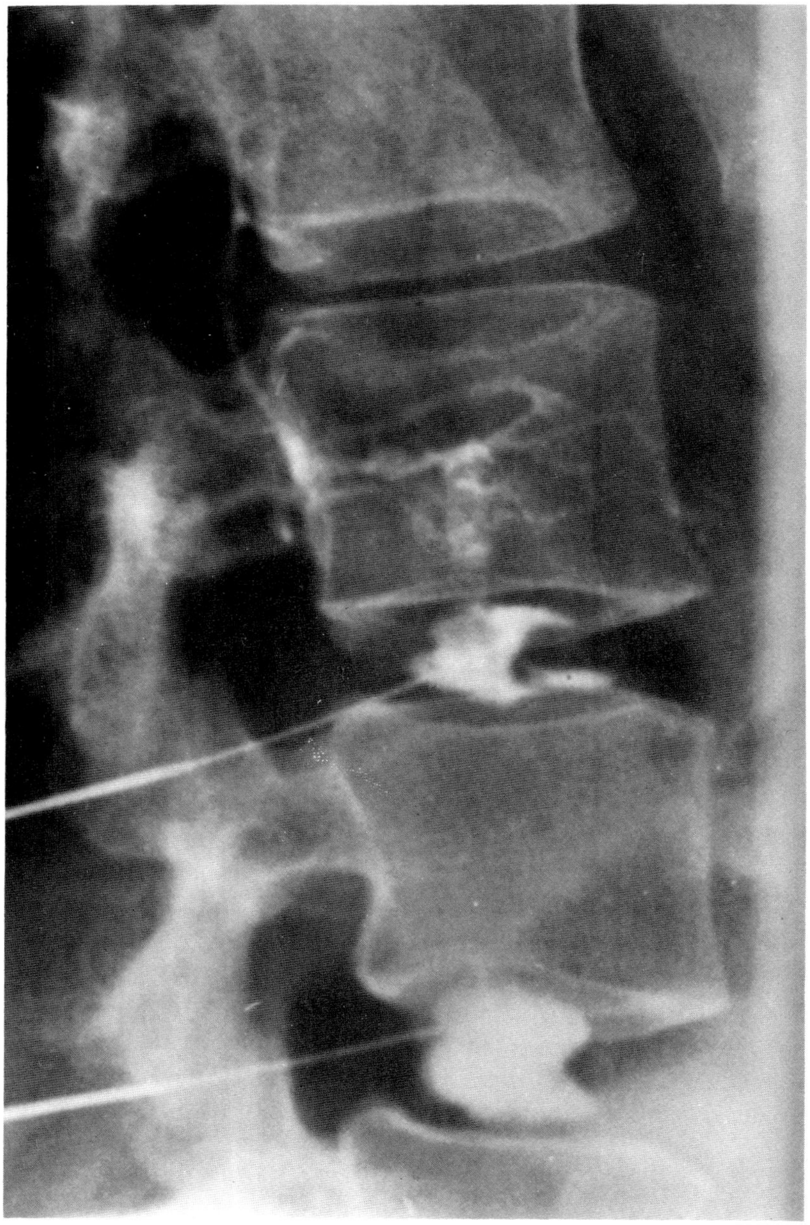

Figure 2.2. A lateral radiograph of the lumbar spine showing discrograms at L3/4 and L4/5. The L4/5 discogram is normal. The L3/4 discogram shows a normal nuclear outline but note the spread of dye into the veins of the vertebral body. Batson's plexus is filled and tributaries of the anterior internal vertebral venous plexus are also filled

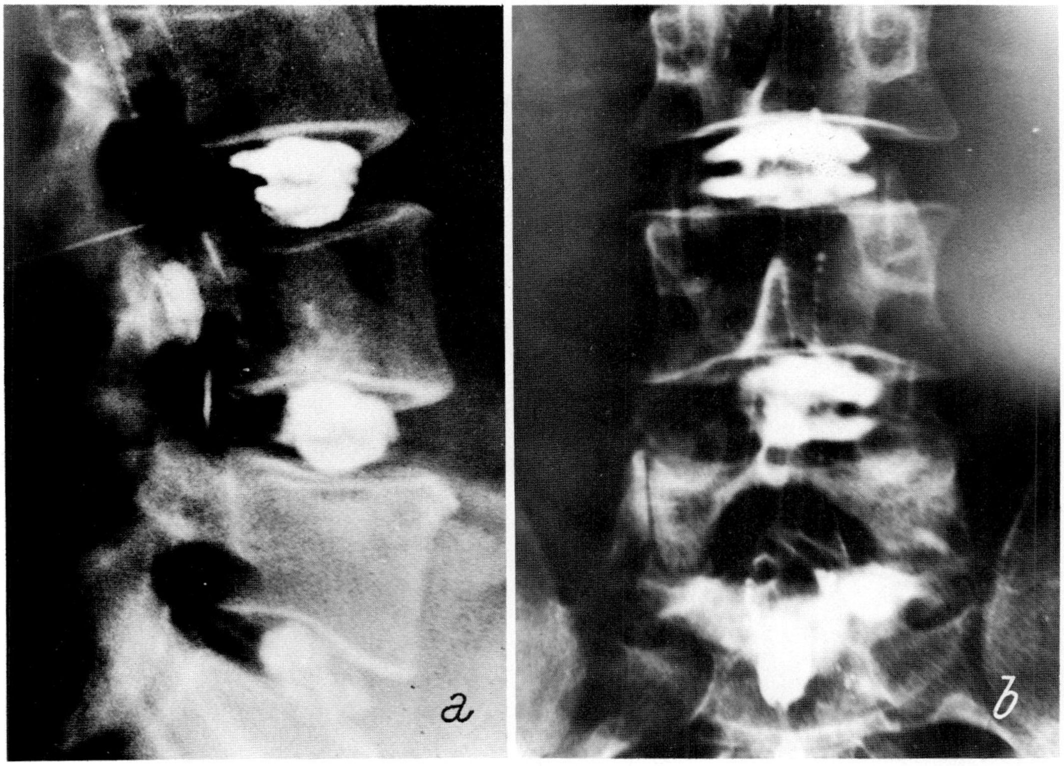

Figures 2.3 a and **b.** Radiographs of the lumbar spine of a man aged 37 years showing discograms at the L3/4, L4/5 and L5/S1 levels. Remnants of myodil are noted in the spinal canal from a previous myelogram performed some years earlier. The volume of dye injected at the L3/4 and L5/S1 disc spaces was approximately 1.9 ml at each disc. The volume injected at the L4/5 level was 4.5 ml. Note the flare in the body of the 4th lumbar vertebra, indicating leakage of dye through the vertebral end-plate cartilage. During injection of contrast medium at the L4/5 disc, the patient complained of severe low back pain similar to that for which he had sought treatment. The discograms appear normal in the antero-posterior view

out of the disc, Nachemson (1969); and (iii) leakage of disc protein and catabolites into the general circulation via vertebral end-plate capillaries, producing features suggestive of auto-immune or hypersensitivity reactions. Some of the patients in this group suffer from profound weight loss and they are found to have abnormalities in peripheral blood smears, with rouleaux formation, altered white cell counts and elevated erythrocyte sedimentation rates (E.S.R.) (Crock, 1970). Gurdjian *et al.* (1961) observed elevations of the E.S.R. in patients who progressed satisfactorily following lumbar laminectomy for herniated intervertebral discs. These authors drew no conclusions about the significance of the observation except in those cases where it remained elevated in the range 80 to 120 mm per hour when aseptic necrosis of the vertebral body adjacent to the area of operation, was noted. Grollmus *et al.* (1974) studied the E.S.R. in 49 patients following lumbar laminectomy, contrasting the findings with those in a group of 25 patients with the syndrome of disc space inflammation. Their observations and conclusions in relation to cases with closed disc space infections were similar to those of Gurdjian *et al.* (1961). However, they noted consistent elevation of the E.S.R. after discectomy in patients whose post-operative

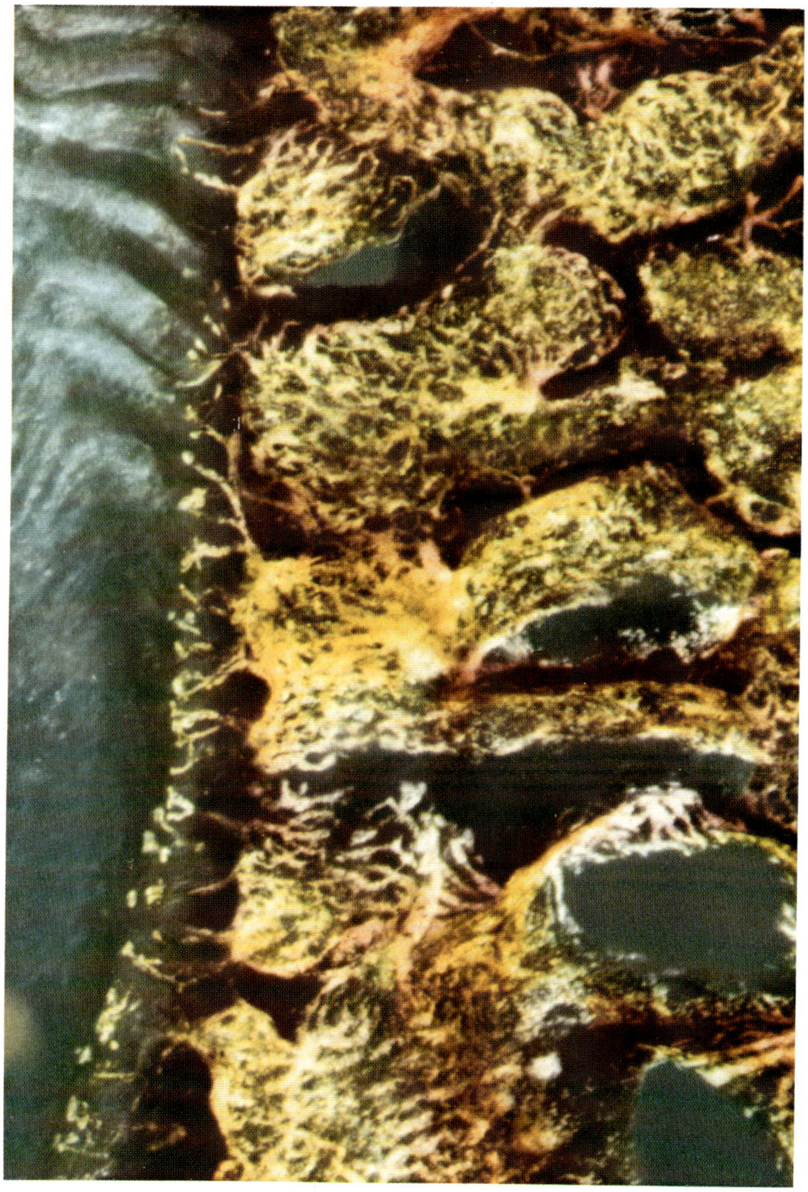

Figure 2.4. A micro-photograph (×60 approximately) showing the capillary bed in the vertebral end-plate cartilage in the lower lumbar ragion in an adult dog. Note the drainage of these capillaries directly into the marrow spaces of the vertebral bodies. *This is almost certainly the pathway for the passage of substances from a damaged "avascular" disc into the patient's immune system.* (Prepared by Drs. H. V. Crock and M. Goldwasser)

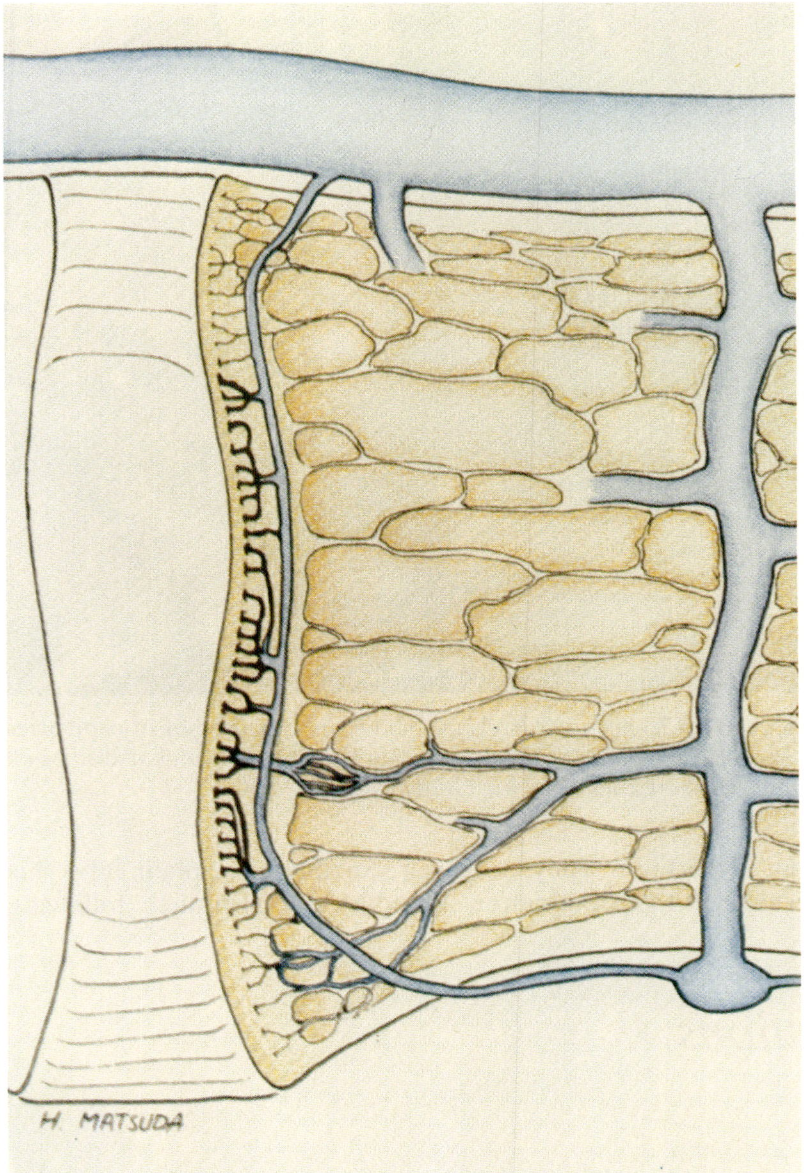

Figure 2.5. A drawing illustrating the methods of drainage of vertebral end-plate capillaries in the dog: (i) either directly into the marrow space veins or, (ii) through a sub-articular collecting vein system into a vertically orientated sub-articular vein system that will drain either backwards into the internal vertebral venous plexus or forward into the external vertebral veins

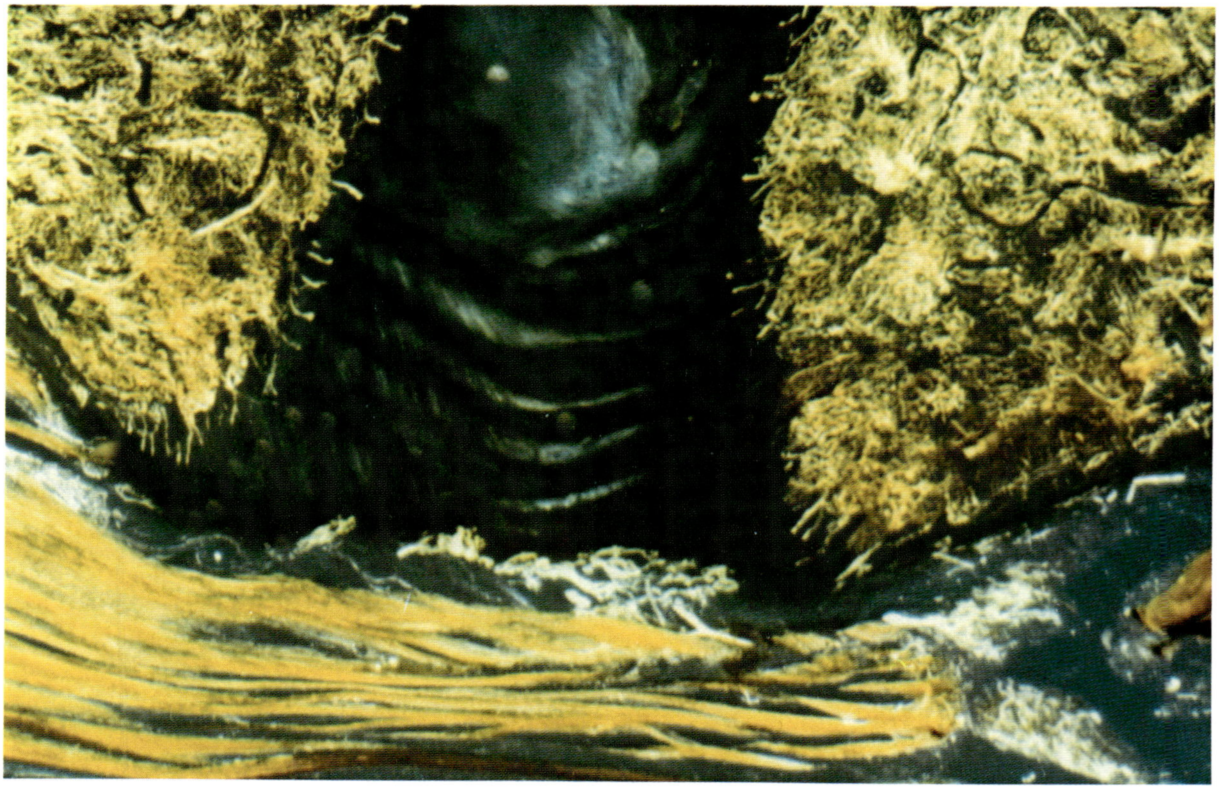

Figure 2.6. A photo micrograph (×20 approximately) to show the distribution of capillaries in the vertebral end-plate cartilages at the anterior disc margin in the lower lumbar disc of an adult dog. (Prepared by Drs. H. V. Crock and M. Goldwasser)

course was otherwise uncomplicated. They, too, were unable to explain fully this phenomenon, but suggested that the examination should be made routinely following operation.

2.3. Investigations

a) Plain X-Ray

Unless clear evidence of vertebral instability can be demonstrated on films taken in flexion and extension, plain X-rays are of no value in establishing this diagnosis (Morgan and King, 1957).

b) Discography

Lumbar Discography was introduced by Lindblom (1948). *This investigation is indispensable in the modern practice of spinal surgery* (Figs. 2.8, 2.9a, b, 2.10a, b). Special needles are required for its performance (Fig. 2.11). Injection of a suitable contrast medium such as Urograffin 60% w/vol should be made through a Luer-lock 1 ml syringe.

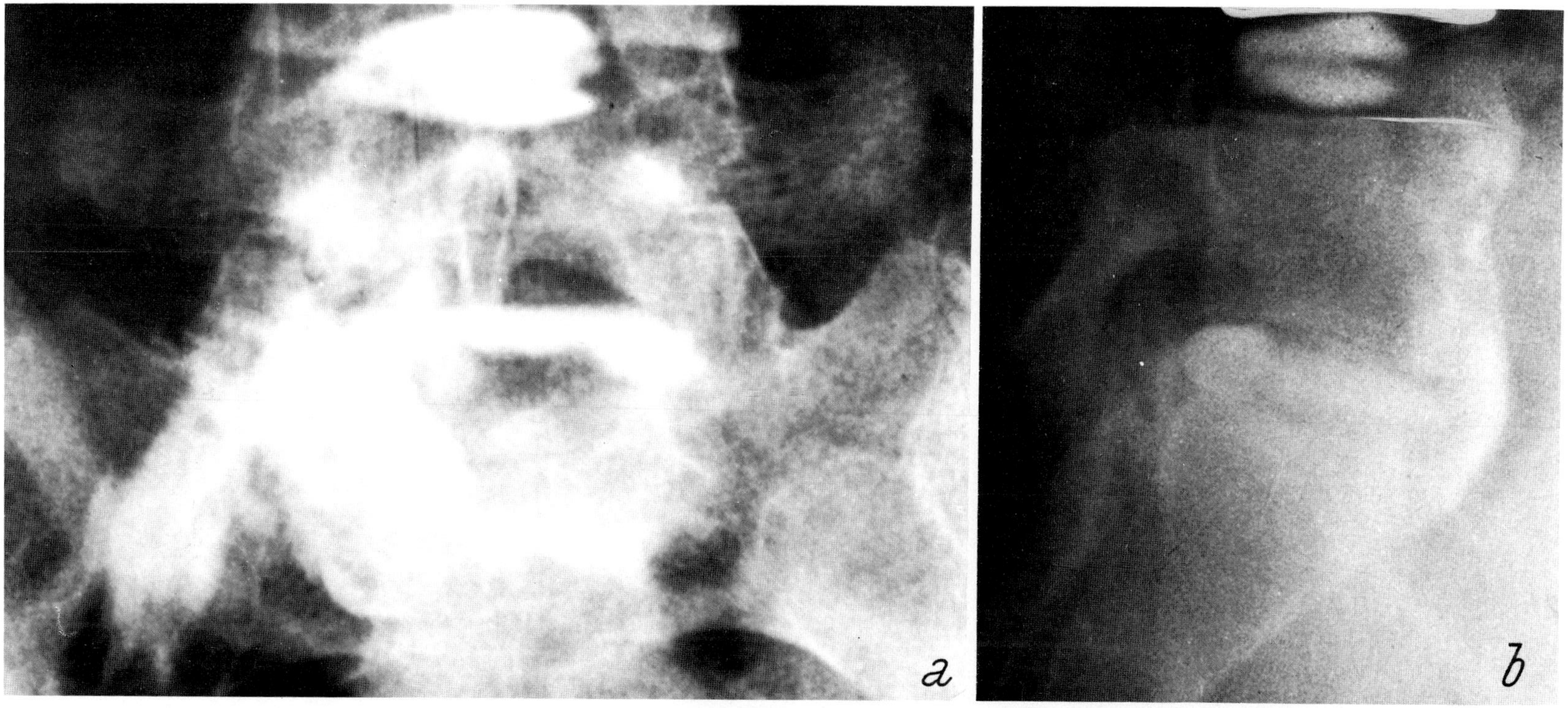

Figures 2.7 a and **b.** Antero-posterior and lateral radiographs of the L 4/5 and L 5/S1 discs in a girl of 17, showing a normal L 4/5 discogram and gross disc disruption at L 5/S1 with antero-lateral leakage of dye. This young lady had been involved in a motor vehicle accident two years earlier and presented with classical features of post-traumatic internal disc disruption, with chronic back pain, referred leg pain, loss of energy, intolerance to physical activity, and profound weight loss

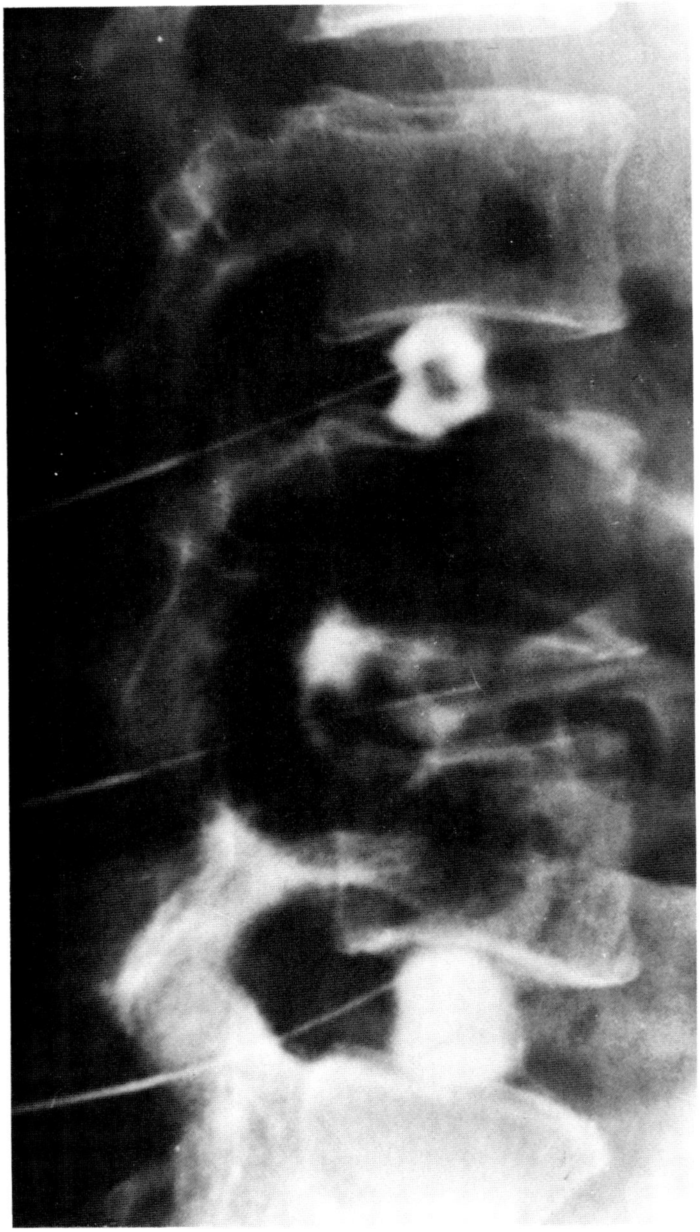

Figure 2.8. A lateral radiograph of the lumbar spine of a man aged 48 years showing normal discograms at L3/4 and L5/S1. 2 ml of dye was injected at each of these disc spaces and no pain was reproduced. At L4/5, 5 ml of dye was injected. Gross disc disruption is shown. The patient's pain was reproduced at the time of injection

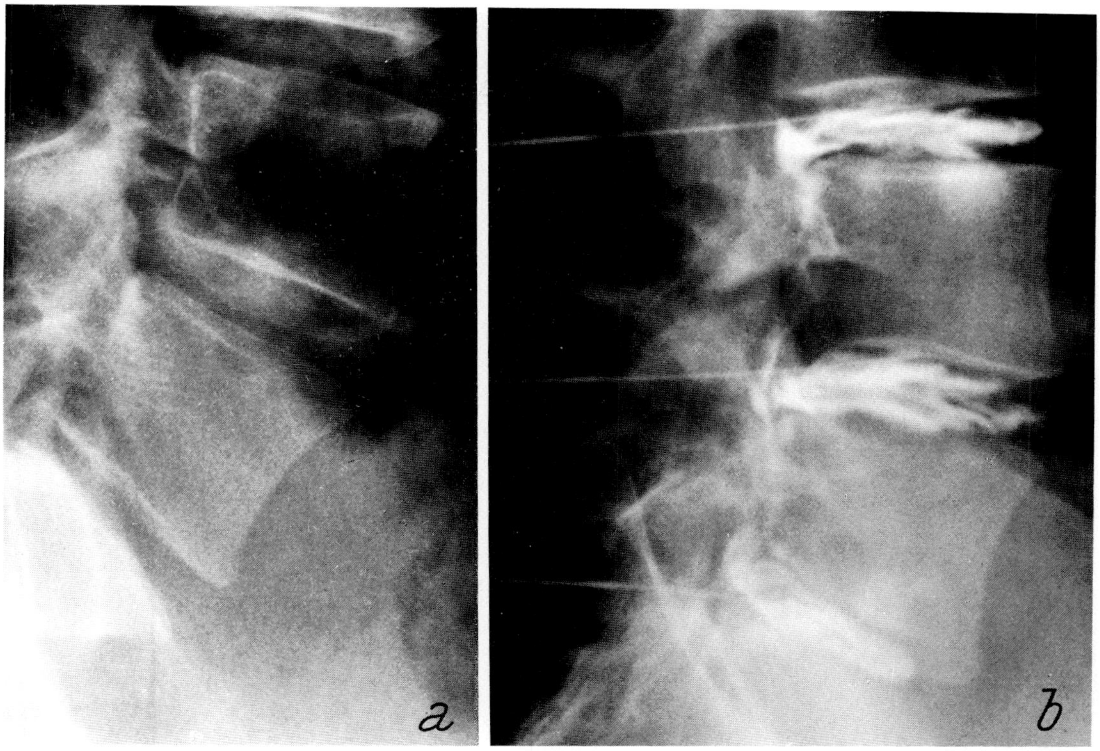

Figures 2.9 a and **b.** Lateral X-rays of the lumbar spine to show the plain film appearance and the gross disc disruption at three levels demonstrated by discography

Many authorities have tended to play down the importance of discography when their personal experience of it is small (Epstein, 1969; De Palma and Rothman, 1970). Some who have firmly advocated the procedure, place undue emphasis on its use in the investigation of suspected cases of disc prolapse when either myelography or C.T. scanning may be used with greater effect (Collis, 1963).

The indications for discography are: (1) in suspected cases of internal disc disruption assessed on the clinical syndrome; (2) in suspected cases of internal disc disruption in patients who have had failed "laminectomies"; (3) as a supplementary test following negative myelography; (4) in some cases of spondyloiisthesis to determine if adjacent discs are disrupted; and (5) to plan the level and extent of spinal fusion in lumbar spondylosis.

Using an image intensifier X-ray machine with video-storage facilities, the needles may be inserted easily into the discs to be examined, the patient being sedated with intravenous diazepam. If this sophisticated equipment is not available, X-rays in two planes should be obtained after the needles have been inserted into the discs. Injections *must never be made* until the needles have been placed accurately in the area of the nuclei pulposi and their positions confirmed by X-rays taken in antero-posterior and lateral views (Figs. 2.12–2.14).

The discogram "guiding needle" should be inserted about four fingers breadth lateral to the spinous process, angled towards the disc space at about 45° to the long axis of the spine. When the discogram needle is passed through the "guiding needle" into the disc, there is a characteristic sensation as though it were being pushed into a

anaesthetic into the disc. Pain emanating from a disrupted disc at the time of discography is not provoked by a rise in intra-discal pressure as it may come on after the injection of as little as 0.3 ml of dye, whereas the injection of 1.5 ml of dye into an adjacent normal disc will be painless. Notes should be made on the ease or difficulty experienced in injecting the dye, on the volume and the pattern of the pain response described by the patient. *In internal disc disruption,* dye spreads beyond the

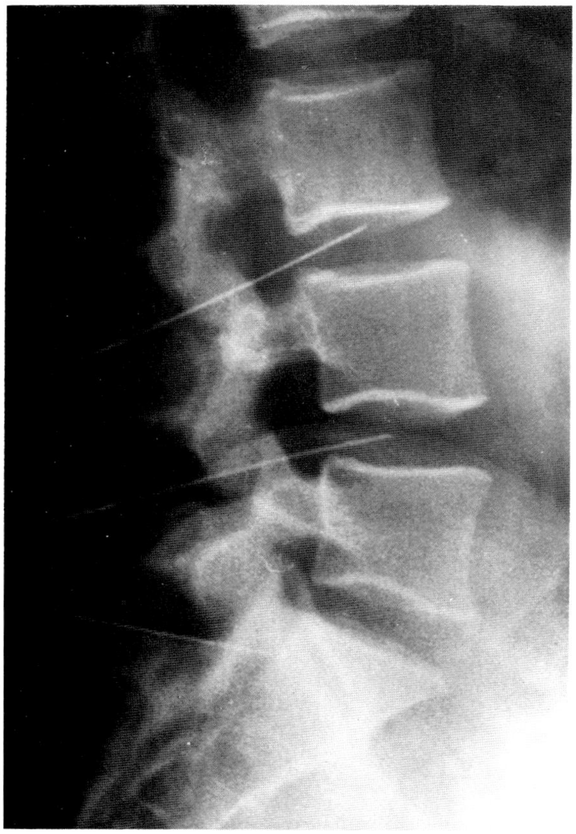

Figure 2.13. A lateral X-ray of a lumbar spine showing control X-rays with needles satisfactorily placed in the lateral view at L3/4 and L4/5 but incorrectly placed at the lumbo-sacral level

normal confines of the nuclear zone, the radiographic patterns of the discogram varying with the anatomy of the disruption of the annular fibres of the disc or with the presence of vertebral end-plate defects (Figs. 2.3a, 2.15a, b, 2.16a–c). *Spread of dye beyond the disc margins and into the spinal canal is a manifestation of abnormal permeability of the annular fibres and should not be interpreted as indicating prolapse of disc material.*

A discogram report should provide the following information:

1. The placing of the needles within individual discs.
2. The type and volume of dye injected.
3. The ease or difficulty of injection.
4. The patient's description of induced pain.

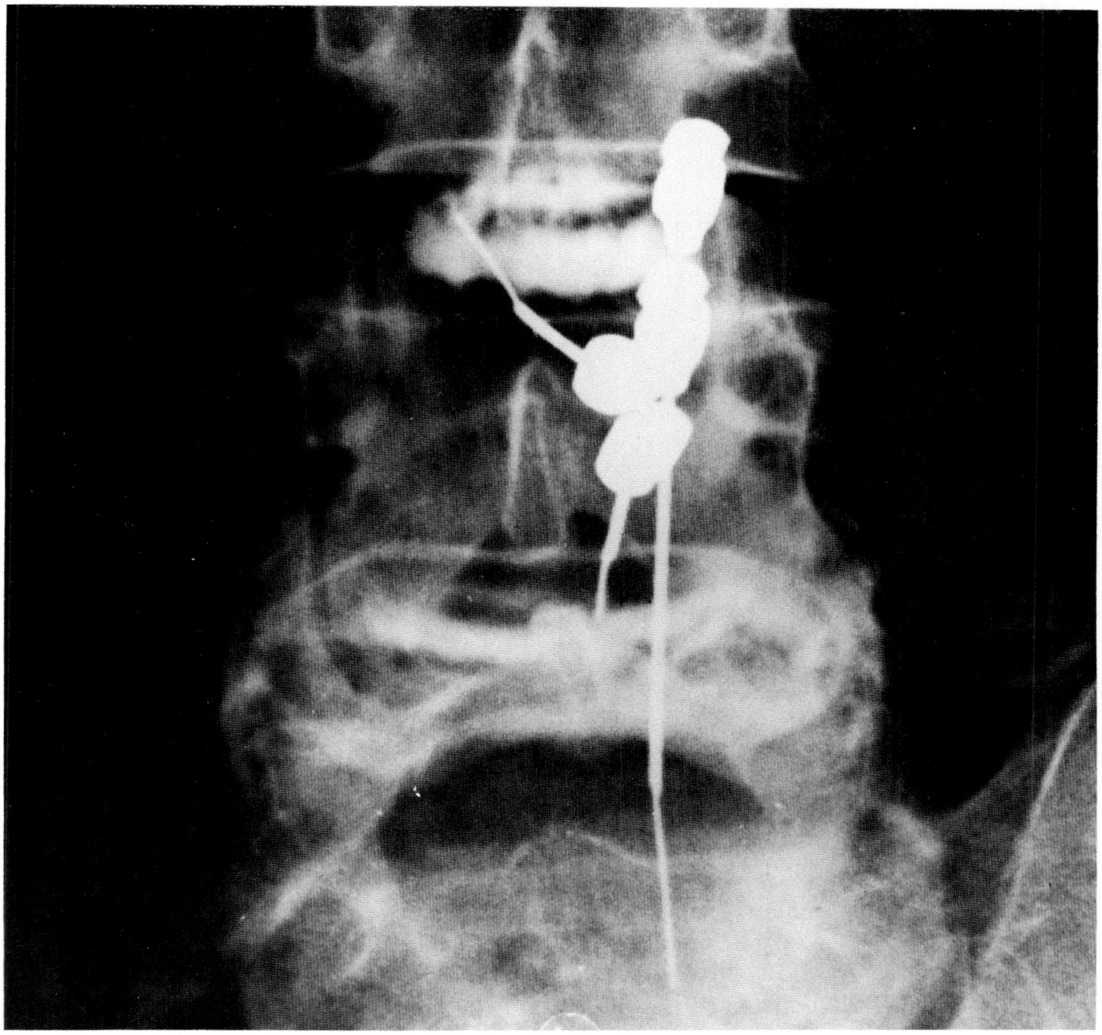

Figure 2.14. An antero-posterior view of the lower lumbar spine showing the disposition of the needles in the intervertebral disc spaces with dye injected at L3/4 and L4/5. If the needles are eccentrically placed in relation to the nuclear zone of the disc, then artefacts will appear when dye is injected

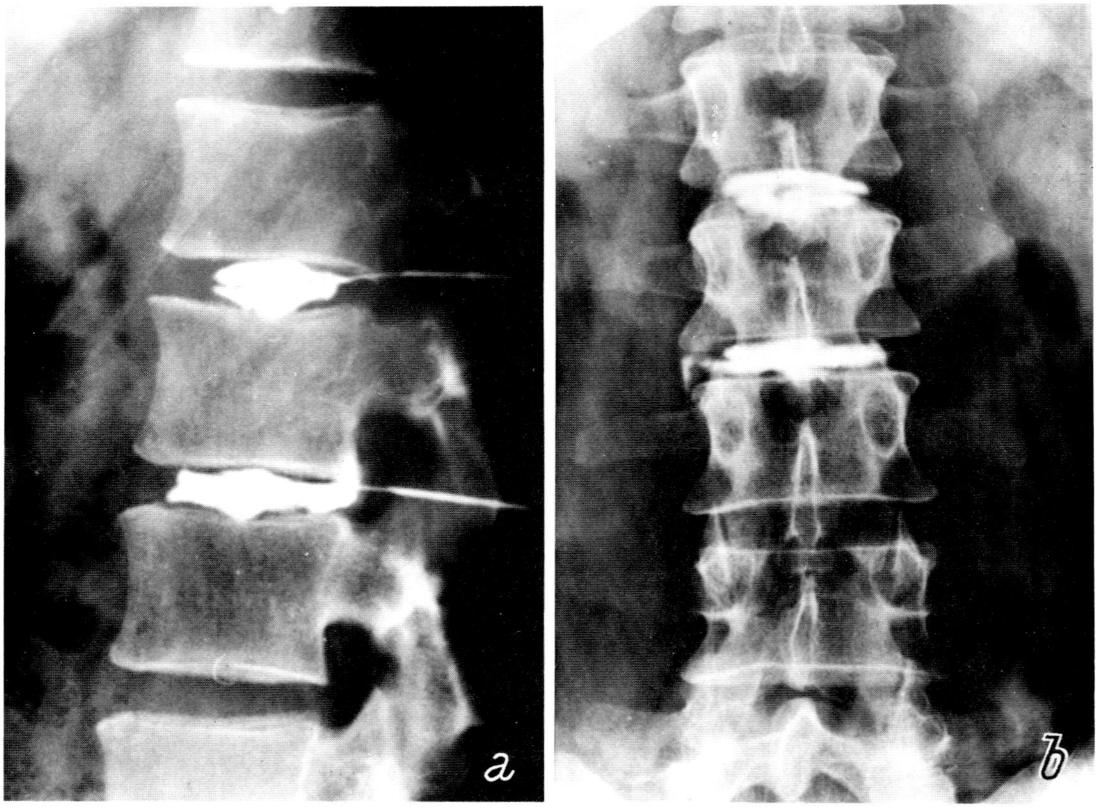

Figures 2.15. **a** A lateral radiograph of the lumbar spine of a man aged 42 years. Discogram needles have been inserted into the discs between L1/2 and L2/3 vertebral bodies, lateral and anterior to the thecal sac. The upper discogram is normal; that at the L2/3 level shows posterior internal disc disruption. **b** Antero-posterior view of the same case

5. The patterns of distribution of the injected dye in antero-posterior and lateral X-rays of the disc space.
6. The volume of corticosteroid injected before the discogram needle was withdrawn.

Excluding technical faults in its performance, chemically induced discitis is the major complication which may result from its use. The latent period between the time of discography and the appearance of discitis varies between three to twelve weeks. For this reason, radiologists rarely see the complication. Having performed discograms personally over a period of ten years, I estimate that this complication may occur in about 1.5–2% of patients on whom the investigation has been performed. *This is one of the causes of excruciating spinal pain* and it is often associated with marked spasm of the paraspinal muscles, causing gross lumbar scoliosis.

Post-discogram discitis responds to rest and corticosteroid therapy, either by intradisc injection or orally (Figs. 2.17, 2.18a, b, c, 2.19a, b). Infection due to introduced bacterial contaminants has been reported, though it is rare (Matsubara *et al.*, 1966). Simple puncture of the disc by discogram needles has no proven complication.

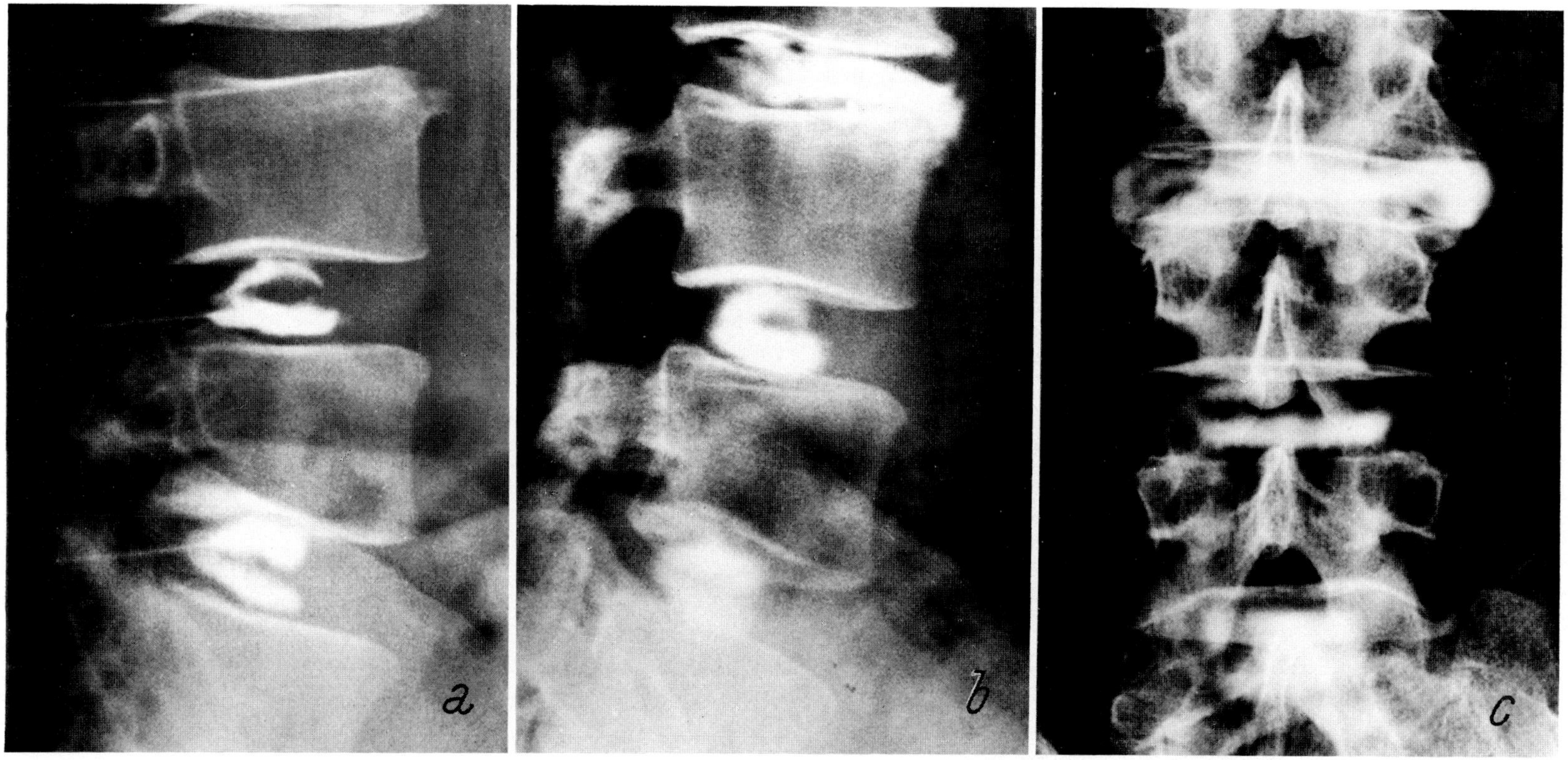

Figures 2.16 a–c. Normal discograms at L 4/5 and L 5/S1, with a needle directed towards the back of the vertebral body of L 3 at the upper part of the picture. In **b** note the gross disc disruption at L 3/4. **c** An antero-posterior view showing normal discograms at L 4/5 and L 5/S1 with marked disc disruption at the L 3/4 level

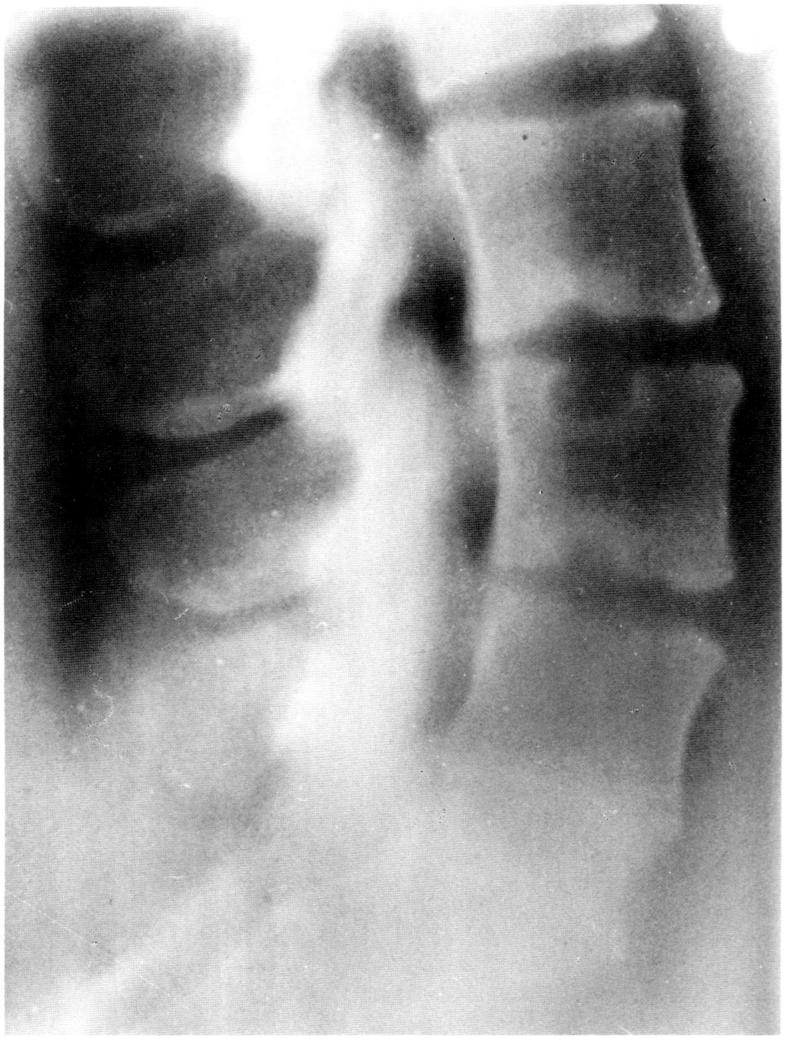

Figure 2.17. A mid-line tomogram of the lower lumbar spine from a man aged 27 years, taken three months after lumbo-sacral interbody fusion. The L3/4 and L4/5 discograms had been normal. Note the changes of vertebral end-plate erosion and loss of disc height typical of post-discogram discitis

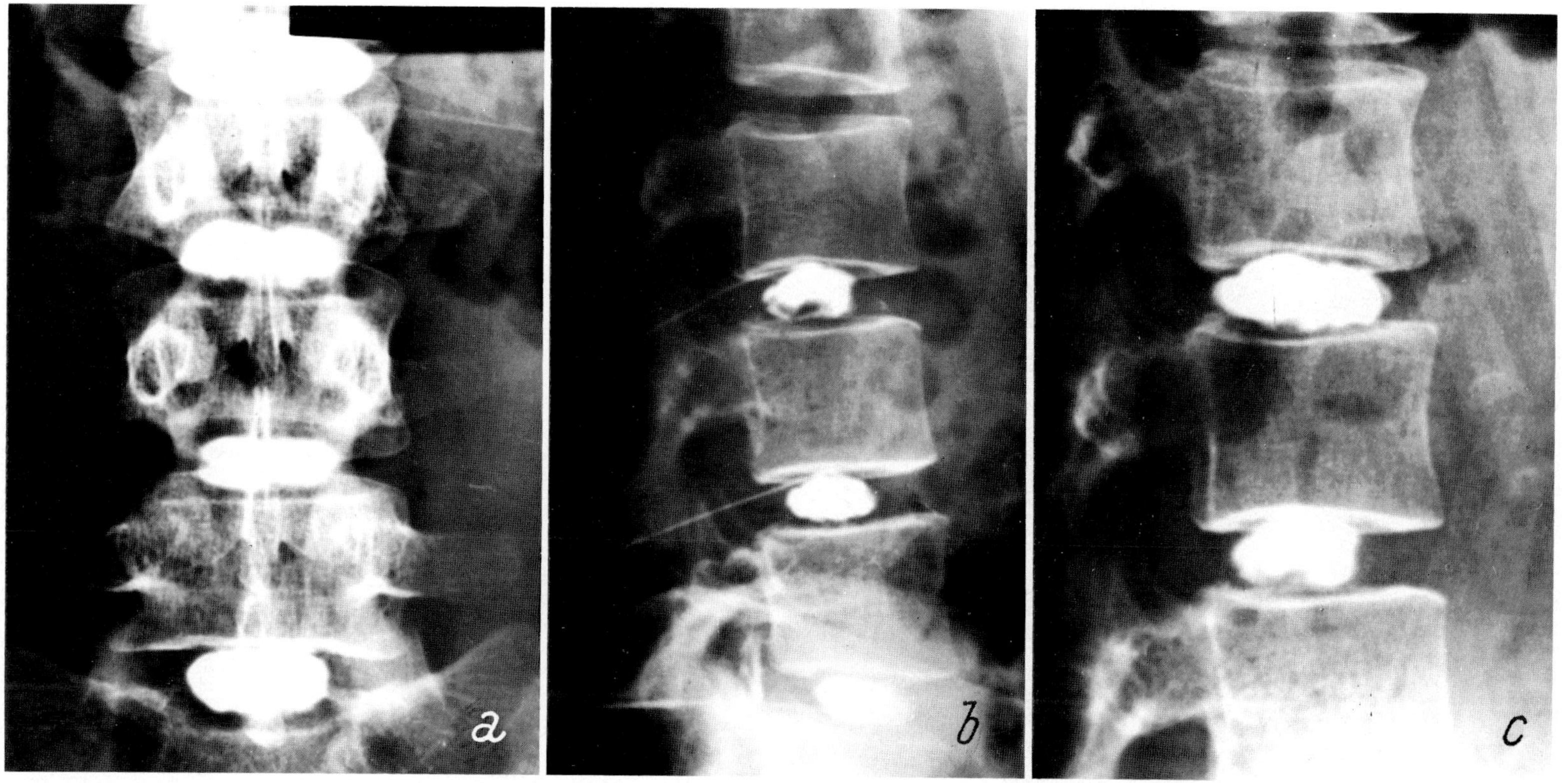

Figures 2.18. **a** An antero-posterior radiograph of the lumbar spine of a woman aged 32 years. The L 2/3, L 3/4, L 4/5 and L 5/S1 discs appear normal. **b** A lateral radiograph showing normal discograms at L 3/4, L 4/5 and L 5/S1. **c** Lateral radiograph showing the L 2/3 and L 3/4 discograms. The L 2/3 disc is disrupted posteriorly, but the L 3/4 discogram is normal

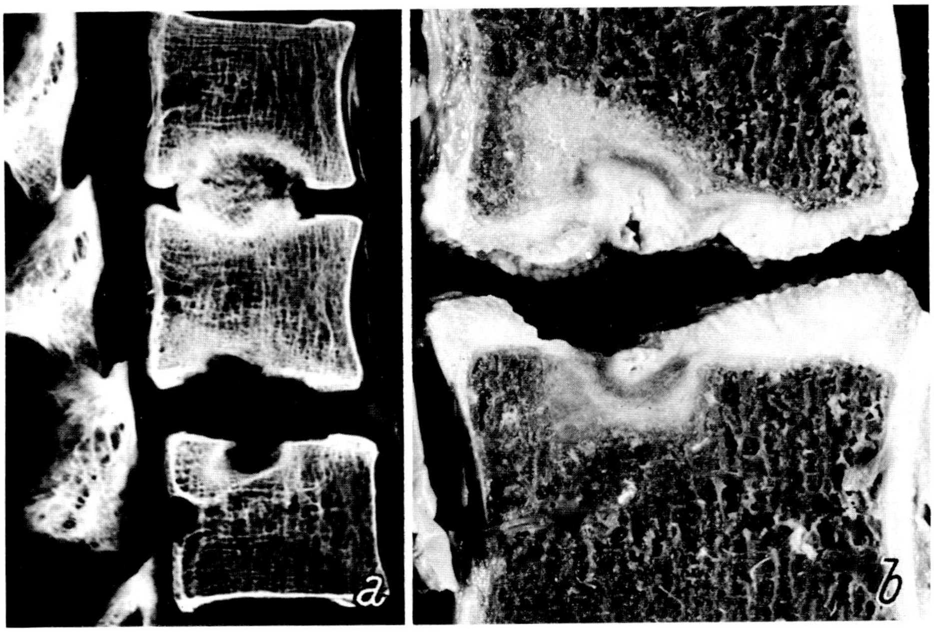

Figures 2.19. **a** X-ray of a thin sagittal section of the lumbar spine taken at necropsy. At L2/3 union of the graft is incomplete. There are erosions of the end-plates of the bodies of the 3rd and 4th lumbar vertebrae with reactive changes in excavated areas of the bodies, resulting from chemical discitis. **b** A detailed photograph of the necropsy specimen at the level of the discitis at L3/4. This patient committed suicide four months after operation for L2/3 interbody fusion

c) Myelography

Myelography has no place in the investigation of internal disc disruption.

2.4. Surgical Treatment

a) Types

Surgical treatment is recommended after the failure of comprehensive conservative treatment. Pain will often subside to tolerable levels after prolonged rest. If re-employment after re-training could be assured–though this is usually not possible in highly competitive industries–then surgery would be indicated less frequently.

Poor results of spinal canal surgery for disc lesions other than for disc prolapse have been reported frequently (Kudelka, 1968). These poor results which are known to follow "negative laminectomies" could be largely prevented by more accurate preoperative assessment including the use of discography. If nothing else, the use of this investigation would restrict the extent of spinal canal exploration, as, often, more than one disc will be inspected in the hope of finding an elusive disc "prolapse". Discography before operation in this case will allow precise definition of the lesion.

Surgical treatment along the following lines should give satisfactory results:

i) Total Disc Excision and Interbody Fusion

Total disc excision and interbody fusion–for single or double level disc disruptions with intractable limb and spinal pain and constitutional symptoms (Fig. 2.1) (Debeyre and Delforges, 1959). In the lumbar region this method may be satisfactory for one or two disc levels, providing:

- the patient is not obese;
- there is no antecedent history of pulmonary embolism or deep vein thrombosis in the legs;
- lumbo-sacral articulation anomalies are not associated with great vein anomalies which may render access to the intervertebral disc space hazardous or impossible; and
- surgical technique is meticulous.

Whereas the operation of lumbar interbody fusion finds a small but undisputed role in the management of failed spinal operations (Sacks, 1965), its real place in the present state of knowledge should be for the primary surgical treatment of non-prolapsing lumbar disc lesions. Cloward (1955) has described a method of inserting grafts between adjacent vertebral bodies via the spinal canal for the treatment of lumbar disc "lesions". The operation which bears his name is not used widely because of the technical difficulties of its execution, although some surgeons still advocate it (Finneson, 1973). Exceptional surgical skill is required for its safe and effective use. For similar reasons, the operation described by Wiltberger (1957, 1958), which involves the insertion of accurately cut dowel grafts between adjacent vertebral bodies via the spinal canal, is rarely used.

When the four prerequisites set out above can be met, anterior lumbar interbody fusion is a satisfactory operation which can be rapidly and safely performed by an extra-peritoneal left-sided abdominal approach, allowing ready access to more than one disc if required. Near-total disc excision can be accomplished by fashioning two parallel dowel cavities into which dowel grafts can be accurately and firmly impacted. The grafts are cut vertically downwards from the anterior third of the left iliac crest. They have tooled cancellous surfaces between the stout cortical tables of the iliac crest and their depth can be determined at will. Inserted parallel to each other with their cancellous faces abutting the prepared cancellous surfaces of the adjacent vertebral bodies, these grafts are ideally situated for rapid vascularization. One cortical surface of each graft on either side of the disc space prevents penetration of any disc remnant which may have escaped removal by curettage before the grafts were inserted, thereby diminishing the risk of non-union.

Anterior lumbar interbody fusion being the operation of choice for the surgical treatment of lumbar internal disc disruptions, the details of technique and assessment of results achieved will be described in detail below.

ii) Bilateral Nerve Root Canal Decompression Laminectomy

Bilateral nerve root canal decompression laminectomy–where single level lumbar disc disruption has been identified by discography in a young patient with predominant referred leg pain without neurological abnormalities or constitutional illness. The aim is to enlarge the nerve root canals, the rationale being to allow the nerve roots to accommodate to the vertebral instability resulting from the disc disruption (Morgan and King, 1957). This operation is described on p. 23.

iii) Posterior Spinal Fusion

Posterior spinal fusion, without spinal canal exploration—for multi-level disc disruption with dominant back pain and insignificant referred leg pain, without constitutional disturbances such as weight loss and psychiatric upsets.

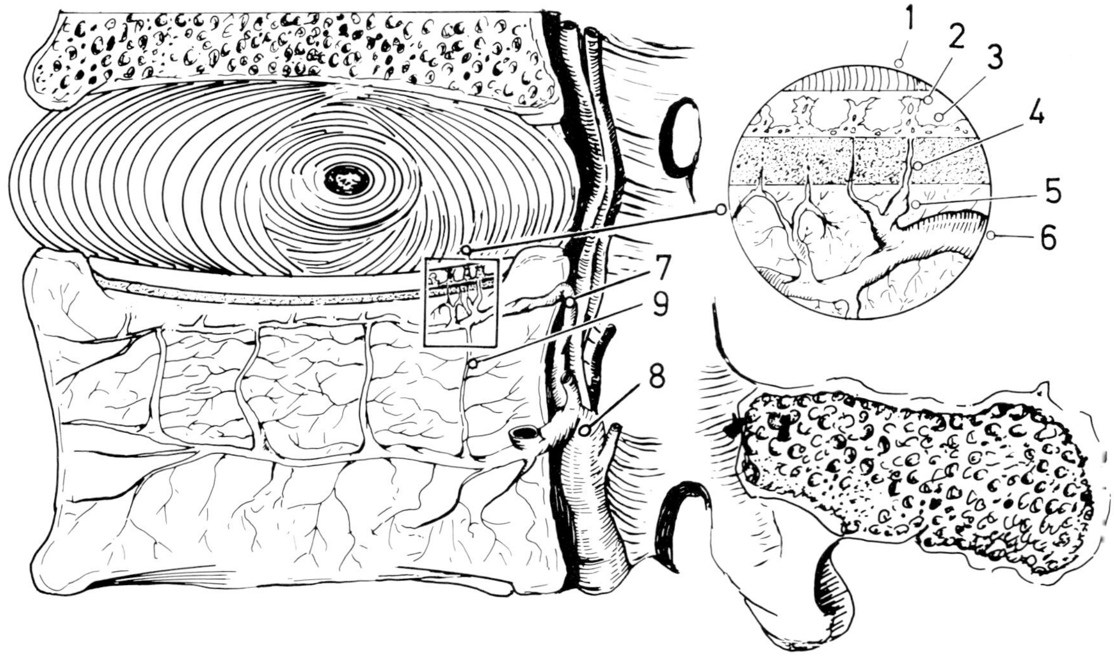

Figure 2.20. A schematic drawing to show the spatial relationships of the veins of a typical vertebral body. **1** intervertebral disc; **2** capillary bed in vertebral end-plate cartilage; **3** sub-chondral post-capillary venous network on the vertebral end-plate; **4** vertebral end-plate perforated by short vertical venous tributaries; **5** vertical tributaries from the sub-chondral post-capillary venous network, draining to the horizontal sub-articular collecting vein; **6** horizontal sub-articular collecting vein; **7** horizontal sub-articular collecting vein joining the anterior internal vertebral venous plexus; **8** basi-vertebral vein joining the anterior internal venous plexus; **9** vertical tributary of the basi-vertebral system of veins

Armstrong (1965) makes sound comments on the selection of posterior spinal fusion operations in his chapter on the operative treatment of lumbar disc lesions. The procedure is most likely to succeed where a single level fusion is required. If fusion is attempted concomitant with spinal canal exploration, methods using other than postero-lateral or inter-transverse-alar grafting are likely to fail. The probability of failure is even higher if posterior fusion is attempted following earlier spinal canal surgery (Adkins, 1955).

The diagnosis of internal disc disruption is most often established by a process of exclusion after months of careful clinical observation. Attention has been drawn to the importance of assessing correctly the role of precipitating trauma. Attention has also been focused on the description of pain and especially on the difficulty which these patients find in describing their limb pain. When first seen their problems are indistinguishable from many of the common short-lived episodes of spinal and limb

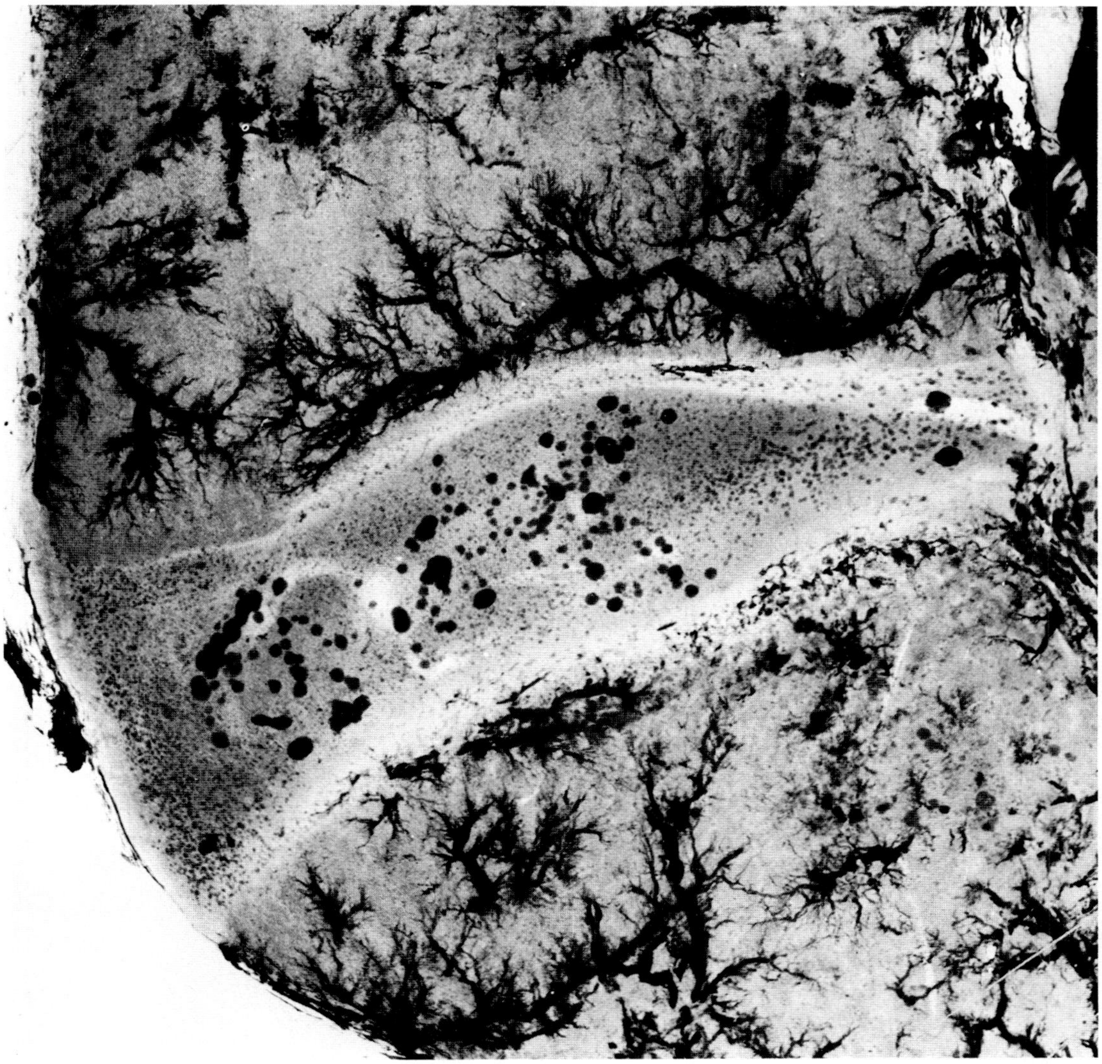

Figure 2.21. A radiograph of a thin sagittal section cut laterally near the vertebral pedicle from the lumbo-sacral junction of a woman aged 67 years. Some fragments of barium sulphate debris have adhered to the cut surface of the disc. The horizontal sub-articular collecting vein system of the vertebral body can be seen running parallel to the vertebral end-plate area on the lower surface of the 5th lumbar vertebra. Nearer the disc, of smaller calibre, running parallel to the vertebral end-plate cartilage, the sub-chondral post-capillary venous network can be seen. It is only partly filled. This system drains by vertical stems through perforations in the vertebral end-plate into the larger horizontal sub-articular collecting vein system. In this specimen only one such stem can be seen joining these two venous channels. [Reproduced by courtesy of the Editor, J. Bone Joint Surg. *55b* (1973), and J. B. Lippincott & Company from: Clinical Orthopaedics and Related Research, No. 115 (1976)]

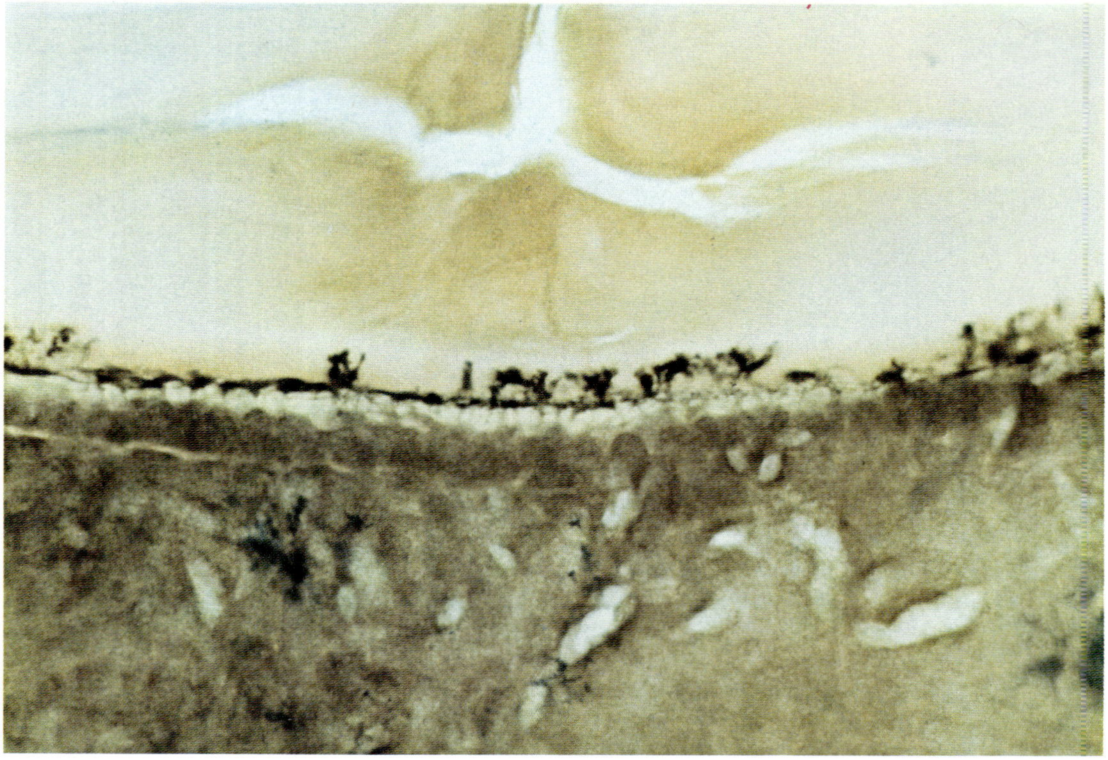

Figure 2.22

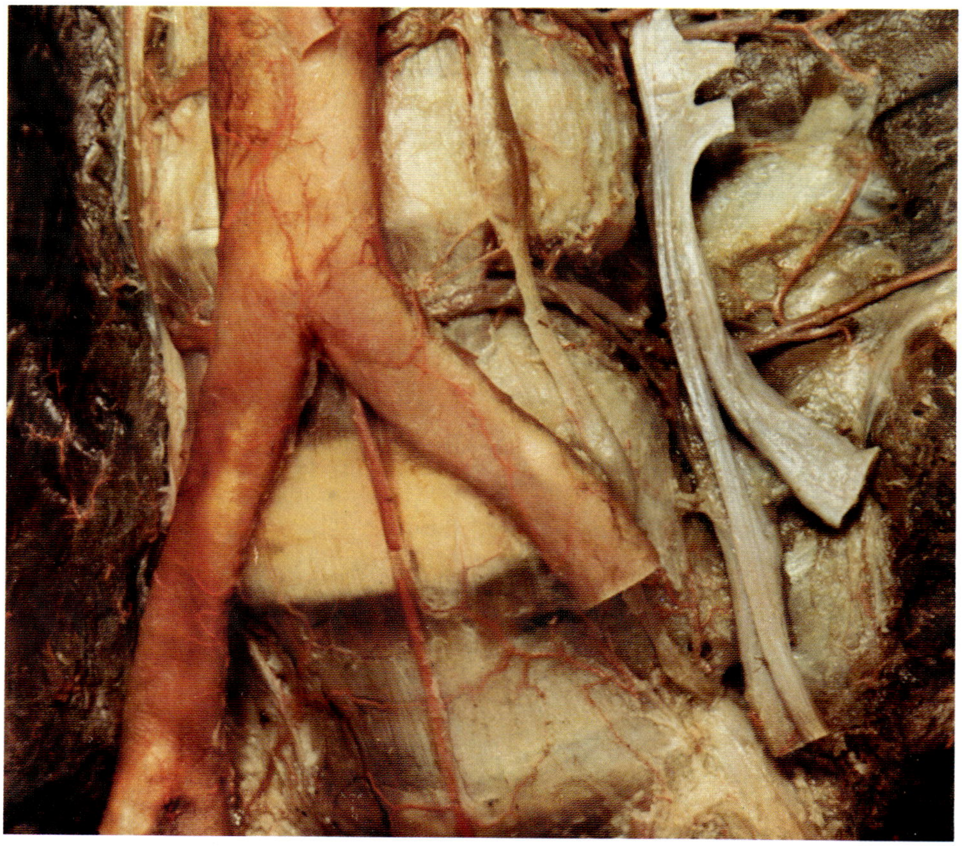

Figure 2.23

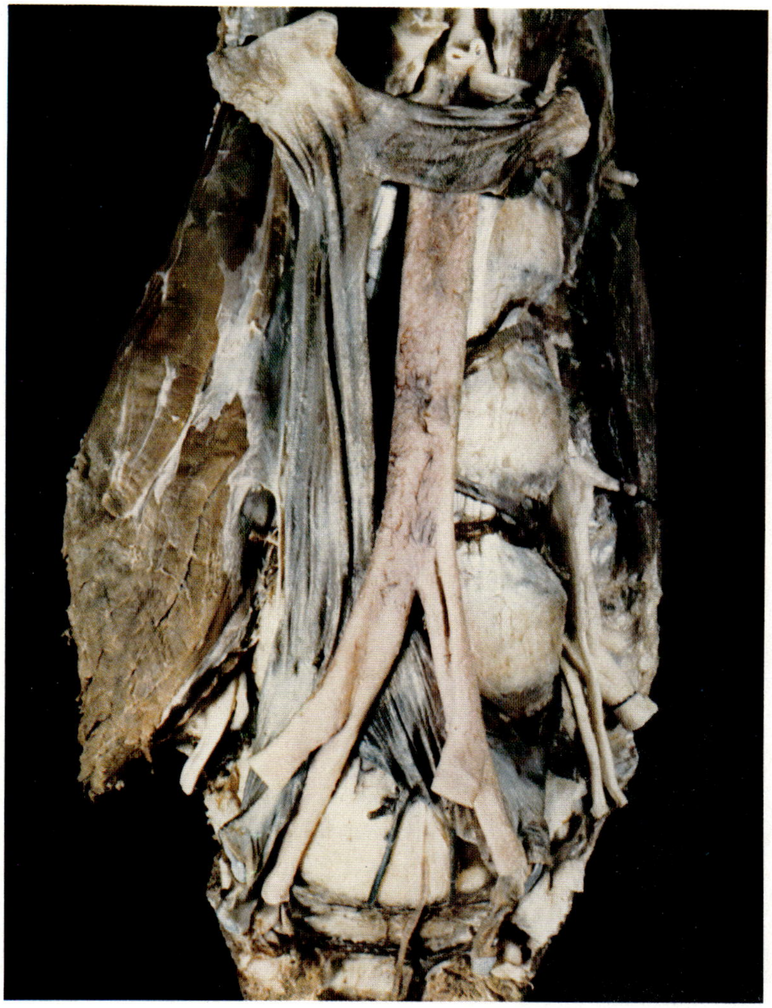

Figure 2.24. A photograph of a dissection to show the aorta and the vena cava in the abdomen. Note the bifurcation of the aorta at the lower border of the 4th lumbar vertebra. The relationship of the common iliac arteries to the common iliac veins is clearly shown. The ascending lumbar vein can be seen in the depths of the dissection, just below the disc between L4 and L5, on the right hand side of the photograph. Note that the left psoas muscle has been removed, so that the lumbar arteries and veins can be seen on the right side of the photograph. See also Fig. 2.36, p. 72

Figure 2.22. A detailed photograph taken from the central area of the disc and vertebral body (500 μm thick) from a woman of 30 years. Spalteholz-cleared specimen (approximately $\times 20$). The demarcation line between the intervertebral disc and vertebral end-plate cartilage is clearly visible. The vertebral end-plate cartilage capillary bed is shown, with vertical tributaries draining to the sub-chondral post-capillary venous network orientated parallel to the vertebral end-plate

Figure 2.23. A detailed photograph of a dissection of the lumbo-sacral junction in an adult, showing the relations of the 3rd and 4th lumbar arteries to the sympathetic trunk and the pattern of branching of the median sacral artery related to the 5th lumbar vertebral body. (Dissected by Dr. S. Sihombing, of Indonesia)

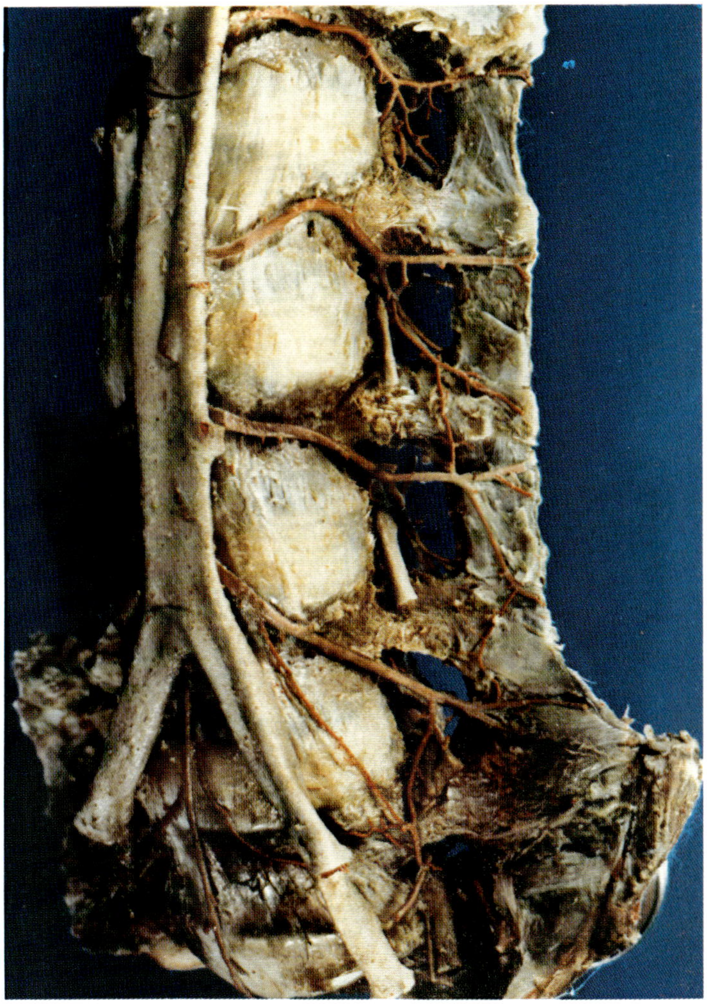

Figure 2.25. A photograph of a dissection of the lumbar vertebral column in an adult viewed from the left side, showing the origins and distribution of the lumbar arteries from the aorta. The median sacral artery is also clearly shown. The psoas muscle has been removed in its entirety

pain for which, in about 80% of cases, no cause is evident (Dillane *et al.,* 1966). However, these patients consistently fail to respond to conservative treatment and often are made worse by standard methods of physical therapy involving exercises or spinal manipulations. Likewise, their symptoms are aggravated by travelling in modern vehicles. It is important to distinguish these cases from disc prolapses in order to reduce significantly the "negative laminectomy" rate which accounts for many of the poor results of spinal surgery for disc lesions.

Certain anatomical factors are pertinent to the interpretation of the causes of symptoms in internal disc disruption. These and others relevant to the performance of interbody fusion operations and to their ultimate success are shown in Figs. 2.20–2.28.

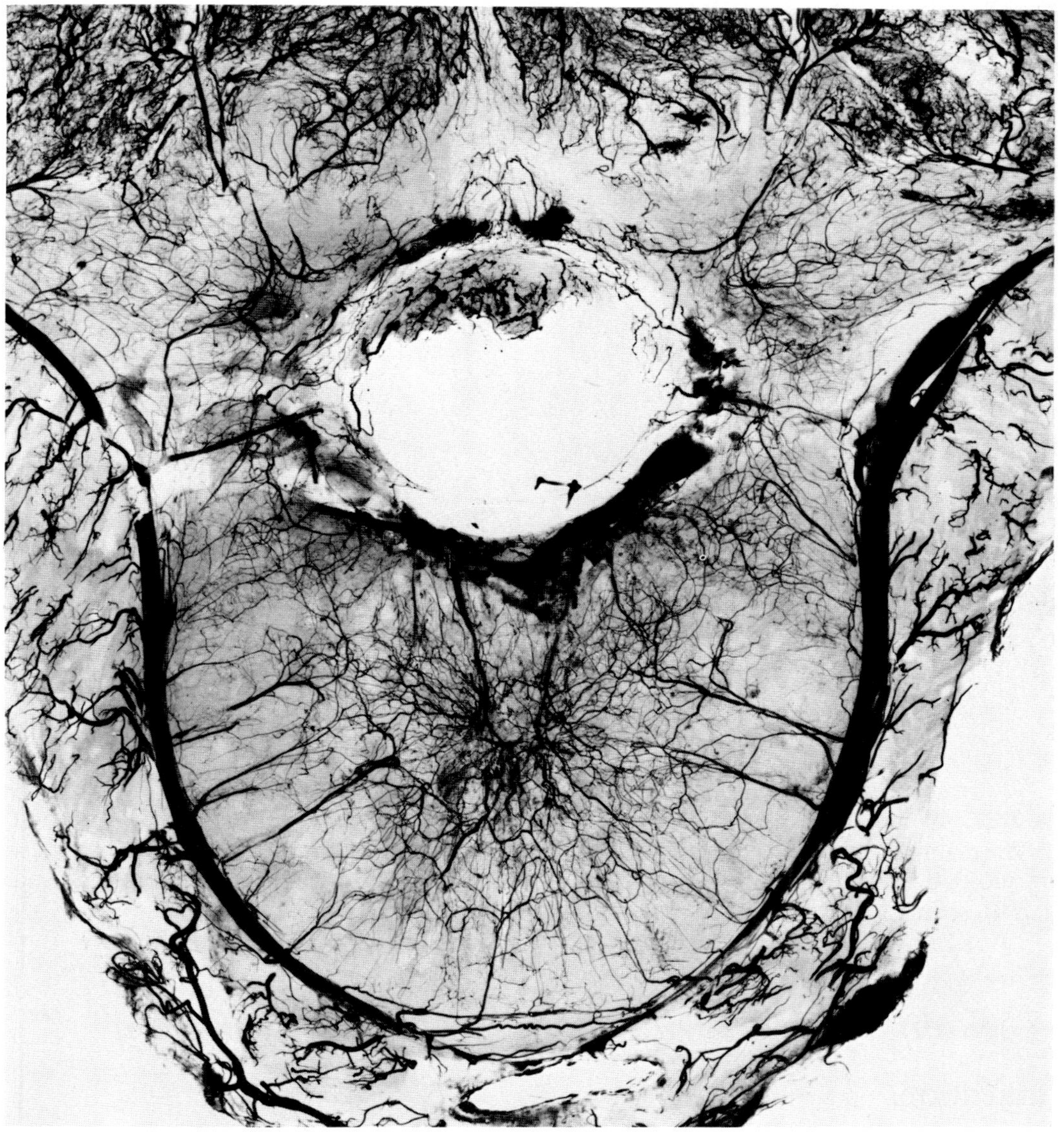

Figure 2.26. A transverse section through the lumbar vertebral body of a child aged 13 years. The radiate distribution of the centrum branches arising from the inner surface of the lumbar arteries on each side has been shown. Note the muscular branches passing directly into the muscles from the outer side of the main trunk of each lumbar artery. [Reproduced by courtesy of J. B. Lippincott & Company from: Clinical Orthopaedics and Related Research, No. 115 (1976)]

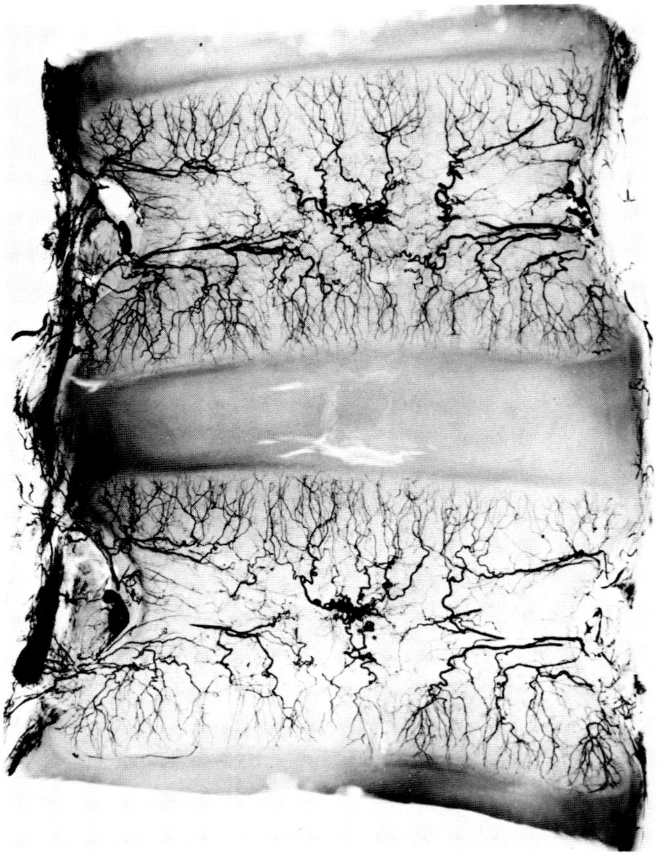

Figure 2.27. A thin coronal section through the centre of two adjacent lumbar vertebral bodies from a male aged 65 years, showing details of the intra-osseous distribution of arteries. [Reproduced by courtesy of J. B. Lippincott & Company from: Clinical Orthopaedics and Related Research, No. 115 (1976)]

b) Technique of Anterior Lumbar Interbody Fusion

i) Indications

The operation of spinal fusion was introduced first by Albee (1911) for the treatment of spinal tuberculosis. Its use was then extended by the application of anterior interbody fusion methods, popularized in Hong Kong by Hodgson and Stock (1956). In selected cases with spinal tuberculosis, anterior interbody fusion still enjoys an undisputed and favoured place in treatment (see p. 233).

The role of spinal fusion in the treatment of disorders of the lumbar spine has remained vexed and confused. Apart from a general agreement on the possible application of spinal fusion in the treatment of spondylolisthesis, there are no clear-cut published statements on indications for the use of spinal fusion techniques. With the decline in the use of fusion operations for major joints in the limbs, there has been a corresponding fall in the number of these procedures applied to spinal problems. In particular, a number of the degenerative disorders of the lumbar spine

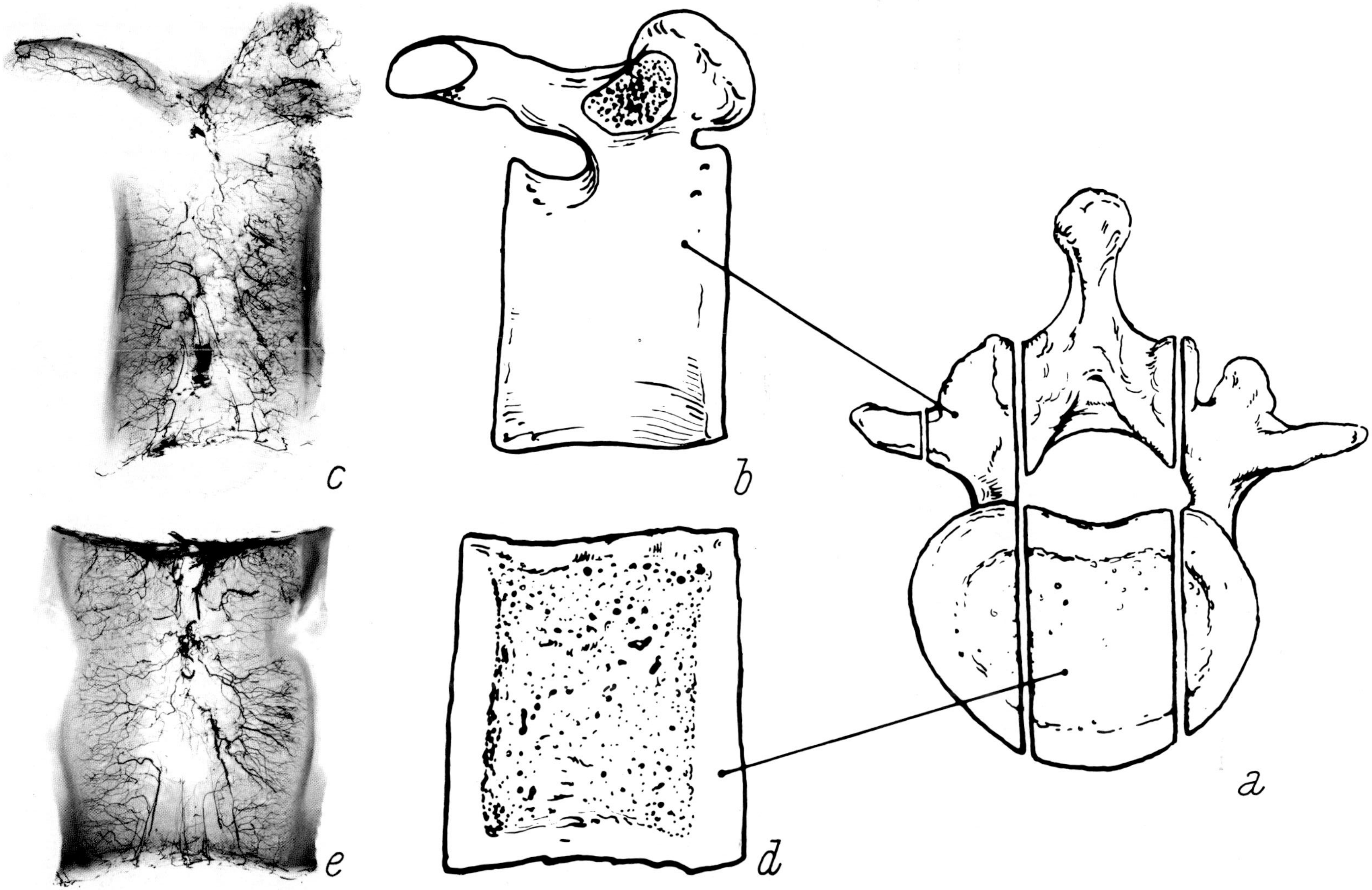

Figures 2.28 a – e. Line drawings **a, b, d** indicating the division of a lumbar vertebra into sagittal sections. Sections **c** and **e** of the specimen alongside show the distribution of arteries within the vertebral body from a male aged 30 years. The feeding branches to the centrum grid can be seen in both sections. [Reproduced by courtesy of J. B. Lippincott & Company from: Clinical Orthopaedics and Related Research, No. 115 (1976).]

now can be more effectively treated by some form of spinal canal or spinal nerve root canal decompression.

In the author's opinion, the present indications for the use of anterior lumbar interbody fusion operations are as follows:

1. For the treatment of other failed spinal operations;
2. for the treatment of certain disc lesions:
   a) internal disc disruption (frequently),
   b) isolated disc resorption (occasionally),
   c) nucleus pulposus calcification (rarely),
   d) disc herniation (rarely);
3. in the management of selected cases of spondylolisthesis;
4. for the treatment of certain spinal infections;
5. for the correction of selected spinal deformities;
6. for the treatment of rare miscellaneous cases, e.g. vertebral body tumours.

The operation of lumbar interbody fusion should be performed ideally with the aid of two competent assistants. Until the orthopaedic surgeon is thoroughly familiar with every aspect of the procedure, he would be wise to work with a general surgeon who has special competence in vascular surgery.

When Sir John Charnley first introduced his operation of total hip joint replacement in the early 1960s, he provoked an angry response from many surgeons by refusing to allow them to obtain the recommended instruments until they had been specially instructed in their use. The wisdom of his early caution doubtlessly served a good purpose in as much as total hip joint replacement operations, performed by otherwise untrained surgeons, can maim. But when anterior lumbar interbody fusion is attempted by surgeons who are not specially trained, the results can be devastating and the patient may lose his life.

ii) General Pre-Operative Preparation

Patients arrive at the operating room with an intravenous infusion inserted. Two or three litres of compatible blood should be available for use during the operation; blood loss at the time of surgery is usually about 300–500 ml, varying with single or double level fusions.

The patient's X-rays, including lumbar discograms when appropriate, should be clearly displayed. Facilities should be available for taking control X-rays on the theatre table when fusions above the lumbo-sacral junction are to be performed. The quality of such films is often poor. Good quality films of the patient's spine must be available in the theatre for comparison with those taken at the time of surgery.

iii) Positioning

For approaches to the lower three lumbar intervertebral discs, patients are placed supine on the operating table. For rarer upper lumbar fusions, they are placed in the lateral position with the left loin uppermost. The surgeon should pay particular attention to the placing of restraining devices and arm supports, ensuring that the patient's trunk is held in a stable position and that undue pressure is not exerted on the peripheral nerves or veins in the legs. Electric calf stimulators are applied.

iv) Abdominal Incision

In the lower lumbar region, oblique, left-sided incisions are made, commencing at the mid-line between the umbilicus and symphysis pubis and extending upwards and laterally, parallel to the level of the iliac crest. The anterior rectus sheath is divided in the line of the skin incision, extending out into the fibres of the external oblique muscle and over the length of the skin incision. At the lateral border of the rectus abdominis muscle, the internal oblique muscle and transversalis fascia are split to identify the extra-peritoneal space. The peritoneum is separated from the inner aspect of the abdominal wall, and these two muscles are further split laterally in the line of the main incision. In obese patients, it is wise to retract the lateral border of the left rectus abdominis muscle, to identify the inferior epigastric vessels. These should be divided between ligatures and the rectus abdominis muscle then divided across transversely to the level of the mid-line; such an incision will allow wide extra-peritoneal approach to the lower lumbar spine. The accompanying illustrations show the steps in the muscle splitting approach devised by Fraser (1982) which allows wide extra-peritoneal approach to the lumbar spine, *without division of the rectus abdominis muscle.* The posterior rectus sheath is also split vertically downwards after retraction of the outer edge of the rectus abdominis muscle (Figs. 2.29–2.32).

The skin incision should be placed nearer the umbilicus if the L3/4 disc is to be approached. Mid-line trans-peritoneal approaches may be indicated for operations at the L5/S1 level in some cases of spondylolisthesis or in very obese patients with high Ferguson angle measurements at the lumbo-sacral junction (Ferguson, 1949).

When the abdominal wall incision has been completed, the peritoneum is separated from the posterior abdominal wall and the psoas major muscle. A small Raytec pack is inserted into the paracolic gutter and pushed upwards for some distance. The ureter can be seen lying adherent to the peritoneum. It is carried forward when a large modified Deever-type retractor is inserted, resting on the anterior surface of the lumbo-sacral disc or on the antero-lateral edge of the L4/5 or L3/4 discs at the anterior edge of the left psoas major muscle, depending on the level to be fused (Fig. 2.33).

v) Haemostasis

The techniques of vessel ligation are vital to the success of exposing the disc spaces at various levels in the lumbar spine and essential for the safe performance of these operations.

Vascular sutures, including 5/0 suture material on atraumatic needles, are required. In addition, long-handled instruments and right-angled artery forceps must be available for use.

When the median sacral vessels have been ligated and divided, small gall bladder dissecting swabs mounted on long-handled forceps are used to clear the loose tissues from the front of the disc space between the limbs of the aortic bifurcation and the right and left common iliac veins, thus clearly exposing the anterior longitudinal ligament (Fig. 2.34). In retro-peritoneal approaches to the L5/S1 disc space, the filaments of the presacral sympathetic plexus are rarely seen; the danger of damaging these nerves in the male has been exaggerated by opponents of this method of spinal fusion (Flynn and Hoque, 1979). The thin anterior longitudinal ligament is then

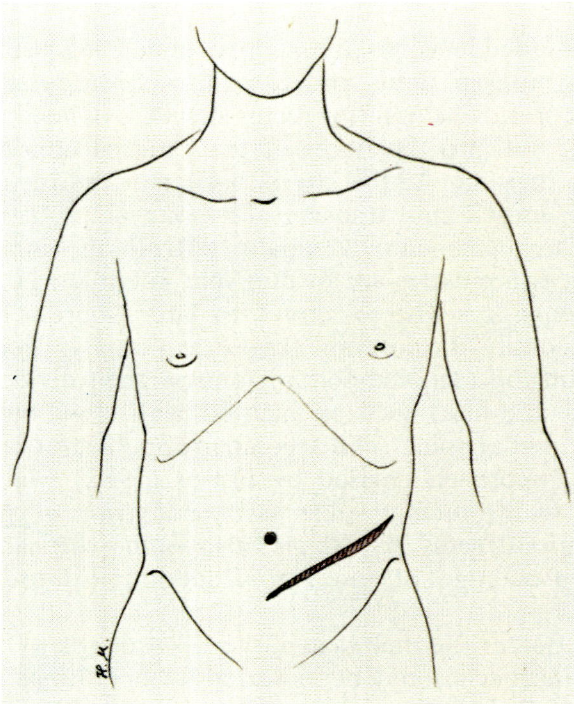

Figures 2.29–2.33. The Fraser Incision

Figure 2.29. A drawing to show the line of the skin incision for a left-sided extra-peritoneal approach to the lower lumbar vertebral column

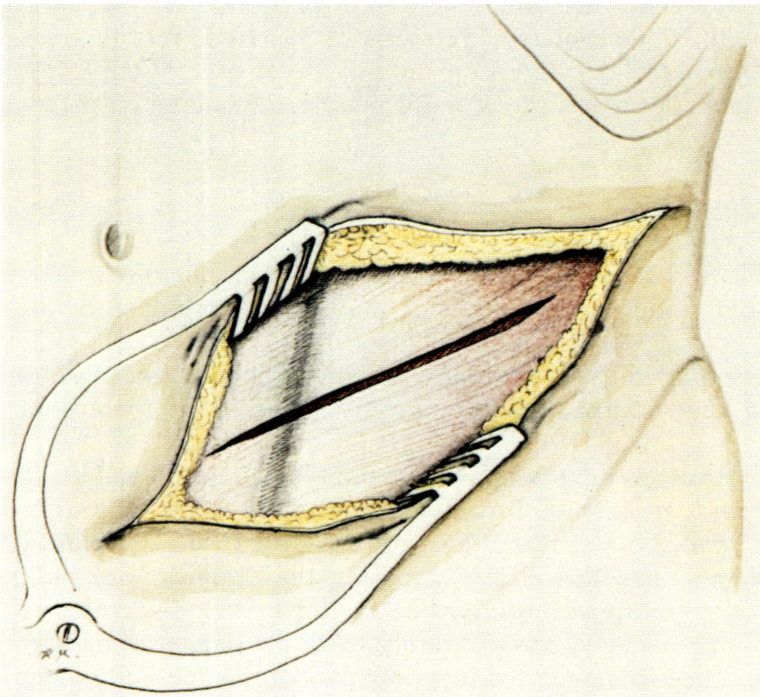

Figure 2.30. A drawing to show the line of division of fibres of the external oblique muscle

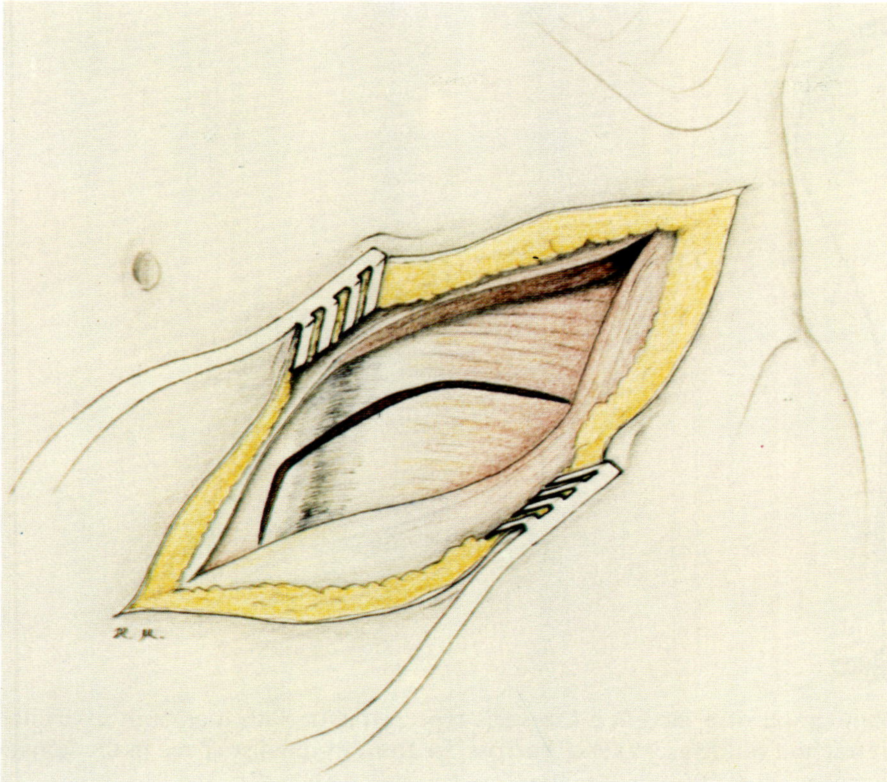

Figure 2.31. A drawing depicting the division of the rectus sheath vertically downwards at its lateral edge

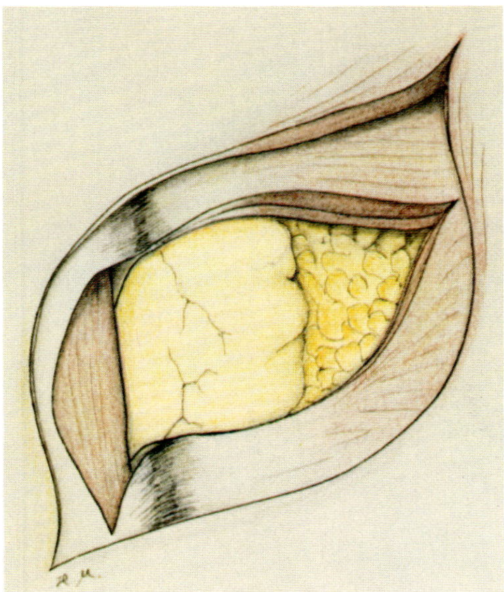

Figure 2.32. A drawing illustrating the splitting of the fibres of the internal oblique and transversalis muscles to expose the extra-peritoneal space on the left side of the abdomen. Division of the anterior layer of the rectus sheath vertically downwards permits wide exposure of the extra-peritoneal space without requiring division of the rectus abdominis muscle mass

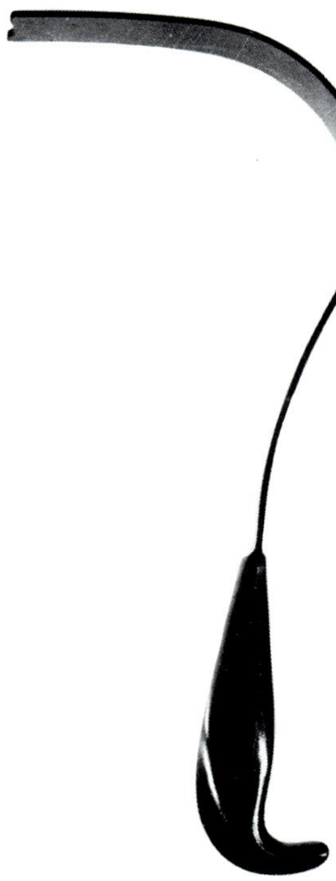

Figure 2.33. A photograph of a modified Deever's type retractor with a smooth excavated end, suitable for retraction of the great vessels across the front of the disc space in the lumbar region

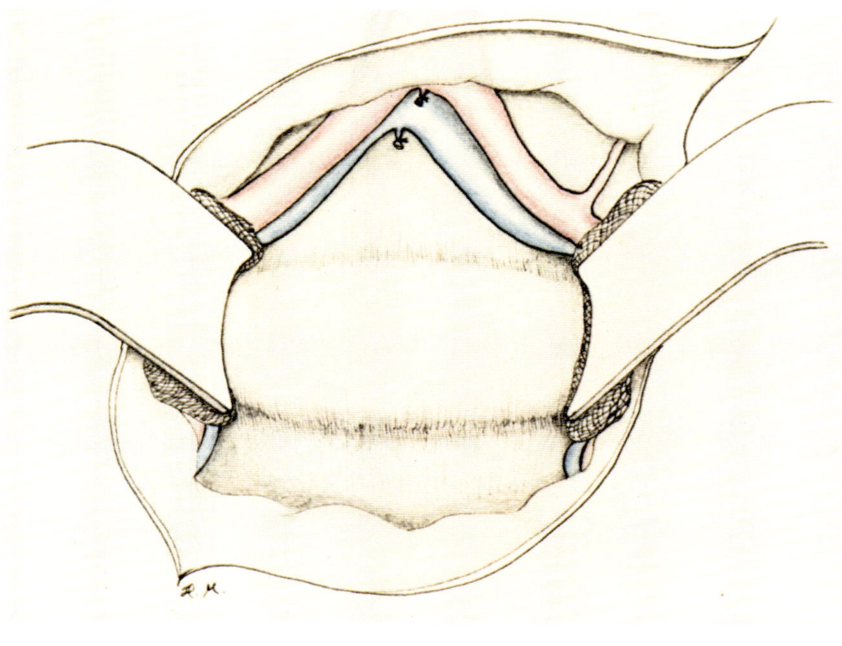

Figure 2.34. A diagram illustrating the use of the retractors at the lumbo-sacral space, with loose Raytec swabs beneath them protecting the walls of the great vessels

divided transversely across the middle of the disc space and the ends are swept upwards and downwards to expose the junction of the vertebral end plate and the disc on either side of the disc space. The cuff of tissue formed by its rolled edges helps to protect the walls of the great veins at the sides of the disc space.

Retro-peritoneal fibrosis is seen without exception when anterior interbody fusion operations are performed following previous explorations of the spinal canal. Of variable density in cases of isolated disc resorption or internal disc disruption, this

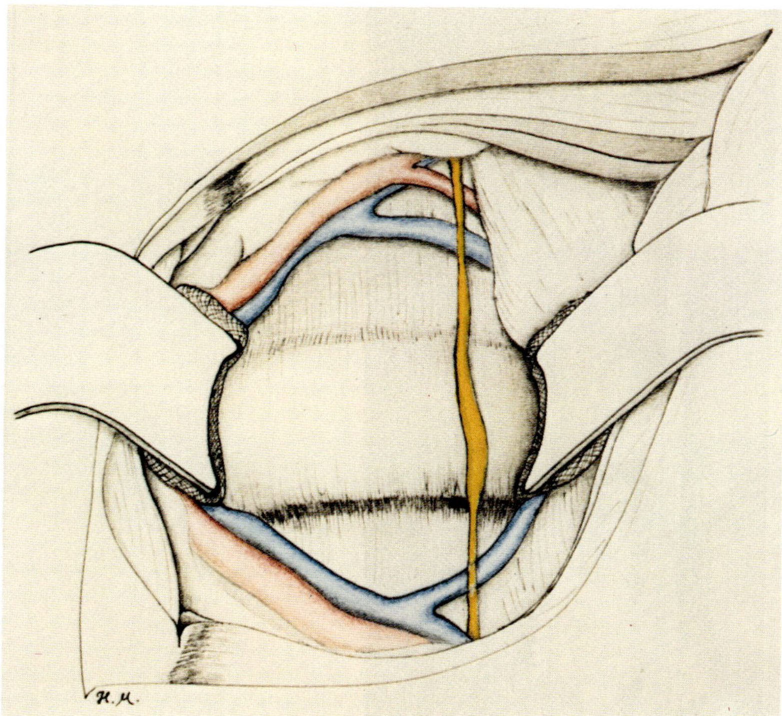

Figure 2.35. A drawing to illustrate the principal anatomical features at the L4/5 level, showing the modified Deever's retractors in place. Note the retraction of the psoas muscle on the right side of the drawing, with the outline of the sympathetic trunk (in yellow) anterior to this retractor

fibrotic tissue may make it very difficult to separate the common iliac veins in the midline, even rendering access to the disc impossible. In such cases damage to the thin wall of the left common iliac vein is likely to occur unless the surgeon is aware of this potential problem. The application of artery forceps or vascular clips–such as Weck clips–to this large thin-walled vein should be avoided. Repair of this vessel requires that the bleeding site be adequately exposed. Digital pressure above and below any tear will control the blood flow to allow identification of the defect in its wall until it can be repaired with a fine atraumatic vascular suture.

The left common iliac vein is sometimes very large–measuring 3 or 4 cm from lateral to medial edge, rendering access to the lumbo-sacral disc between the medial edges of the right and left common iliac vessels impossible. In such circumstances, the medial border of the left psoas muscle should be retracted carefully. Un-named

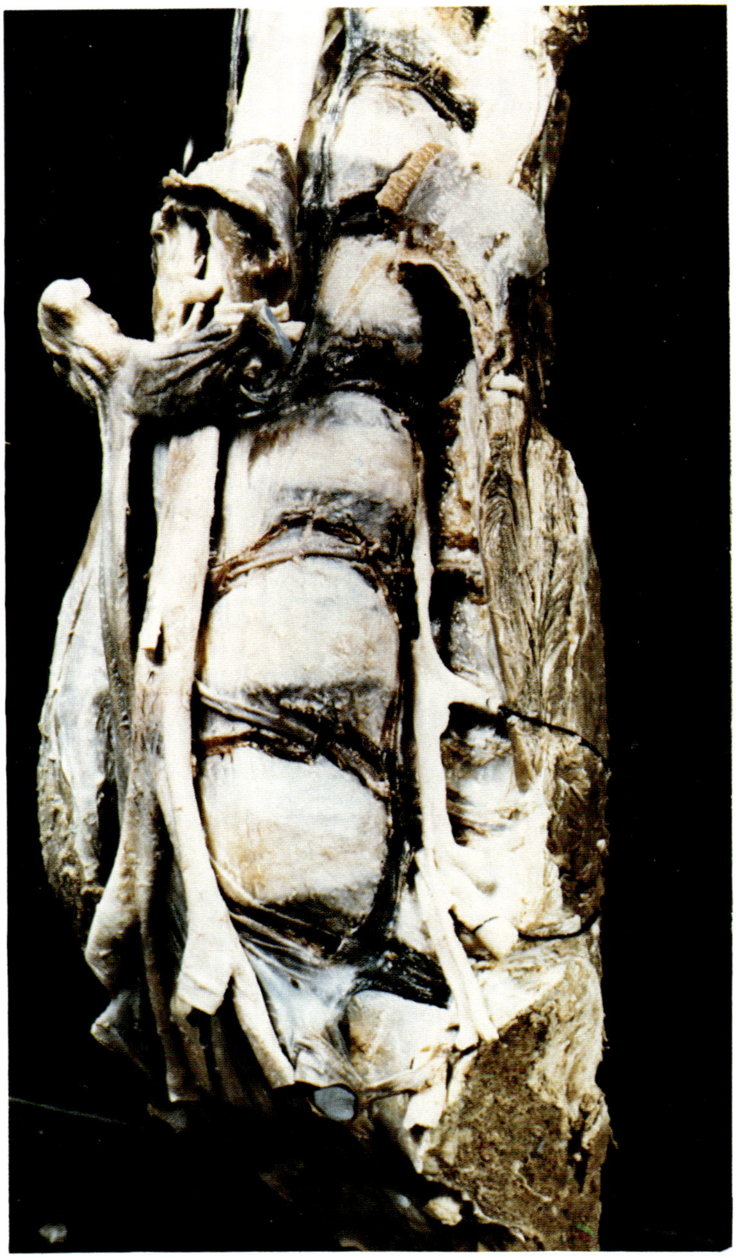

Figure 2.36. A photograph of the left side of the specimen illustrated in Fig. 2.24 to show the arrangement of the left ascending lumbar vein in relation to the left common iliac vein

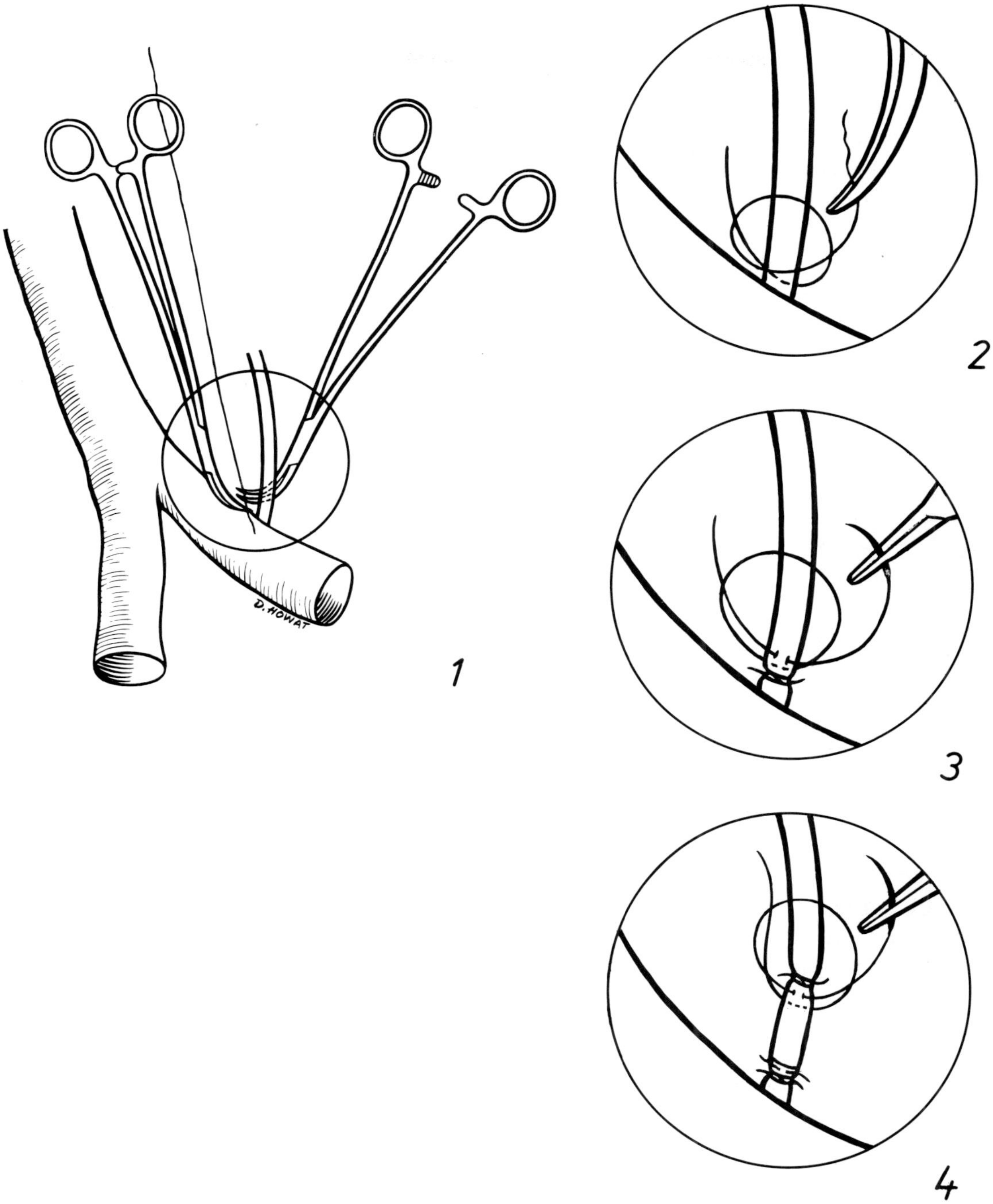

Figure 2.37. **1** A drawing to illustrate the passage of a ligature beneath the ascending lumbar vein on the left side. **2** Tying the ligature on the ascending lumbar vein adjacent to its entry point into the left common iliac vein. **3** Showing the passage of *a transfixion circumferential locking suture* beyond the first tie placed on the ascending lumbar vein near its junction with the left common iliac vein. **4** Showing the insertion of *a transfixion circumferential locking suture* further along the course of the ascending lumbar vein. The vessel is divided then between these four ligatures, without risk of slipping of the ties after the vessel has been cut

arteries and veins often pass into the muscle directly from the lateral walls of the adjacent left common iliac artery and vein. These small vessels can cause troublesome haemorrhage. They should be carefully isolated and coagulated with diathermy well clear of their origins from the great vessels, before being divided.

The lateral wall of the left common iliac vein should then be exposed by careful blunt dissection aided with the use of a sucker to remove surrounding loose fat. The left sympathetic nerve trunk should be identified and regional lymphatic channels coagulated before the edge of the left common iliac vein can be clearly seen. The ascending lumbar vein will be seen at this stage and the decision taken to ligate and divide it, depending on its length. If it becomes tightly stretched, preventing retraction of the common iliac vein across the front of the L5/S1 disc space, it must be divided. Details of this manoeuvre are outlined below.

To expose the disc between the L4 and L5 vertebral bodies, it may be necessary to ligate and divide the left ascending lumbar vein. The sympathetic trunk is first identified where it lies along the anterior margin of the psoas major muscle, on the side of the vertebral body (Fig. 2.35). The fibres of the fibrous arcade, which attach the psoas muscle to the superior and inferior vertebral margins at the disc space, are divided and the psoas muscle is retracted laterally.

The ascending lumbar vein is often quite large, with a diameter at its entry point into the lateral wall of the left common iliac vein of between 3 and 5 mm (Fig. 2.36). The techniques for the safe handling, dissection and ligation of this vessel are among the most critical manoeuvres to be performed in the whole of this operation. Whether or not ligation is required depends on the length of the vessel and its site of entry into the left common iliac vein. This vein is usually surrounded by fatty tissues from which it must be dissected free. This can be done by using a blunt probe and a smooth-ended fine sucker.

The vessel is ligated with sutures of 3/0 black silk, just beyond its entry point into the left common iliac vein and again, further along its course, deep to the psoas muscle. It is essential to lock these black silk sutures on to the wall of the ascending lumbar vein with 5/0 sutures, transfixing its wall and encircling the vessel adjacent to each suture. The vessel is then divided between these locking sutures with a fine scalpel blade, mounted on a long handle. With these precise manoeuvres safely completed, the great vessels may then be retracted towards the mid-line from the antero-lateral surface of the L4/5 disc space (Figs. 2.35, 2.37).

Exposure of the L3/4 disc space can be achieved often without division of any significant vessels; although, on occasions, the lumbar vessels lying on the side of the body of L4 may need to be separately ligated near the anterior margin of the psoas major muscle before the great vessels can be safely retracted from the antero-lateral surface of this disc.

Exposure of upper lumbar discs is best done with the patient in the lateral position on the operating table and with the incision running through the bed of the twelfth rib to allow extra-peritoneal exposure of the upper lumbar vertebral column.

vi) Preparation of the Interspace for Graft Insertion

The preparation of dowel cavities in the intervertebral space is carried out with the use of special cutters supplied in six sizes for use at any vertebral level. Each cutting cylinder has circumferential markings clearly visible on its external surface. These rings are separated from each other by 5 mm (Figs. 2.38, 2.39).

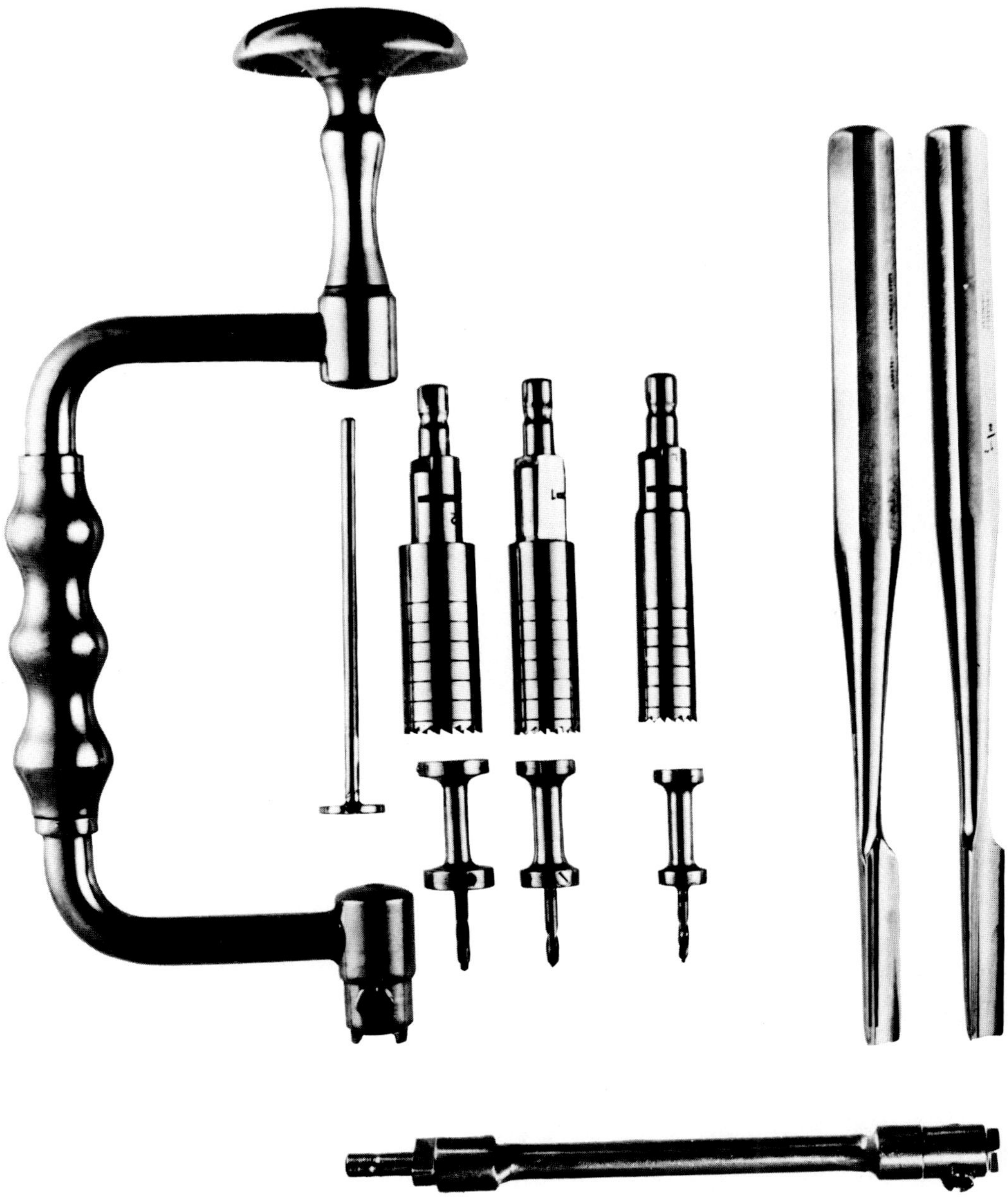

Figure 2.38. A photograph showing a modified Hudson brace and three dowel cutting instruments, with starter centre pieces and one graft ejector. On the right side, note the special gouges which are used with the cutters. At the bottom of the picture, an extension piece is shown for use during lumbar interbody fusion operations. These instruments are manufactured exclusively by the Thomson and Shelton Instrumentation Company, 6119 Danbury Lane, Dallas, TX 75214, U.S.A.

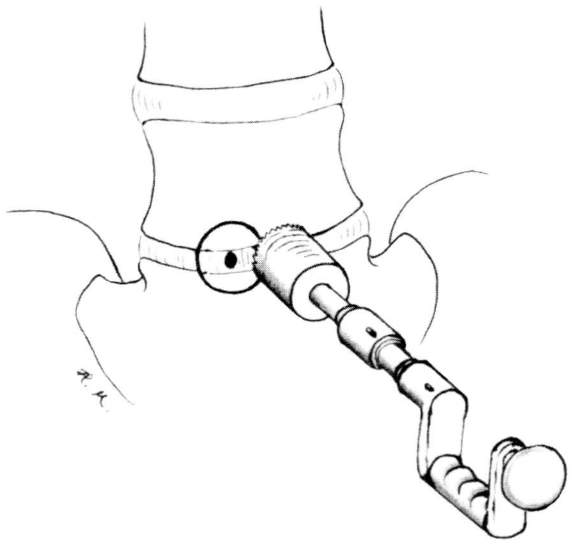

Figure 2.39. A drawing to illustrate the use of the Hudson brace, with the extension piece and the cutter, to prepare a dowel cavity at the lumbo-sacral junction

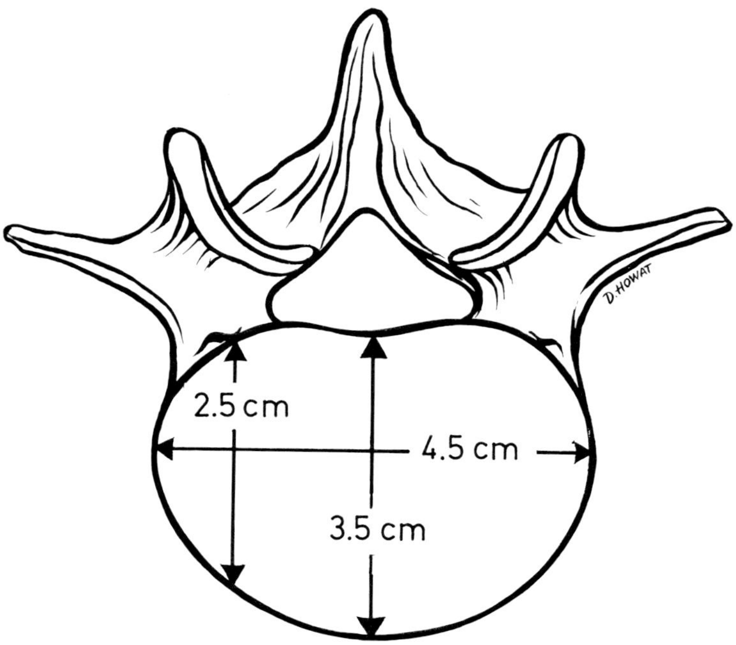

Figure 2.40. A drawing to illustrate the measurements of the L5 vertebral body in an adult of average size

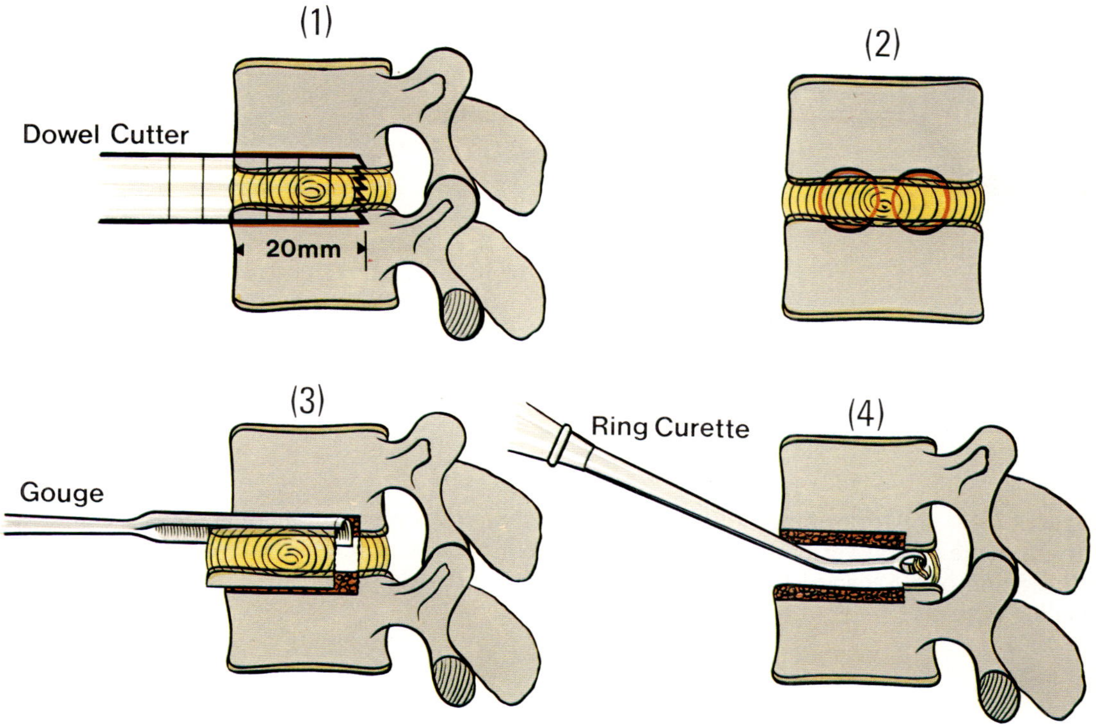

Figure 2.41. Lower lumbar dowel cavities. **1** The use of a dowel cutting instrument in the lumbar spine. **2** The antero-posterior orientation of two dowel cavities in the lower lumbar area. **3** The use of the special gouge to displace the disc and adjacent fragments of the vertebral bodies. **4** The use of the ring curette for the removal of vertebral end-plate and disc tissue remnants from the interbody space

In due course, *grafts are cut using the cutting cylinder that is one size larger than that used to cut the intervertebral dowel cavities.* When the cutting instruments are in use in the disc spaces, the surgeon must at all times have the undivided attention of his two assistants, to ensure that the great vessels are protected from injury. Specially modified Deever's retractors, which have smooth excavated ends, are held in place with loose Raytec swabs positioned to prevent the edges of the great vessels or adjacent soft tissues from herniating beneath them.

The surgeon must be thoroughly familiar with the measurements of the intervertebral space in each patient when preparing the dowel cavities. Measurements of the vertical height of the disc space and the antero-posterior depth should be available from preoperative roentgenograms. In addition, it is to be noted that the antero-posterior measurements vary, being greatest in the mid-line and smallest laterally because the shape of the disc bearing surface of the vertebral body is oval, not rectangular (Fig. 2.40).

When the parallel plugs of the adjacent vertebral body fragments and the intervening intervertebral disc have been displaced from the interspace using a gouge specially tooled to match the size of the cutter (Figs. 2.41, 1–4), the disc remnants are then removed from the interspace with rongeurs. In addition, vertebral end-plate remnants should be removed with ring curettes (Figs. 2.42a, b). Aided by the use of a vertebral spreader, it is possible to remove the bulk of the disc tissue and vertebral

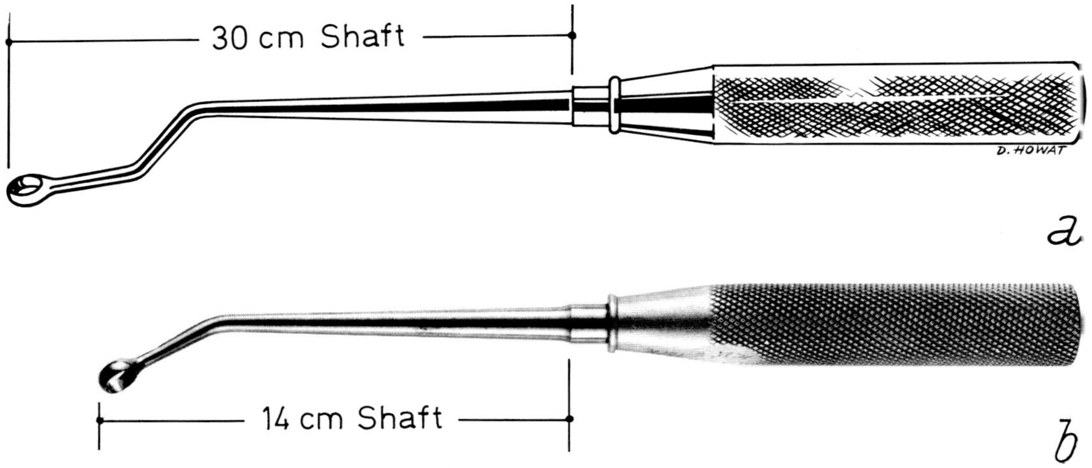

Figures 2.42. **a** A drawing of a long handled ring curette with a double-angled shaft, suitable for curettage of the vertebral end plate and disc remnants in lumbar interbody fusions. **b** A photograph of a Cloward-type ring curette with single angle on the shaft, suitable for use in smaller patients

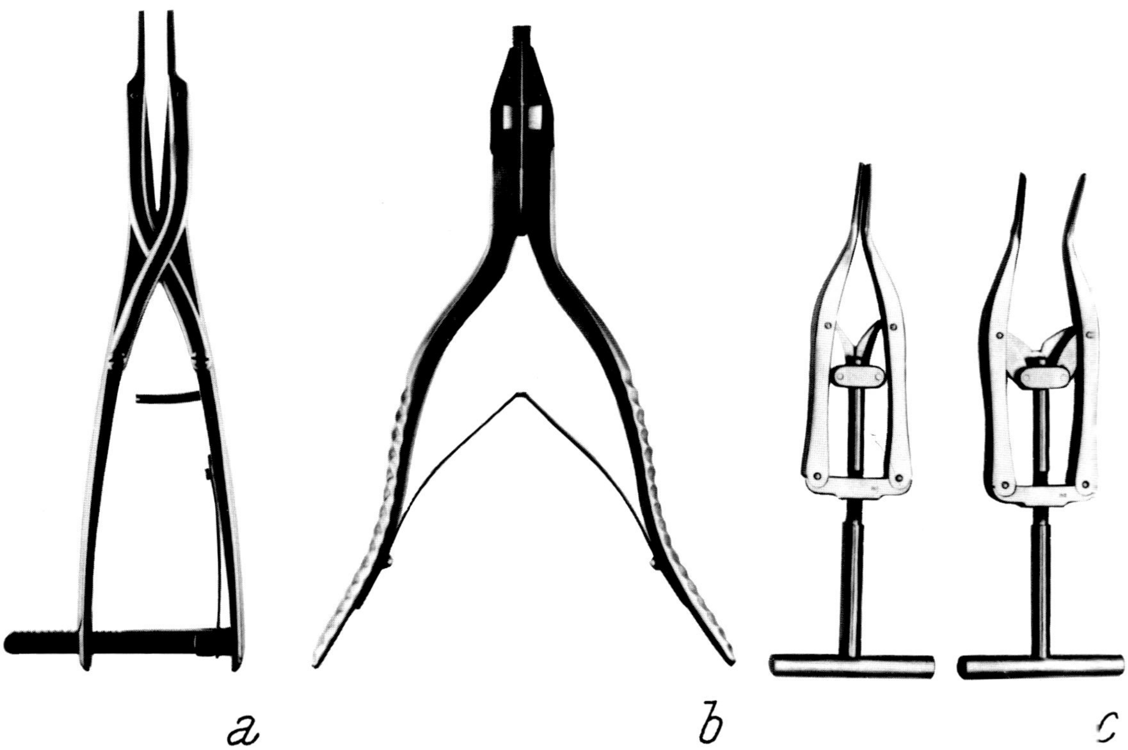

Figures 2.43 a–c. Photographs of different types of vertebral spreaders. The central instrument is of Cloward design and is not self-retaining. It is suitable for use in interbody fusions, though it was not designed for that purpose. The instruments in **a** and **c** are of Japanese design

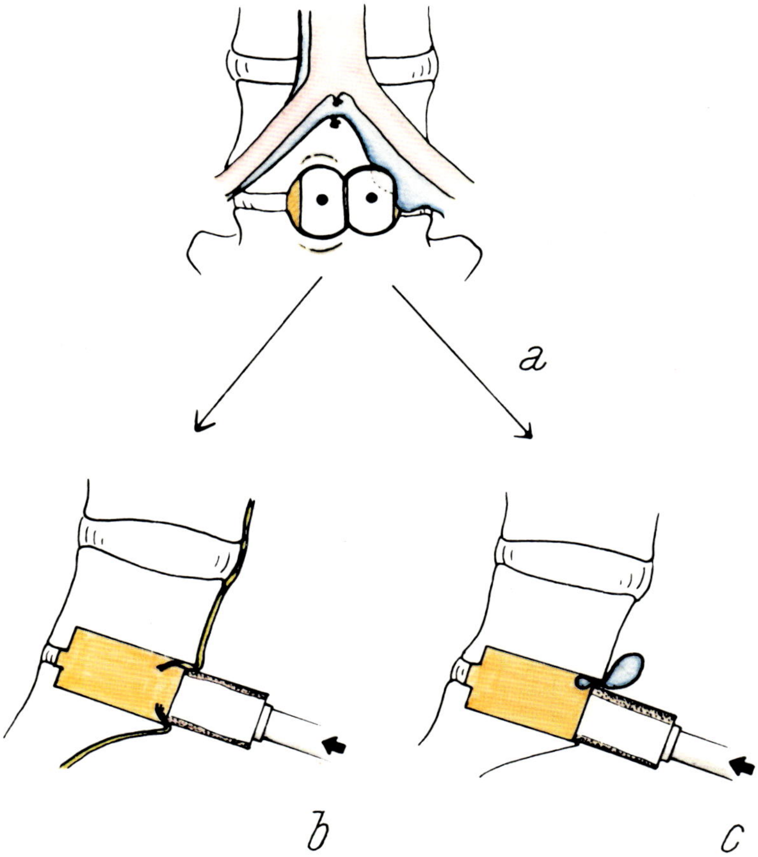

Figures 2.44. **a** Drawing illustrating the entrapment of part of the medial wall of the left common iliac vein after graft impaction. **b** A lateral view of the lumbo-sacral space depicting the rolling inwards of the free margins of the anterior longitudinal ligament during graft impaction. This should be avoided by proper retraction of all soft tissues adjacent to the dowel cavity before grafts are impacted. **c** A lateral view of the lumbo-sacral space demonstrating the hazard of trapping the medial edge of the left common iliac vein during graft impaction. This problem should be avoided at all times by careful retraction of the vessels at the time of graft impaction

end-plate cartilages from the interspaces (Figs. 2.43a–c). However, during these manoeuvres the surgeon must avoid penetrating the spinal canal or damaging the great vessels, which may have slipped out from beneath the retractors (Figs. 2.44a–c).

The graft beds prepared by this method are well-vascularized. Indeed, one of the great advantages of this operation is that the blood supply of the vertebral bodies is not disturbed; thus, vascularization of appropriately placed grafts is assured (Crock and Yoshizawa, 1977).

Graft Preparation

The use of autogenous bone grafts is strongly recommended. The left iliac crest is exposed by retracting the infero-lateral edge of the abdominal incision. A

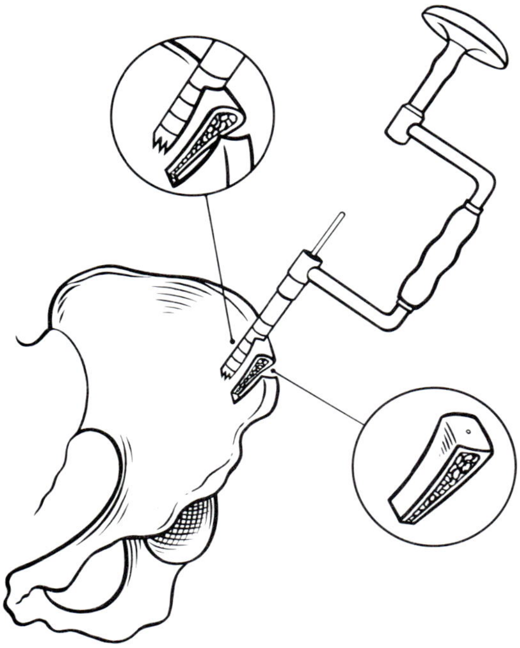

Figure 2.45. Drawing to illustrate the method of cutting grafts from the anterior third of the iliac crest. Each graft has two tooled cancellous surfaces and stout cortical faces on three sides

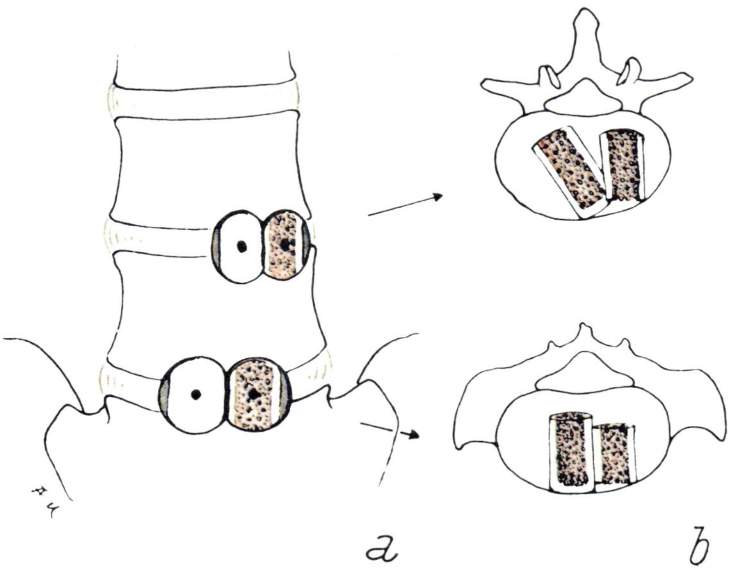

Figures 2.46 a and **b.** Drawings illustrating the orientation of grafts in the intervertebral spaces at L5/S1 and L4/5

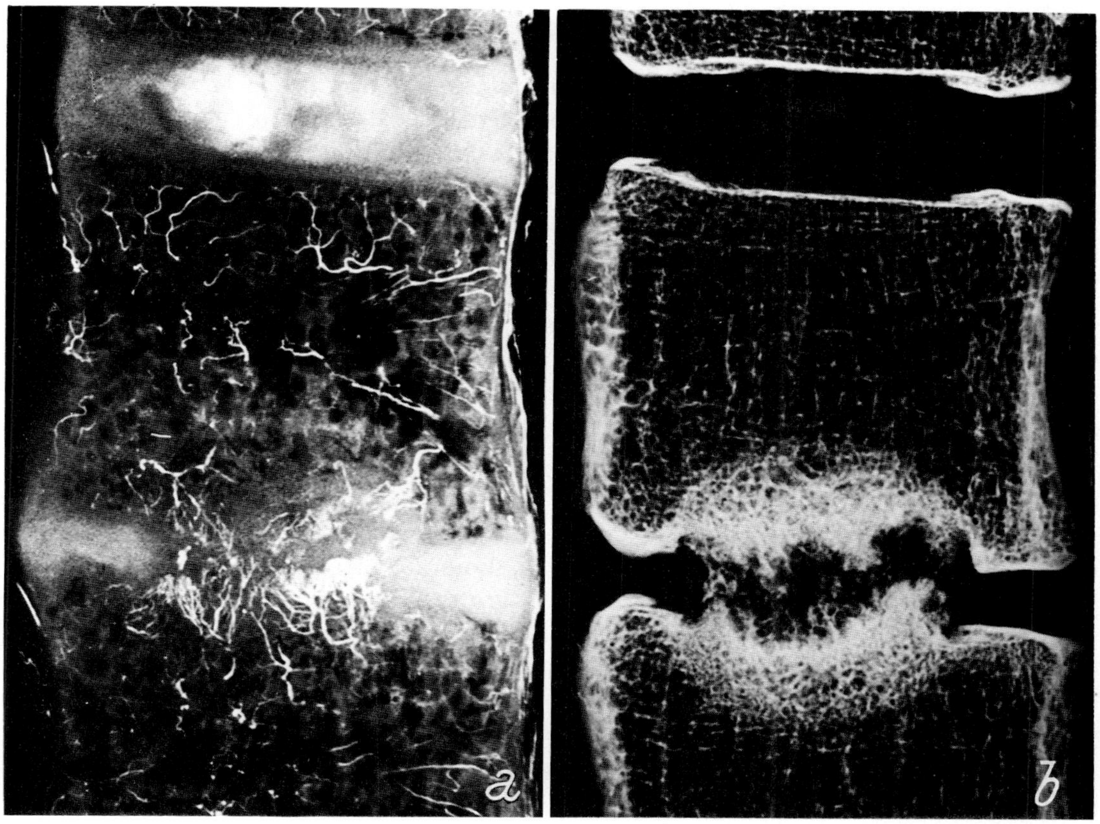

Figures 2.47. **a** Photograph of a thin sagittal section of the lumbar spine taken at necropsy. The L1/2 disc is shown at the top of the specimen. At L2/3, vessels in the interbody graft can be seen. On the right, tufted vessels abut against invading disc tissue. Centrally, the graft is vascularized. **b** At the L2/3 level, union of the graft is incomplete, and the cancellous bone of the graft has been infiltrated by disc tissue remnants

supplementary incision is then made running along its upper border. *Dowel cutting instruments one size larger than those used to prepare the dowel cavities in the intervertebral space, are then used to cut grafts from the iliac crest,* passing vertically downwards to the required depth. Grafts of 2.5–2.8 cm in depth are of satisfactory size in most patients. On occasion, cancellous chips may be cut from the bony fragments of vertebral bodies obtained from the dowel cavities. (These fragments may be used to supplement the iliac crest grafts in larger patients.) The iliac crest grafts have three cortical faces and two "tooled" cancellous faces (Fig. 2.45). They are designed to be impacted adjacent to each other with the cortical faces orientated laterally in the disc space and the cancellous surfaces facing the vertebral bodies (Figs. 2.46a, b). Purely cancellous grafts inserted into the intervertebral disc space have been shown by Crock (1976) to be liable to invasion by disc remnants, thus predisposing to non-union (Figs. 2.47a, b). This complication has been largely obviated by the use of grafts cut from the anterior iliac crest in the manner just described.

vii) Graft Impaction

In the last phase of this operation, the intervertebral disc space is again carefully exposed by the assistants. A vertebral spreader is inserted into one of the dowel cavities and opened to allow a final inspection of the interspace. *The depth of the dowel cavity is checked with a depth gauge and ruler* and the first graft then impacted. This is a potentially dangerous manoeuvre as the edge of a great vessel may become trapped between the graft and the wall of the dowel cavity. Successful retraction at this critical stage of the operation calls for strict attention to detail.

Following impaction of the first graft, the vertebral spreader is removed from the second dowel cavity and the second graft is then impacted. Some haemorrhage will occur from the site; but this is never severe and usually ceases in two or three minutes.

Attention is finally focussed on the donor site. If two grafts have been cut from the iliac crest then *the bony defect is filled with orthopaedic bone cement* before the wounds are closed in layers with suction drainage. Small cavities are curetted out between the cortical faces of the iliac crest at the anterior and posterior limits of the pelvic defect left after removal of the dowel grafts. Bone cement pushed into these cavities helps to maintain the stability of the newly moulded "pelvic crest" and diminish pain in the post-operative period.

The method of operation described here has been used by the author at St. Vincent's Hospital, Melbourne, since 1961. Of approximately 1,000 operations performed in 20 years, three patients have died. Two of these died in the post-operative period of acute coronary occlusion; the third committed suicide four months after operation.

No significant urologic complications have been encountered with this method of spinal fusion. Retention of urine occurs in some patients, but its management only rarely involves the use of a catheter for one or two days. In most cases bladder function is restored after the use of one or two doses of Urecholine (Merck, Sharp & Dohme).

In exposing the lumbo-sacral intervertebral disc space in the male, the use of diathermy in the presacral area has been avoided. The author is aware of complaints of sterility in only two patients, both of whom were psychiatrically disturbed and both of whom had complained of impotence before operation.

viii) Post-Operative Care

Patients are nursed supine with one or two pillows, and rolled from side to side several times a day with a pillow placed between their legs. We recommend the use of beds which can be tilted vertically to allow patients to stand and to get out of bed with little assistance from the nursing staff. Intravenous therapy is continued until bowel sounds are heard or flatus has been passed.

Prophylactic anticoagulant therapy with subcutaneous calciparine (Heparin, Difrex Australian Laboratories Pty. Ltd., Glebe Street, Glebe, N.S.W.) is administered until patients have become fully mobile.

Spinal supports are fitted within a few days of operation and worn for three or four months afterwards.

ix) Complications

1. Deep vein thrombosis

This is a major problem. An important step in its prevention is to avoid entrapping the edge of a great vein during graft impaction (Figs. 2.44a–c).

2. Non-union of grafts

a) The use of purely cancellous grafts may lead to non-union following infiltration of the grafted bone by reactive disc tissues which also prevent vascular penetration of the graft (Figs. 2.47a, b).

b) Special surgical techniques will be required to prevent non-union in the following circumstances:

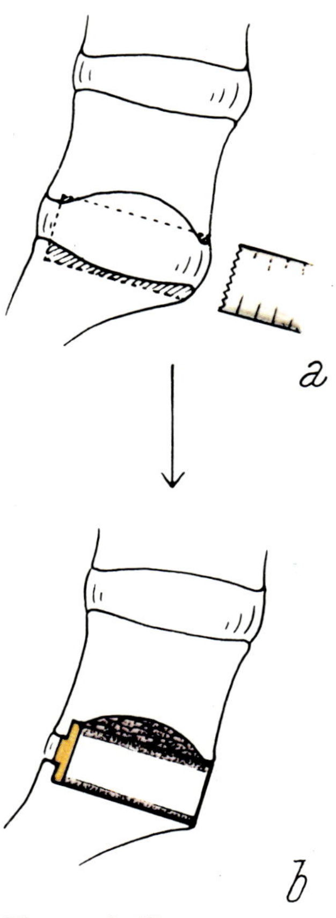

Figures 2.48

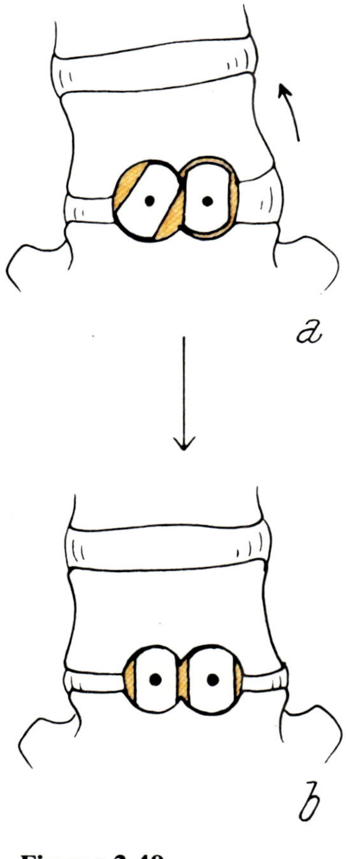

Figures 2.49

Figures 2.48. **a** A drawing of a lateral view of the lumbo-sacral space to illustrate the problem created when the vertebral end-plate of L5 is "ballooned". A cutter then fails to remove the "ballooned segment" when it is inserted in the course of preparing the dowel cavity. **b** A drawing to show that the area needs to be separately prepared with a curette and grafted with cancellous chips before the dowel graft is impacted

Figures 2.49. **a** A drawing to illustrate the point that the graft which has been inserted eccentrically–as on the left-hand side–distorts the outline of the other cavity so that the second graft will not fit firmly into it. **b** A drawing to demonstrate the correct placing of grafts parallel to each other, so that each fits snugly in the intervertebral space

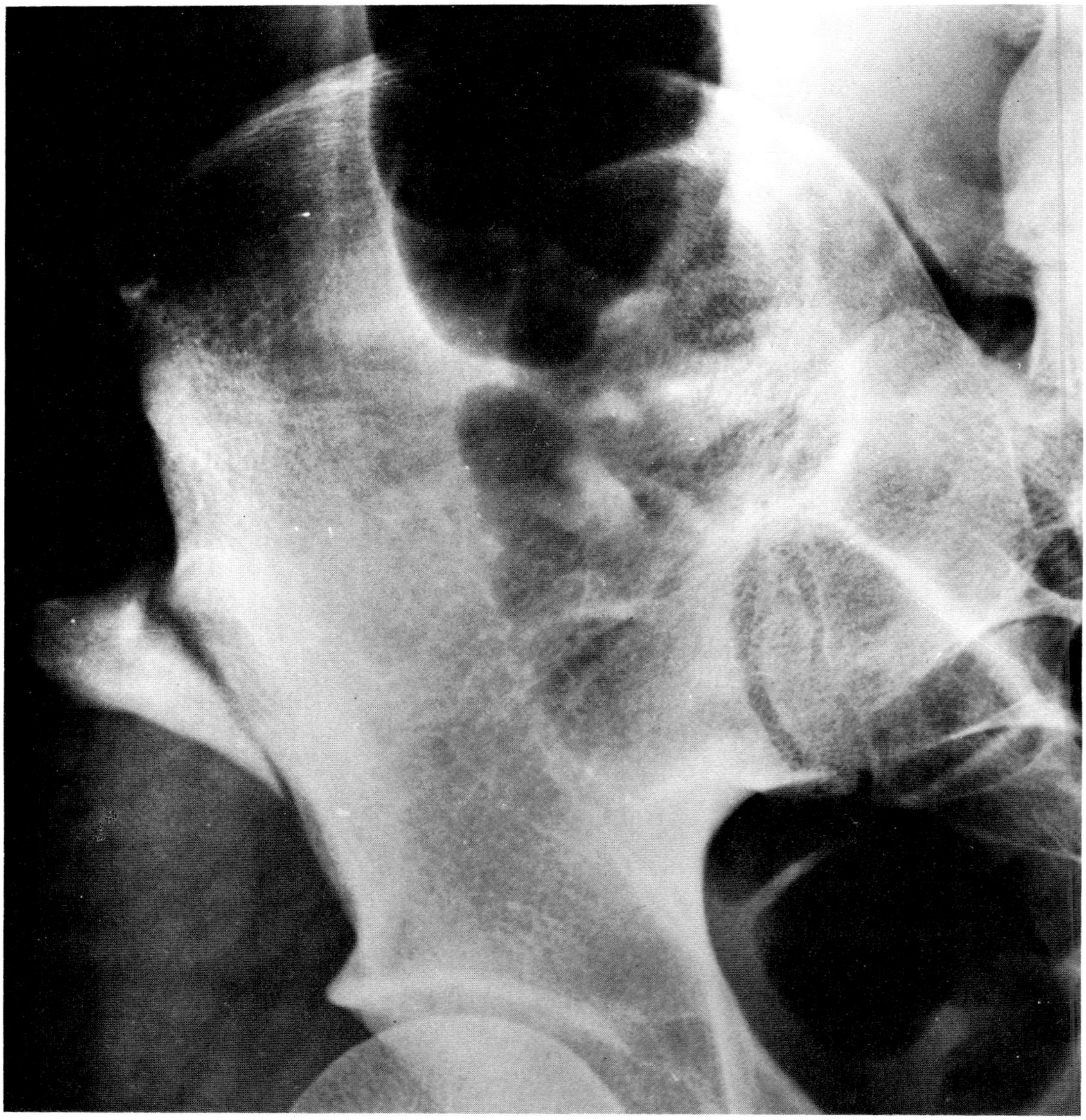

Figure 2.50. A radiograph of the ilium to show a fracture in the region of the anterior-superior iliac spine which occurred following removal of grafts for interbody fusion

i) When the vertebral end-plates are widely separated. The disc tissues should be excised with a scalpel and the vertebral end-plate cartilages curetted. The disc space is thereby narrowed. A dowel cutter of appropriate size should then be selected. The starter centre piece should be removed and the cutter, affixed to the extension piece alone should be placed across the disc space and tapped into place with a hammer. The Hudson brace is then fitted and the cutter oscillated, at first counter-clockwise, then clockwise, until an accurate circular dowel cavity is cut between the vertebral bodies.

ii) When the vertebral end plates are of irregular shape, the cutters may fail to remove a segment of vertebral end-plate cartilage. This area should be identified, by using a *dental mirror*. After curettage of the "uncut" vertebral end-plate remnants, cancellous chips should be placed in the cavity, preliminary to graft impaction (Figs. 2.48a, b).

c) During impaction, care should be taken to avoid rotation of the graft. If this occurs, the dimensions of the second dowel cavity will be larger than required and the second graft will fit loosely (Figs. 2.49a, b).

3. Infection at the graft site

This is a rare complication after interbody fusion operations. If it occurs it may be very serious. Management of this problem is discussed on p. 262.

4. Iliac crest fracture (Fig. 2.50)

5. Post-operative entrapment of the lateral cutaneous nerve of the thigh

Meralgia paraesthetica due to fibrosis around the iliac crest donor site occurs occasionally. Symptoms may be relieved by local steroid injections, though sometimes surgical release of the entrapped nerve may be necessary.

c) Results of Anterior Interbody Fusion

With the use of a technique that allows repeated, reproducible accuracy, lumbar interbody fusions can be achieved in a high percentage of cases in a wide range of disorders of the lumbar spine.

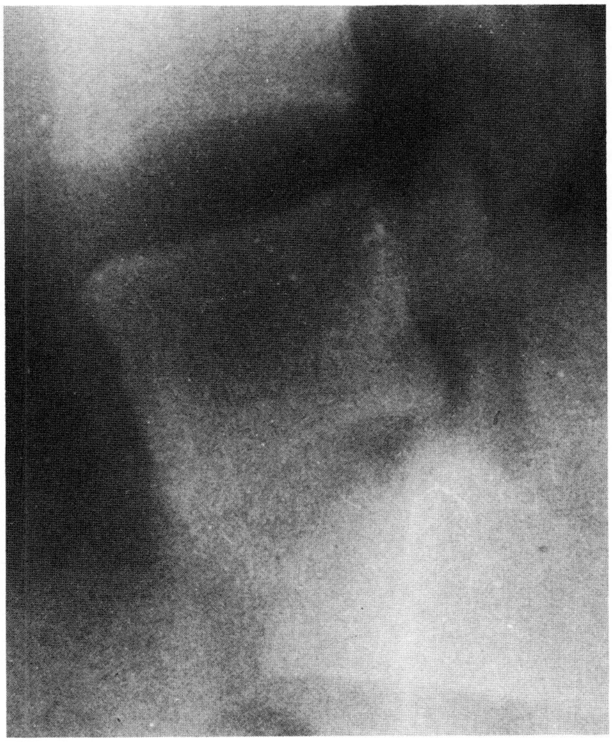

Figure 2.51. A tomogram of the lumbo-sacral junction to show the appearance of an interbody graft inserted three months previously

The results of 150 anterior lumbar interbody fusion operations performed by two surgeons in Australia (H.V. Crock and G.M. Bedbrook) were published by Fujimaki *et al.* (1982).

The data on these patients was gathered, analyzed and classified into three groups: Group I (84 cases): those patients in whom their first and only spinal operation had been an interbody fusion; Group II (38 cases): those patients in whom interbody fusion had followed some other spinal operation; and Group III (28 cases): those patients in whom supplementary operations had been performed following lumbar interbody fusion operation.

The results, including information on occupation, time lost from work and on ultimate re-employment are listed for each group in Table 2.1.

The radiological assessment in these cases is set out in Table 2.2 (Figs. 2.51–2.58).

Table 2.1. Summary of findings

Group	Occupation		Time off (months)	Resumed same occupation	Commenced other occupation	Did not return to work
	Non-sedentary	49	11.8	39	7	3
1	Home duties	18	3.3	16	1	1
	Sedentary	17	7.4	17	0	0
		84				
	Non-sedentary	23	24.0	14	6	3
2	Home duties	7	5.6	6	0	1
	Sedentary	8	6.5	7	0	1
		38				
	Non-sedentary	19	16.5	10	3	6
3	Home duties	5	11.5	3	1	1
	Sedentary	4	12.5	2	0	2
		28				

Table 2.2. Radiological assessment

	Group	G.M.B.	H.V.C.
1.	84 Cases	26 cases	58 cases
	Union	24	56
	Non-union	2	2
2.	38 Cases	16 cases	22 cases
	Union	16	21
	Non-union	0	1
3.	28 Cases	8 cases	20 cases
	Union	8	19
	Non-union	0	1
Total Union		48 (96%)	96 (96%)

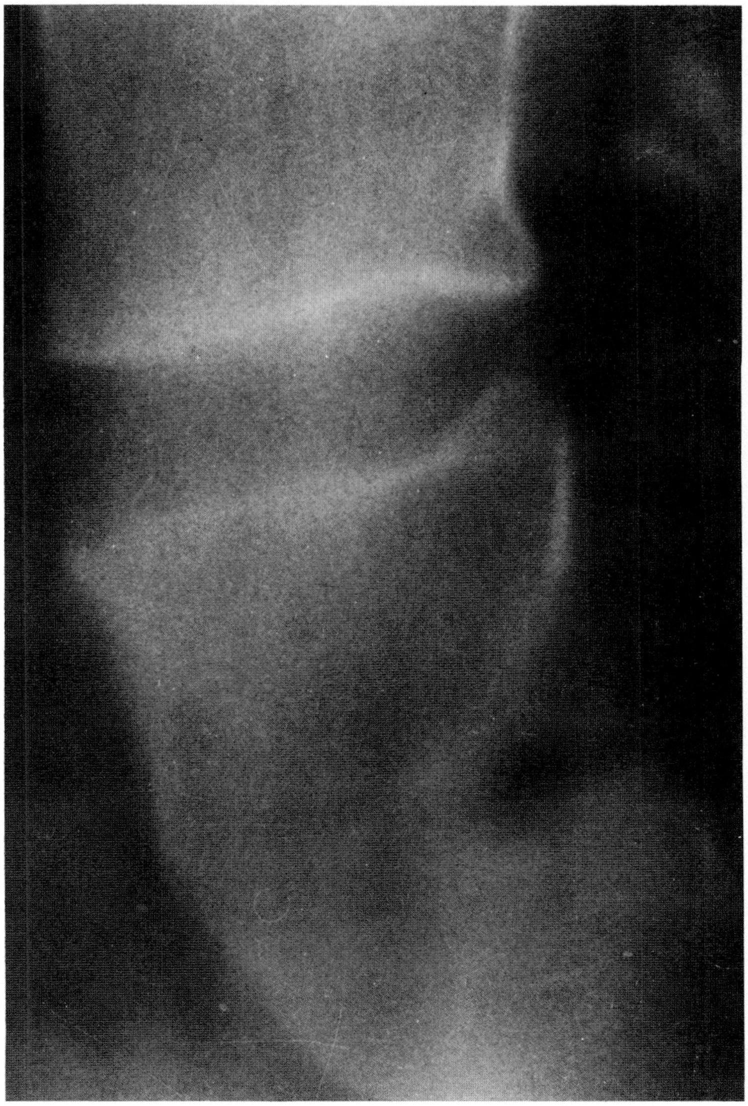

Figure 2.52. A lateral tomogram to show an L5/S1 anterior interbody fusion in a male aged 30 years, taken nine years after anterior fusion

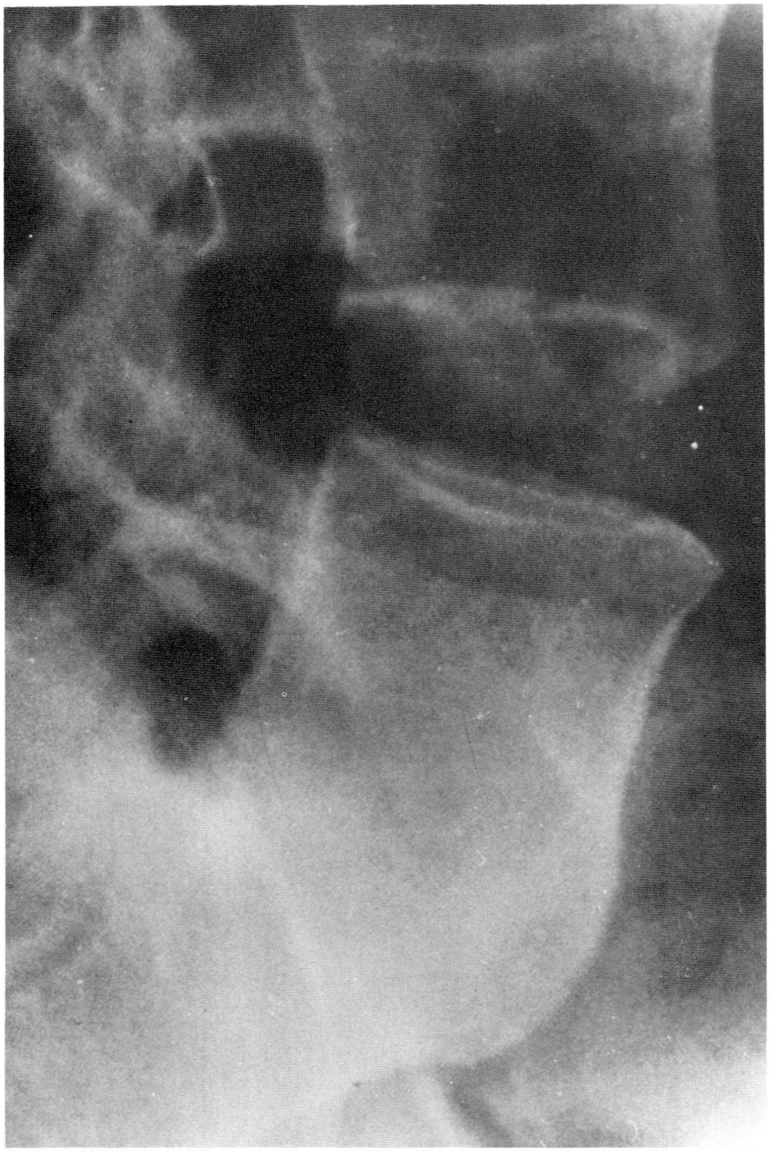

Figure 2.53. A lateral radiograph of the lower lumbar region showing sound L5/S1 interbody fusion ten years after surgery, with a normal L4/5 space above the fused level

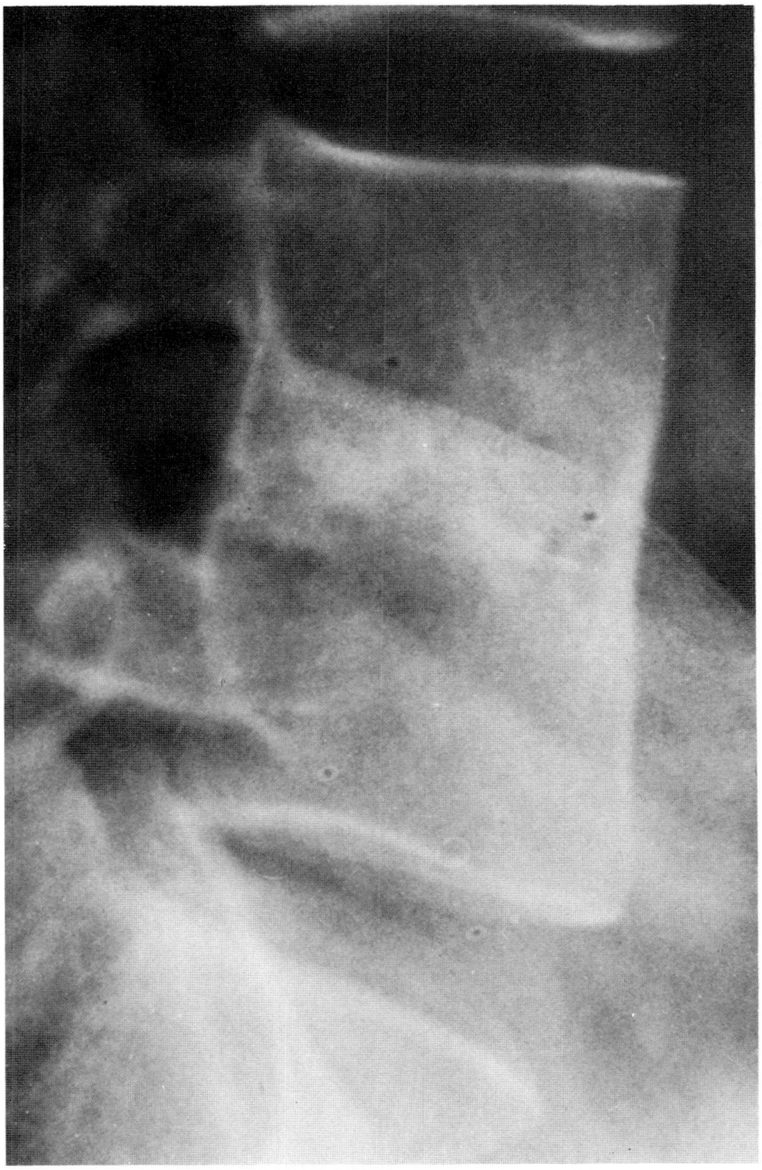

Figure 2.54. A lateral view radiograph showing an L4/5 interbody fusion in a 46 year old woman ten years after operation

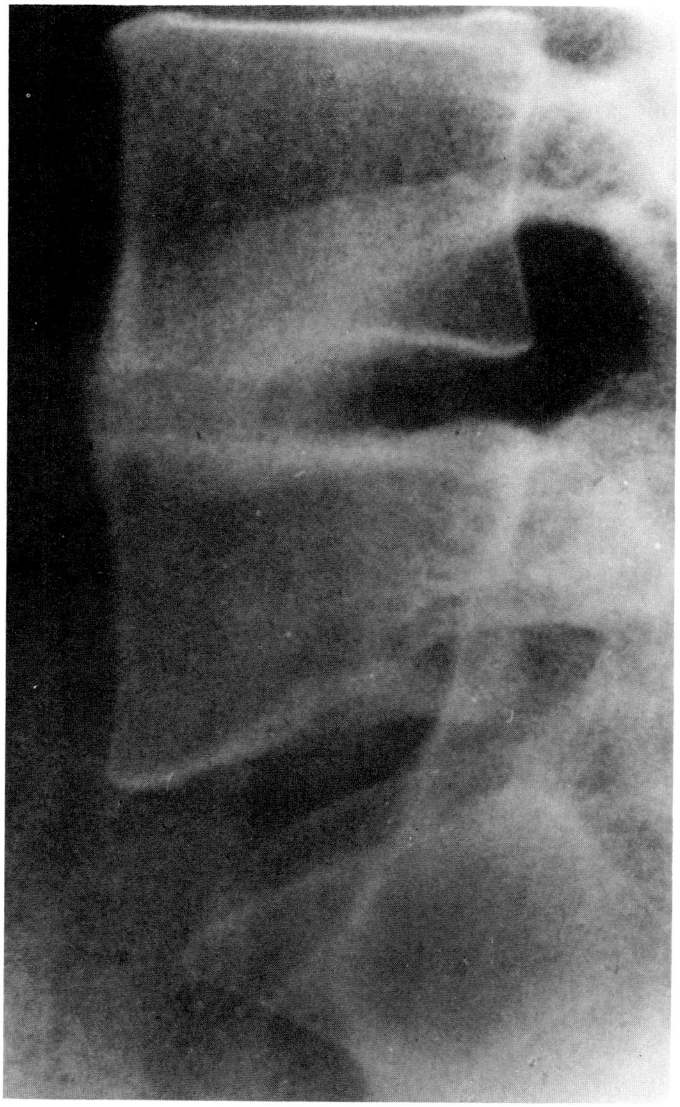

Figure 2.55. A lateral radiograph showing an L4/5 interbody fusion five years after operation

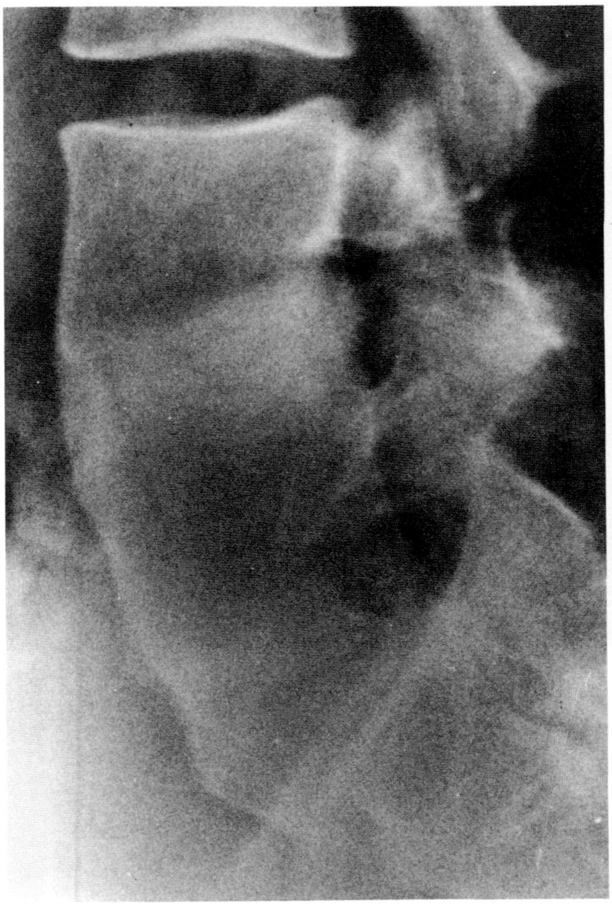

Figure 2.56

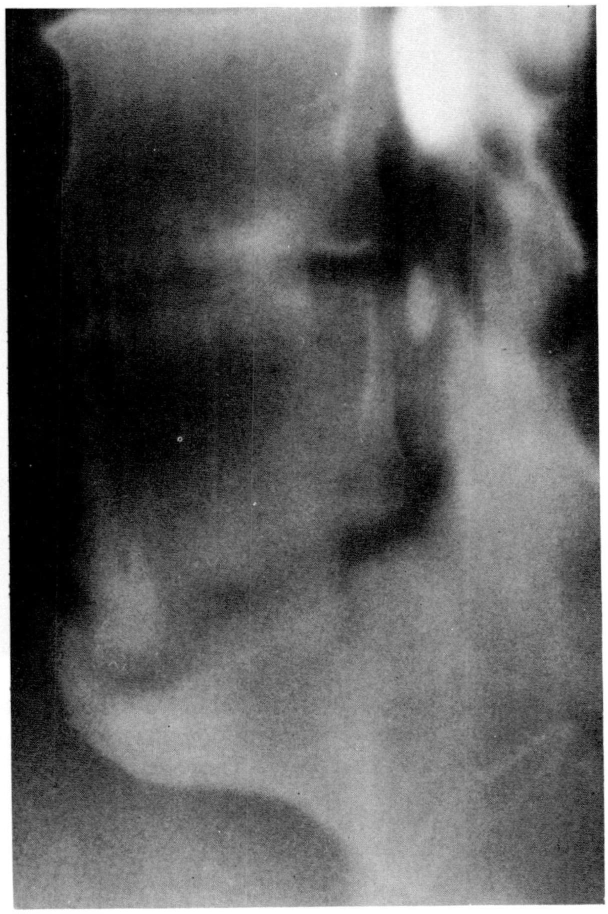

Figure 2.57

Figure 2.56. A lateral radiograph showing L4/5 and L5/S1 interbody fusions in a 48 year old man five years after operation

Figure 2.57. A lateral radiograph of the lower lumbar spine showing a sound L4/5 interbody fusion and an un-united L5/S1 interbody fusion, with sclerosis anteriorly in the intervertebral disc space

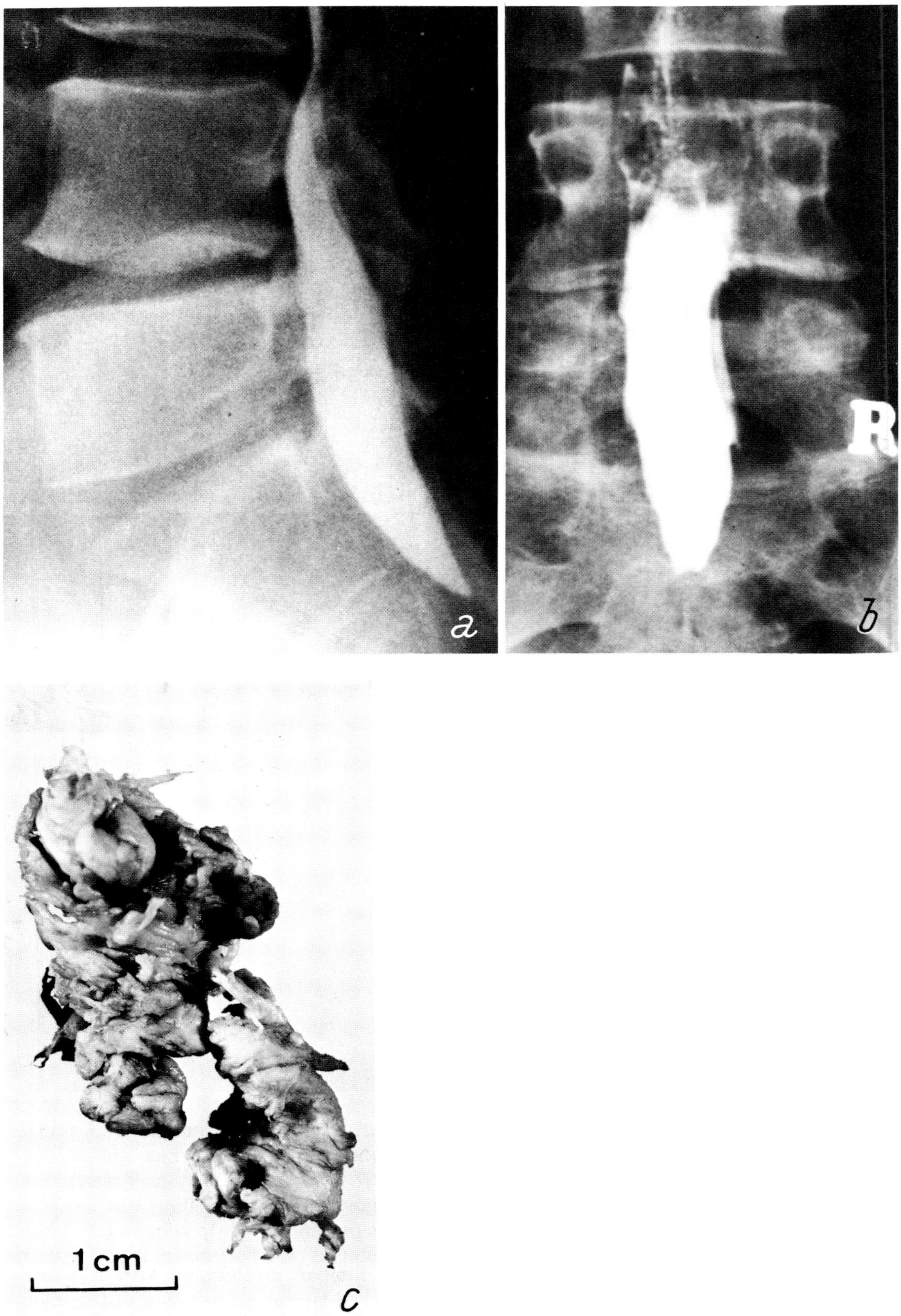

Figures 3.5

3

Lumbar Disc Prolapses

3.1. Introduction

Despite the fact that Mixter and Barr published their description of rupture of the intervertebral disc with involvement of the spinal canal in 1934, confusion still exists about the diagnosis of this lesion and there is often uncertainty about which cases should be treated surgically. Even from the vast literature on this subject a synthesis of practical guidelines to diagnosis and surgical management can be made only with difficulty.

Careful neurological examination is the corner-stone of clinical diagnosis, though it may not be possible to distinguish between disc prolapses at the L5/S1 or L4/5 levels on neurological grounds.

Lumbar disc prolapses requiring surgery are not common. For example, in my own clinic, among 150 cases requiring spinal operations in a six month period during 1981–1982, only four cases were found to have frank disc prolapses.

In operations for suspected disc prolapse where none is found, and following which the patients' symptoms are worse, further investigation will often reveal an unrecognized lesion within the spinal canal, such as some other intervertebral disc disorder–post-traumatic internal disc disruption, or spinal canal or nerve root canal stenosis.

When a surgeon operates on a patient for suspected disc prolapse, but does not find one, he may consider that the exposed disc is unduly soft on palpation or merely bulging. Should he proceed to incise the annulus fibrosus and to remove some portion of disc tissue, the patient's symptoms will usually be worse after the operation (see pp. 47, 56, 245).

Against this background, what then constitutes a useful guide to the management of lumbar disc prolapses?

These lesions are characterized by the escape of disc tissues beyond the normal confines imposed by the intact outer annulus fibrosus and vertebral end-plate cartilages. Synonyms for disc prolapse in common usage include slipped disc, herniated intervertebral disc, protruded intervertebral disc and ruptured disc.

In the lumbar region, disc prolapses are most commonly seen at either the L4/5 or L5/S1 vertebral interspaces or at both of these levels. Higher in the lumbar region they may present with unusual symptoms and signs mimicking intraspinal tumours. In this region they are rare and usually occur in elderly people (Aronsen and Dunsmore, 1963).

The initiating factors are probably multiple, but trauma may precipitate the prolapse. The physical force of the precipitating trauma is often mild, though its influence varies inversely with the extent of pre-existing pathological changes in the affected disc. In normal discs, tensile forces of considerable magnitude (60–80 kg/cm^2) exist in the posterior part of the annulus; this fact gives strong support to the mechanical theory of the production of ruptures of the posterior annulus (Nachemson and Morris, 1964). In young subjects, heavy lifting while bending may lead to the formation of a small prolapse, whereas in older patients massive disc sequestration may follow simple bodily movements such as bending or twisting of the spine. Disc prolapse may be a complication of posturing of the trunk under anaesthesia for other surgical procedures, such as gall bladder, renal or gynaecological operations.

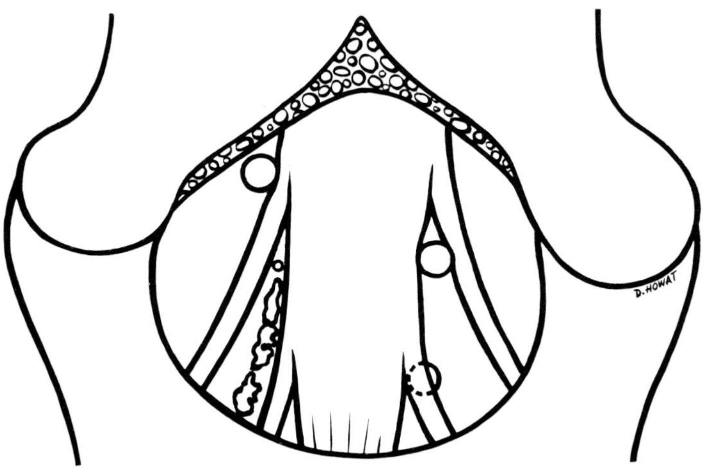

Figure 3.1. A drawing depicting the four common types of disc prolapses found in the lower lumbar region. On the left side a para-rhizal prolapse is shown at the top. Below this, migrating sequestrated disc fragments are shown with a small circular annular defect above them. On the right side an axillary prolapse is illustrated at the top and lower down a sub-rhizal prolapse

3.2. Pathology

The pathological features of disc prolapse have been described by many writers (Coventry *et al.,* 1945; Reynolds and Katz, 1969; Taylor and Akeson, 1971). The characteristics of prolapses vary with the physical qualities of the affected disc tissue. In young persons, discrete, small, rounded, firm or fluctuant protrusions are found with stretched but intact annular fibres and, when incised at operation, only a small quantity of disc tissue may escape and be removed, leaving in the disc a defect which

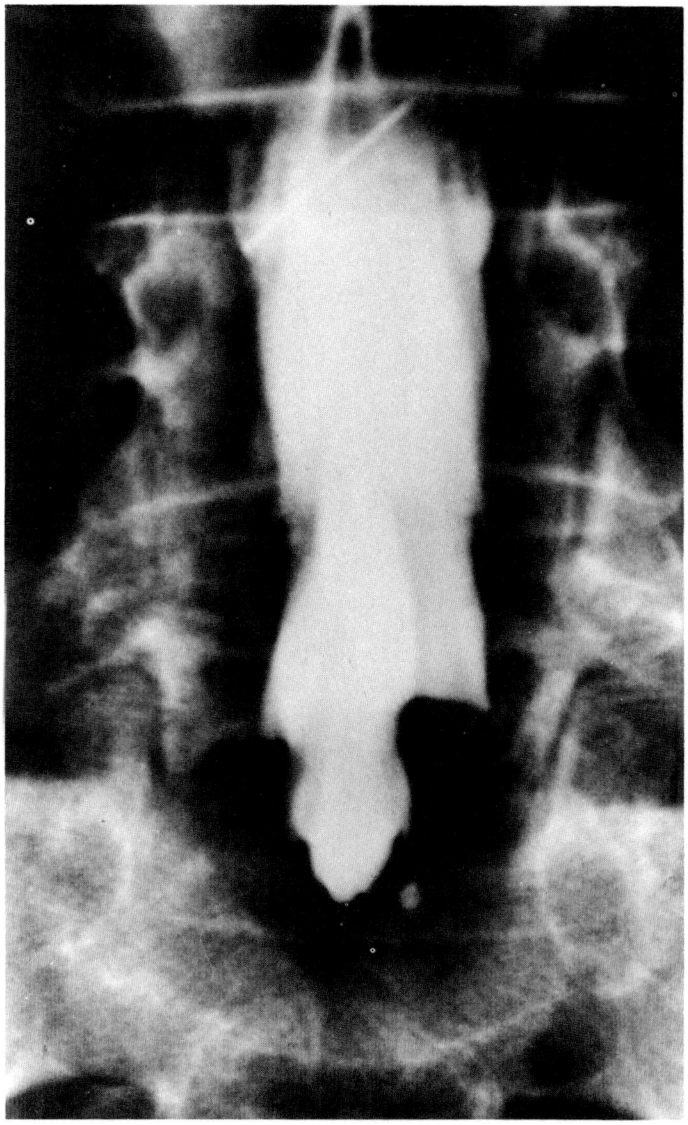

Figure 3.2. An antero-posterior radiograph of a lumbar myelogram in a woman aged 53 years, showing a defect at the L5/S1 level. At operation a sequestrated fragment of disc tissue was found in an axillary position, lying between the inner aspect of the 1st sacral nerve root sheath and the lateral margin of the dural sac

admits neither curettes nor disc rongeurs easily. The consistency of such discs is often described as rubbery. Some degenerate annular fibres are usually found with the extruded nuclear tissue in these cases (Fig. 3.2).

Extrusion of variable quantities of disc tissue (1.1–13.5 g) into the spinal canal may be seen when gross degenerative changes have occurred in the disc as a whole. The description of "sequestrated disc fragments" is then applied. The components of such fragments may include nuclear, annular and end-plate material (Figs. 3.3a–d).

Between these two extremes, a variety of pathological changes may be noted. Incomplete sequestration may be associated with marked peri-neural fibrosis, a

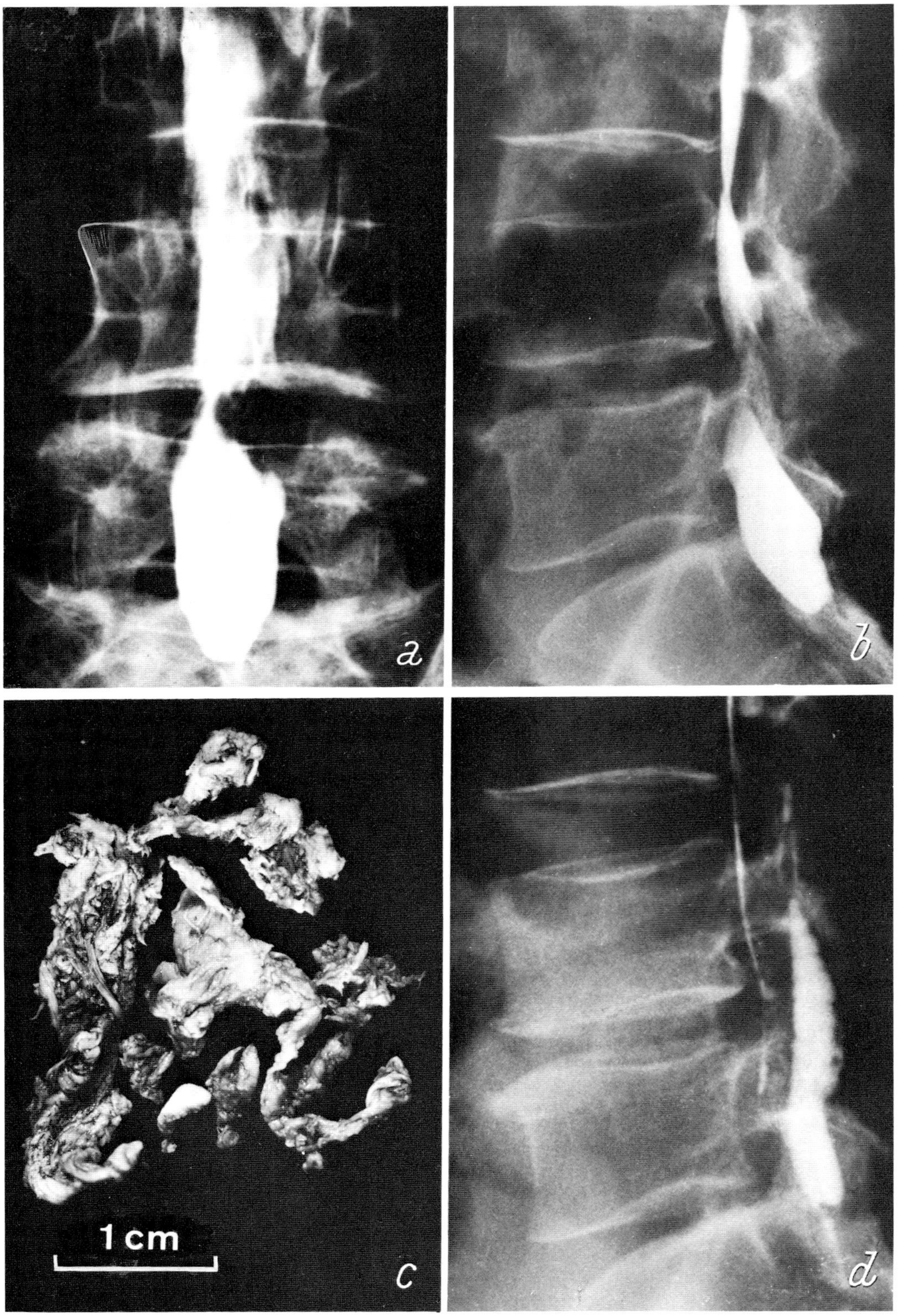

Figures 3.3 a–d. Massive disc sequestration following twisting of the lumbar spine-treated by disc excision and posterior interbody fusion. A 53 year-old male jeweller suffered from intermittent back pain for 13 years. While using a powered floor-sanding machine, he twisted his spine and suddenly developed severe left-sided sciatica. **a** and **b** Antero-posterior and lateral radiographs of the lumbar myelogram, showing a large filling defect at the L4/5 disc space. **c** The sequestrated disc fragments removed at operation. **d** Lateral radiograph taken after operation showing the restored normal outline of the dural sac. Bone grafts are seen between the vertebral bodies of L4 and L5; they were inserted through the spinal canal following disc excision

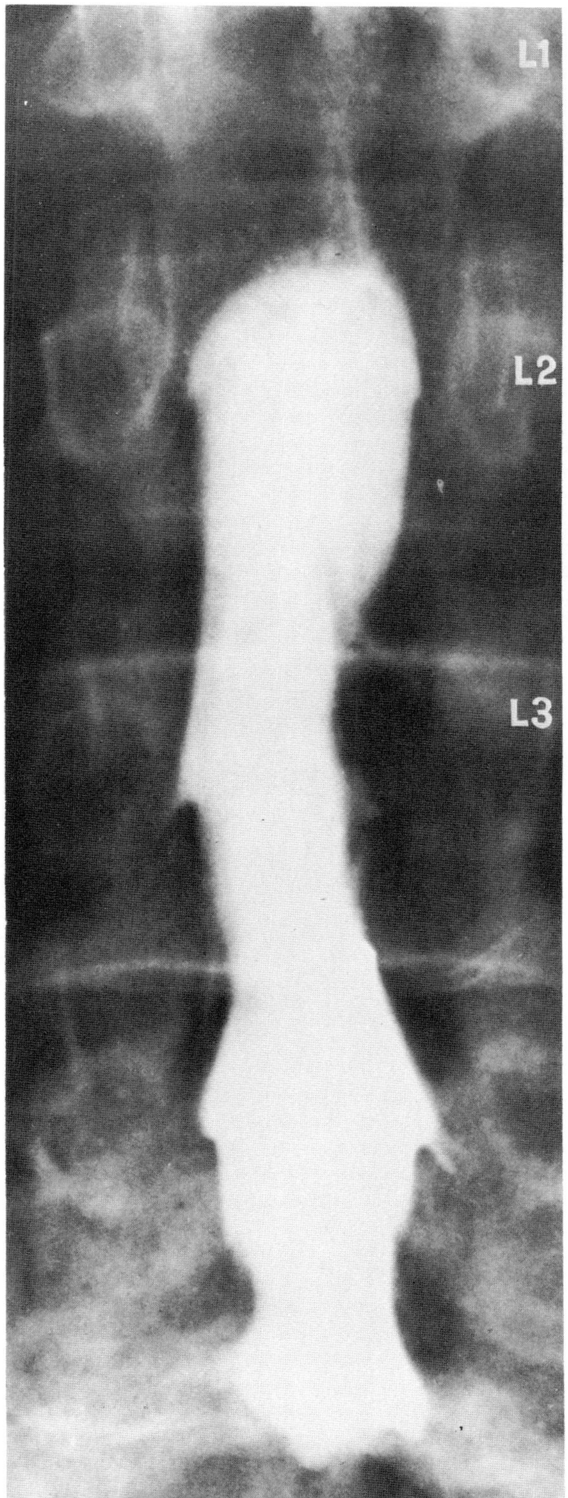

Figure 3.4. Antero-posterior radiograph showing a lumbar myelogram with a massive migrating sequestrated disc from L2/3, producing marked lateral deformation of the myodil column. The patient was a 52 year-old dentist

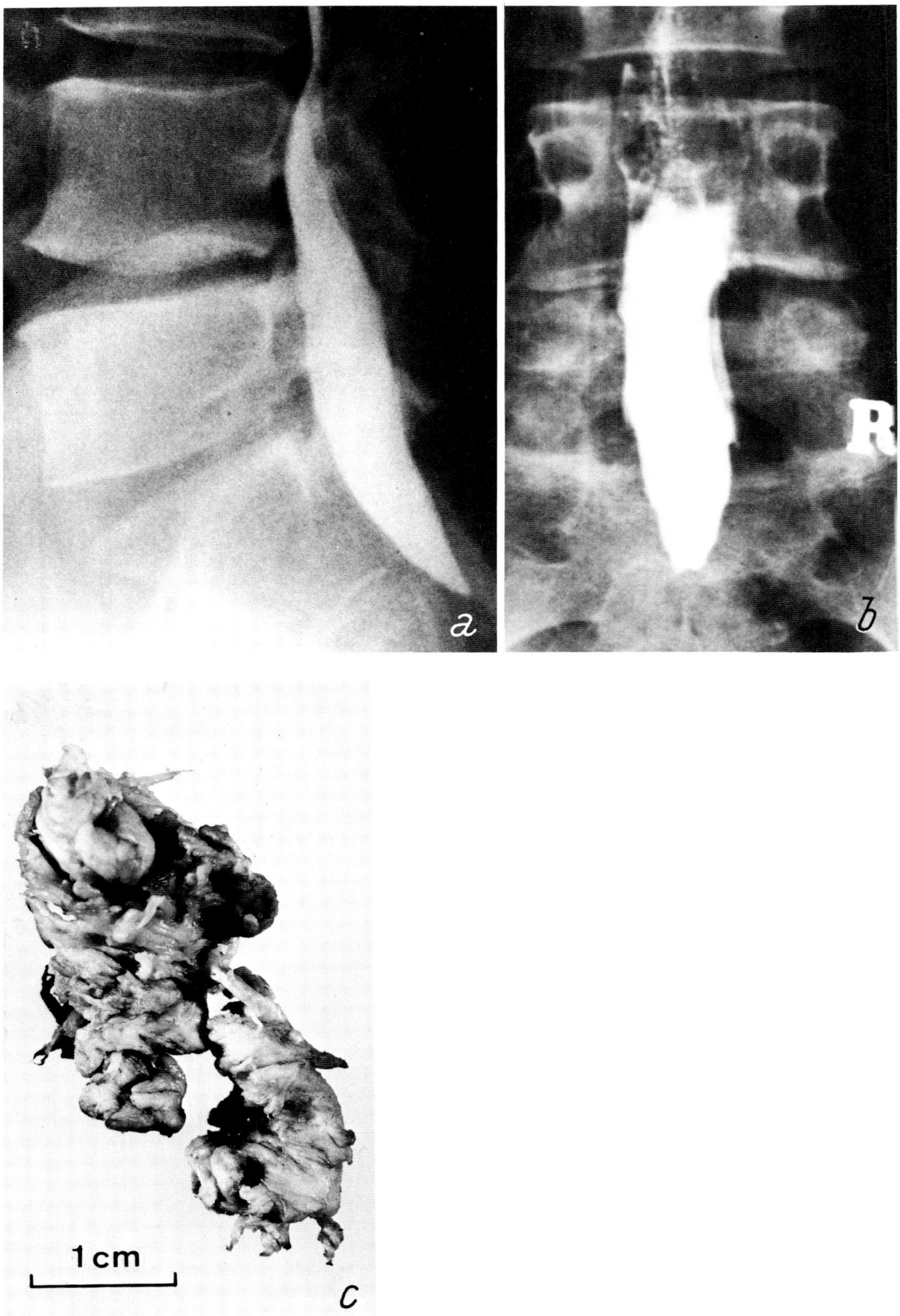

Figures 3.5

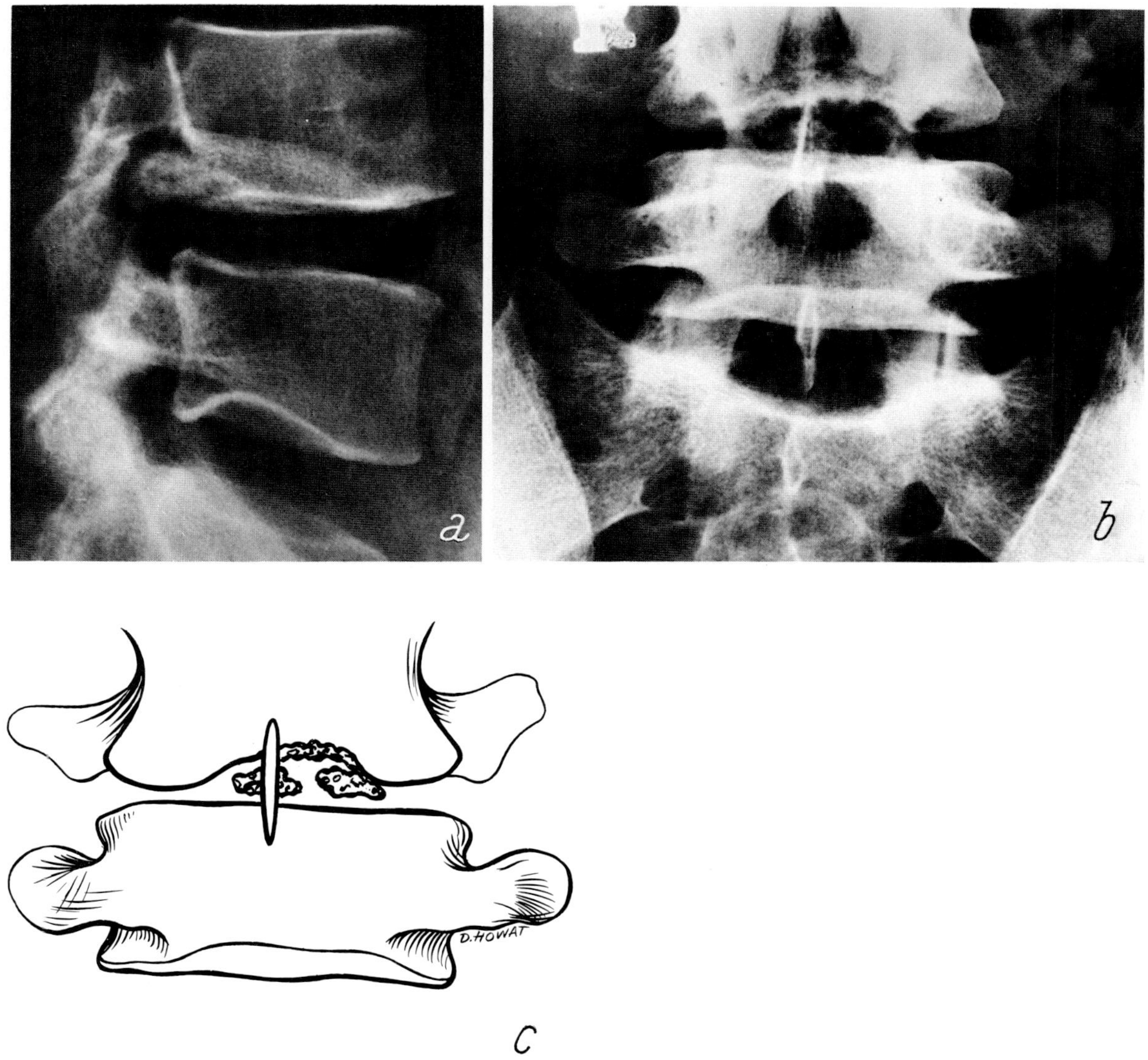

Figures 3.6 a–c. Intra-spongeous disc herniation with fracture of the vertebral body margin and sequestration of disc fragments into the spinal canal. **a** Lateral radiograph. A large bony fragment separated from the postero-inferior margin of the 4th lumbar vertebral body. It projects into the spinal canal. **b** Antero-posterior view. The L4/5 disc space is narrowed and tilted. There is a defect in the central zone of the vertebral end-plate area of the 4th vertebral body. Below this, two bony fragments can be identified. These findings were confirmed at operation. **c** Drawing of the position of these fragments. (Courtesy of Mr. K. Mills)

Figures 3.5 a–c. Sequestrated L4/5 disc with migrating fragments. **a** and **b** Lateral and antero-posterior radiographs of the lumbar myelogram of a woman, aged 39 years, who had severe right-sided sciatica. The deformation of the dural sac is consistent with the presence of migrating sequestrated disc fragments. It is best seen in the antero-posterior view. **c** The photograph shows the appearance of the sequestrated disc material which was removed at operation, orientated to correspond with its position *in vivo*

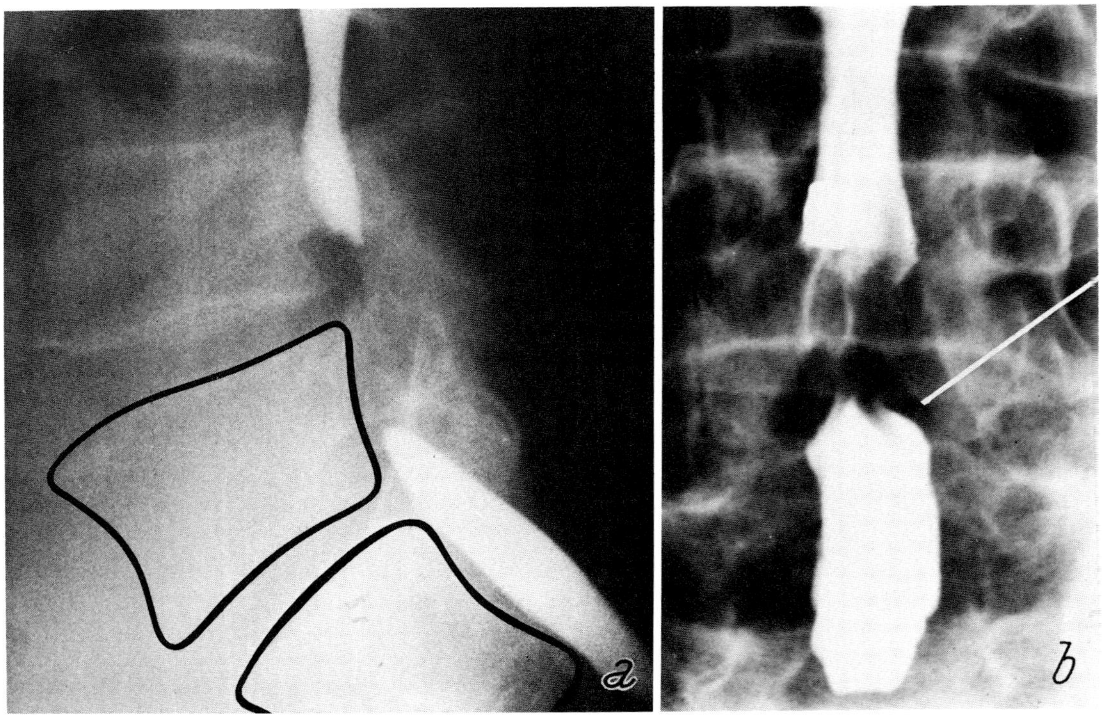

Figures 3.7 a and **b.** Disc prolapse into a congenital narrow lumbar canal. A 62 year-old man (weight 110 kg) lifted a bag of cement, flexing and rotating his spine. He developed back pain and severe bilateral leg pain; these symptoms were relieved following excision of a small disc fragment and bilateral nerve root canal decompression laminectomy. **a** Lateral and **b** antero-posterior radiographs of the lumbar myelogram, showing gross obstruction of the iofendylate column. Note the symmetrical indentation at the upper end of the lower iofendylate column in (b) (marker), suggesting the association of true spinal stenosis. (Courtesy of Mr. B. Davie)

finding related to physico-chemical changes in the disc (Nachemson, 1969). Calcified nuclear tissue may herniate; or calcification may occur in prolapsed tissue leading occasionally to erosion of the dural sac (Blikra, 1969).

A sequestrated fragment may migrate to another level from the disc of its origin, leaving a clearly defined oval defect in the posterior annulus (Figs. 3.4, 3.5). Sequestrated disc tissue may present posterior to the dural sac (Hooper, 1973).

Rarely, disc tissue may prolapse into the vertebral bodies and re-enter the spinal canal, pushing ahead of it a small fragment of vertebral end-plate bone and cartilage (Figs. 3.6 a–c). Knowledge of the varying relationships which prolapsed disc tissue may bear to the neural contents of the spinal canal is essential to the understanding of the varied clinical pictures which many present (Fig. 3.1).

In a sub-rhizal prolapse, the disc fragment lies anterior to the affected nerve root, and this usually causes severe pain with objective motor and sensory signs distally, in the part of the limb supplied by the compressed nerve root (Fig. 3.1).

Prolapses situated between the dural sac and the nerve root sheath–axillary prolapses (Fig. 3.1), or those lying on the outer side of the nerve root sheath–para-rhizal prolapses, may produce symptoms of severe sciatica without abnormal objective physical signs.

Centrally placed prolapses or a large migrating sequestrated fragment in the spinal canal may give rise to physical signs including bowel or bladder dysfunction and neurological signs or symptoms which vary from day to day in one leg or the other. In the lumbar region, cauda equina claudication with the onset of buttock or leg pains after walking short distances may also be found (Verbiest, 1955).

In considering this pathology, the clinician should always give some thought to the shape and size of the patient's spinal canal (Figs. 3.7a, b).

3.3. Clinical Features

The classic features of lumbar scoliosis, depression of one or more reflexes in the affected limb, muscle weakness or wasting, gross limitation of straight leg raising and the finding of areas of impaired sensation over affected dermatomes are all well known.

Perhaps less well appreciated is the reported observation that the pattern of pain radiation into the leg does not differ appreciably in L4/5 and L5/S1 disc lesions. In fact, clinical signs caused by lumbar disc prolapses may be misleading. Brown and Pont (1963) observed in a review of 570 patients that the ankle jerk may be absent in cases of prolapse at L4/5 or at L3/4. They found that sensory changes in the foot were more accurate aids in diagnosis than were changes in the leg as a whole.

In eliciting the physical sign of limitation of straight leg raising as an index of sciatic nerve irritation, attempts to lift the leg quickly from the extended position, with the patient supine, frequently evoke such a painful response that the straight leg can be raised only a few degrees from the examination couch. On the other hand, if the knee and hip are cautiously flexed and the knee then extended slowly with the examiner's thumb in the popliteal fossa exerting some pressure on the terminal branches of the sciatic nerve, and these manoeuvres are combined with dorsi-flexion of the foot, even minor degrees of sciatic nerve irritation can be appreciated. This is commonly known as Lasègue's sign. A patient with convincing sciatica is unable to sit upright with both knees fully extended. In the presence of sciatic irritation he will automatically flex the hip and knee on the affected side when attempting to adopt this posture. This has been described as the "bath-tub sign" by Pennybacker (1959).

Changes in the clinical features referred to above are all important in assessing the progress or failure of recovery of sciatica due to disc prolapse. *Of particular importance is the severity of pain, especially when it reaches a level which consistently disturbs sleep at night.*

3.4. Investigations

a) Plain X-Rays

These X-rays always provide essential information on the bony anatomy of the vertebral column, particularly in regard to the arrangement of laminae and the site of the lumbo-sacral junction. They are also important for the exclusion of other lesions such as spondylosis which may cause confusion in diagnosis. Usually they do not provide any useful guide to the site of prolapse, although there may be exceptions; for example, where there has been marked disc degeneration leading to disc space narrowing on one side, as viewed in the antero-posterior projection, the prolapse may be found on the wider side of the disc space.

b) Myelography

Widely diverging views are held on the proper role of myelography in the investigation of lumbar disc prolapses (Epstein, 1969; De Palma and Rothman, 1970). Hudgins (1970) states that its sensitivity is about 75% (25% false negative), and its specificity is roughly 90% (10% false positive). He claims that in patients with good neurological signs or a crossed Lasègue's sign, the predictive value of a normal myelogram is less than 50%.

Myelography probably should be used as a routine pre-operative investigation in cases of suspected disc prolapse. This investigation is invaluable in the investigation of any atypical case and is especially useful in cases of suspected disc prolapse where there is advanced spondylosis shown on the plain X-rays, or in the presence of bony anomalies such as lumbar sacralization. In these cases, myelography will aid in the diagnosis of associated spinal canal stenosis (Fig. 3.7), or it may help to identify the level of origin of a large disc sequestrum (Fig. 3.4). The introduction of water-soluble myelographic media such as metrizamide in recent years has greatly enhanced the accuracy of diagnosis.

c) C.S.F. Examination

Some authors recommend routine examination of the C.S.F. in the investigation of disc lesions, to test its dynamics and contents (Mercer and Duthie, 1964), while others with extensive experience in the management of spinal conditions rarely do so (Armstrong, 1965; Northfield and Osmond-Clarke, 1967).

The normal protein content of C.S.F. lies between 15 and 40 mg/ml (Bickerstaff, 1973). In lumbar disc prolapses rises up to 100 mg/ml may be seen, with figures as high as 1,000 mg/ml in the presence of marked spinal block. However, many would hold the view that changes in the protein content are rarely of practical use in diagnosis. Johnson (1972) discusses the mechanisms of absorption of C.S.F. and states: "It appears that a subsidiary pathway is via the large spinal veins around the emerging nerve roots." Abnormalities of serum albumin may be found in collagen diseases, those changes being reflected in the C.S.F. with the appearance of abnormal albumins, "para-albumins", in it. With advances in the understanding of C.S.F. physiology, it is logical that surgeons should make greater use of more recent biochemical techniques of analysis of this fluid, especially in some of the non-prolapsing varieties of disc lesions discussed in this chapter. Whenever myelography is undertaken, a sample of C.S.F. should be obtained for cytological and chemical testing.

d) Epidurography

The injection of contrast media into the epidural space has been advocated for the demonstration of small disc prolapses. This has been used in assessing non-operative methods of treatment. The poor quality of published illustrations indicates that there are grave limitations to the use of this investigation (Mathews, 1972).

e) Discography

This investigation finds restricted use in the diagnosis of disc prolapses. In atypical cases of severe sciatica with minimal abnormal physical signs and normal myelographic findings, a discogram may help to clarify the diagnosis (Wilson and McCarty, 1969).

f) Intra-Osseous Spinal Venography

Intra-osseous spinal venography has not been used widely in the English-speaking world. German observers claim that when it is used with tomography it is just as reliable as myelography in the diagnosis of lumbar disc protrusion and prolapse. The special value of this procedure is noted in acute cases of massive midline prolapses involving the cauda equina (Vogelsang, 1970).

g) Electrodiagnostic Tests

Technical and interpretative difficulties in the use of electromyography have been described by Simpson (1972). More recently, Japanese workers have developed new methods using fine electrodes for nerve root stimulation in the lumbar region, recording evoked potentials with promising results in the identification of nerve root irritation of differing types (Matsuda *et al.,* 1979).

3.5. Indications for Surgical Treatment

Absolute indications for operations are:

a) Major neurological deficits. Cases of acute cauda equina compressions due to massive disc sequestration or the prolapse of a small fragment of disc tissue into an abnormally small lumbar spinal canal (spinal canal stenosis) may call for spinal canal decompression involving, if necessary, trans-dural excision of disc fragments (Fig. 3.22).

b) Persistent or recurrent pain, with or without abnormal physical signs, in the legs. This is the most common indication for surgery after an adequate trial of conservative treatment.

c) Progressive neurological deficit, such as paraparesis or foot drop may strengthen indications for operative intervention.

d) Persistent spinal deformity, such as lumbar scoliosis or marked lumbar flexion deformity may be found in certain cases of lumbar disc prolapse or spinal tumour.

3.6. Treatment for Lumbar Disc Prolapses

a) Discussion

i) Surgery

In the lumbar region, a limited unilateral inter-laminar approach may suffice for the removal of discrete small rubbery disc prolapses, but it can only be recommended in young people. Where disc sequestration has occurred or in cases where rather desiccated disc tissue is found, more extensive intra-disc space curettage should be carried out and at the same time a careful bilateral nerve root canal decompression performed. Such a procedure performed at the time of laminectomy for disc fragment excision, reduces the late problems of recurrent nerve root irritation that may arise from nerve root canal stenosis on one or both sides, resulting from secondary disc space narrowing. In these circumstances, there is little justification for extending the operation to include posterior spinal fusion (Spurling, 1949). Indeed, the failure rate is high, graft resorption being very common when inter-laminar fusion has been attempted after exploration of the spinal canal. In addition, late spinal canal stenosis may lead to recurrent symptoms which are difficult to manage. Postero-lateral inter-transverse fusion is more reliable in these circumstances if spinal fusion seems warranted because of gross vertebral instability (Watkins, 1959).

From the point of view of the relief of sciatic pain, recent long term reviews indicate that "laminectomy" alone will produce good results (Jackson, 1971; Naylor, 1974), variations in the actual technique of laminectomy exerting little effect on the outcome.

Where most of the disc remnants are removed in some cases of massive disc sequestration, gross vertebral instability can occur. Posterior interbody spinal fusion performed through the spinal canal, either by the technique described by Cloward (1952) or that recommended by Wiltberger and Abbott (1958), offers a solution to a difficult problem (Fig. 3.3d).

Numerous reviews analyzing the results of various forms of treatment for disc prolapse and spondylosis in the lumbar region are available. Basically it is impossible to compare series published by different authors for two reasons: firstly, because indications for operation vary so widely; secondly, because the operative techniques and pathological findings described are also variable.

Authors everywhere agree on a number of matters:

- compensation patients always respond more slowly to treatment than do private patients;
- the results of simple disc fragment excision for frank disc prolapse are good in more than 80% of cases;
- prolonged paralysis before operation will not remit completely following it; and
- paralysis seen for the first time after operation usually remits rapidly and completely.

ii) Chymopapain

Intra-discal injection of chymopapain (Discase), a proteolytic enzyme, was introduced into clinical practice in 1963 for the treatment of disc prolapse (Smith and

Brown, 1967). Clinical diagnosis is confirmed by discography, following which the enzyme preparation is injected through the discogram needle.

Biochemists have been sceptical of its use because of the difficulty of standardization of the enzyme preparations and the potential for damage of tissues other than nucleus pulposus, should it escape from the intervertebral disc space (Lowther, 1972). Chymopapain nonetheless found its way into quite wide use especially in some parts of the U.S.A. and Canada. The difficulties in assessing its efficacy in treatment have been highlighted by MacNab (1973), because there is no general agreement on clinical syndromes presented by a disc herniation. He quotes the following results assembled from a nationwide review undertaken by Lyman Smith in 1972: in 2,557 patients there was marked improvement in 1,769 (70%), slight improvement in 340 (13%) and no improvement in 448 cases (17%).

b) Technique

i) Pre-Operative Preparation

Full blood examination, including blood grouping and sedimentation rate should be performed. It is wise to insert an intravenous infusion in all patients before operation for disc disorders, though blood transfusion is rarely indicated.

X-rays of the patient's spine should always be available in the operating theatre.

The use of prophylactic antibiotic chemotherapy may be indicated if there has been an antecedent history of serious infection, including previous wound infections.

ii) Anaesthesia

General anaesthesia with muscular relaxation and mechanical ventilation is most commonly employed. Cardiac monitoring is recommended in older patients or whenever it is known that the patient has particular cardiac problems.

iii) Positioning

Of all the factors which may be critical to the success of this operation, none is more important than the position in which the patient is placed before operation commences. A variety of suitable postures is shown in the following illustrations (Figs. 3.8–3.11).

Prone Position

The most versatile and easily managed is the *prone position.* A supporting sponge rubber U-piece is simple to construct and inexpensive. The right arm is shown dependent and supported on a well-padded arm rest which is suspended below the level of the table. Ulnar neuritis may occur unless the arm is carefully postured in this way. The left arm may rest by the patient's side. The table is angled in the centre. The surgeon's assistant and other observers will have unobstructed views of procedures throughout the course of the operation. The entire range of surgical manoeuvres that may be required for the execution of even the most complex operation, including trans-dural excision of prolapsed disc tissue, can be

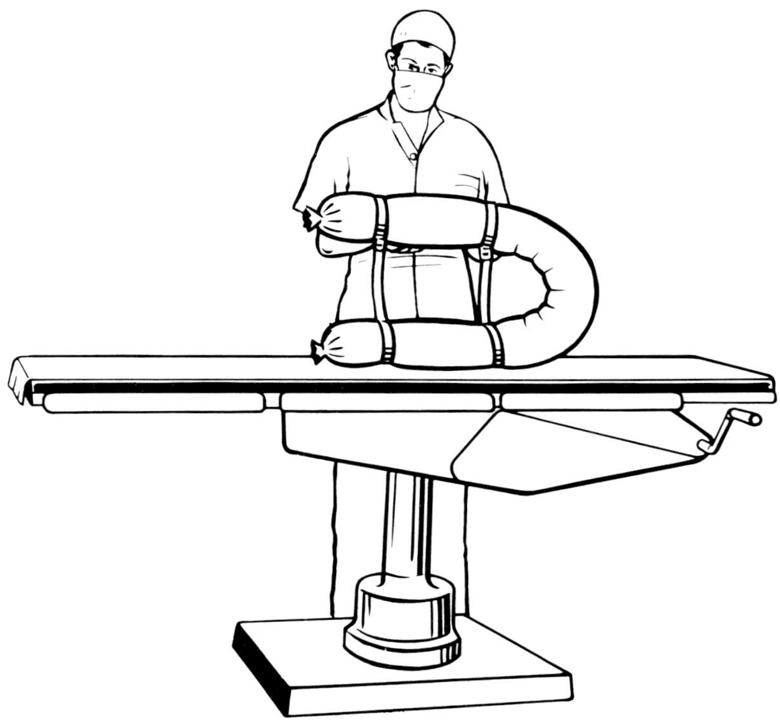

Figure 3.8. A drawing illustrating a simple supporting sponge rubber "U"-piece

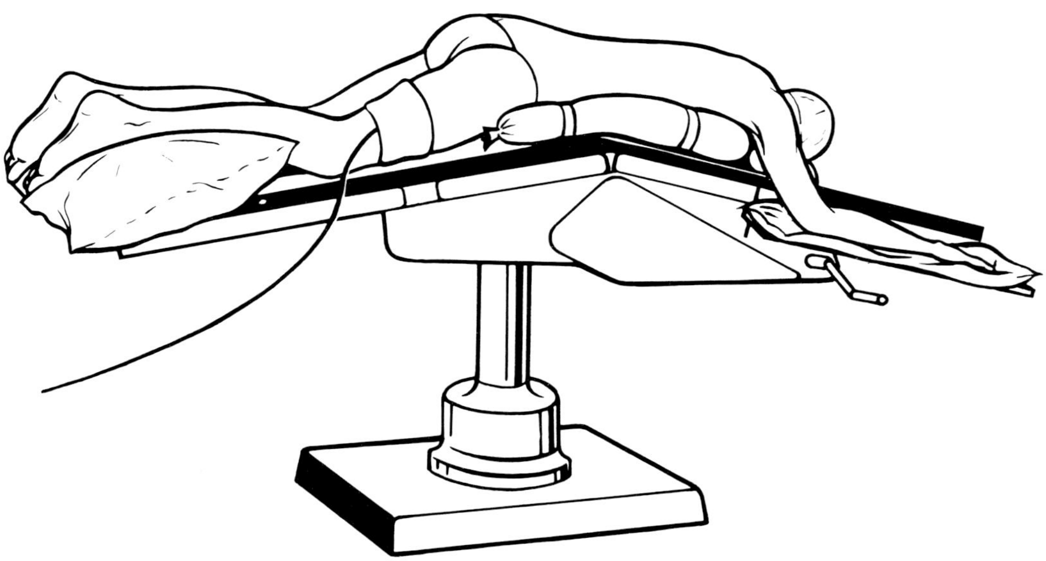

Figure 3.9. The posturing of the patient on this "U"-piece. The right arm is shown dependent and supported on a well-padded arm rest which is suspended below the level of the table. Ulnar neuritis may occur unless the arm is carefully postured in this way. The left arm may rest by the patient's side. The table is angled in the centre

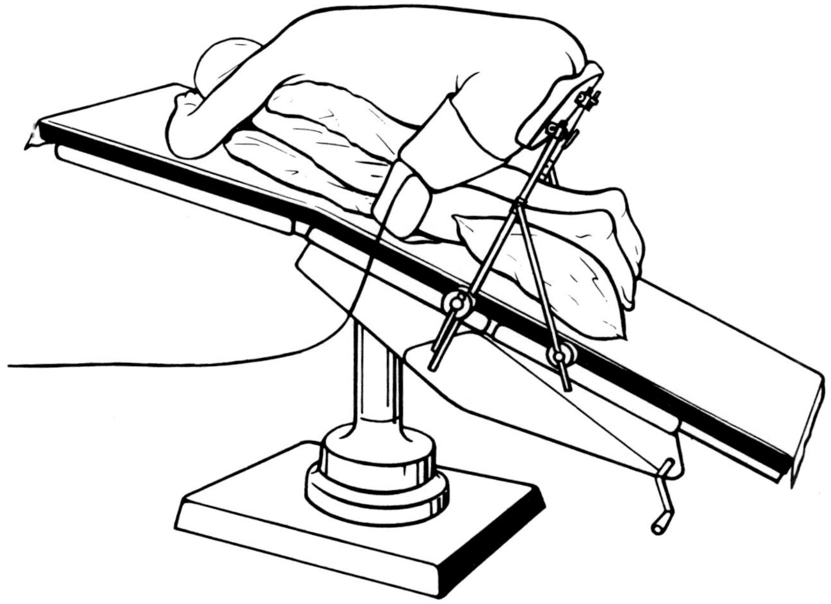

Figure 3.10. A drawing depicting the jack-knife or kneeling position. A simple frame is used to support the buttocks

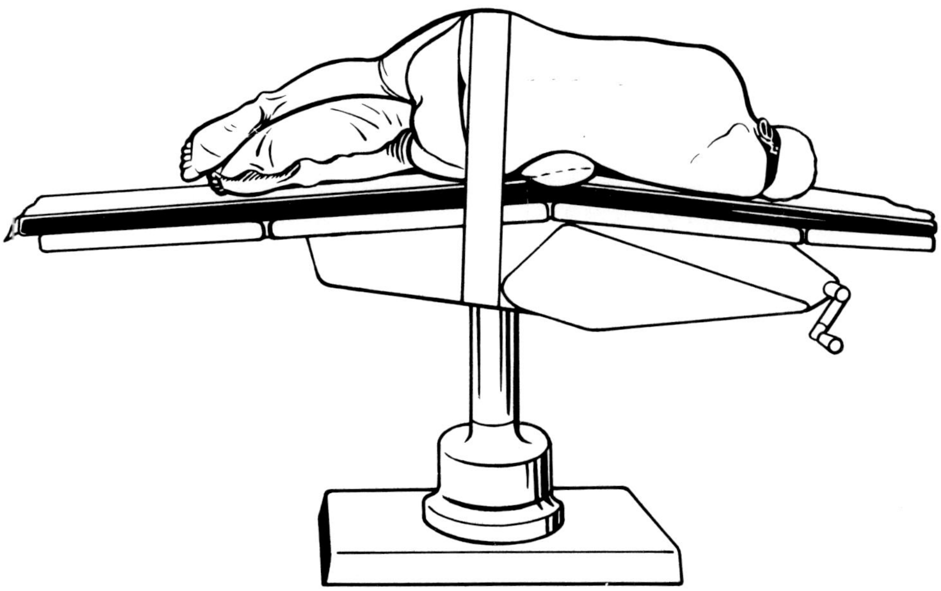

Figure 3.11. The lateral position. The use of this position can be recommended in special circumstances, for example, when the patient is extremely obese or when there are special chest problems which may complicate anaesthesia. Note the pillow between the patient's legs, the restraining strap crossing the iliac crest, the sandbag placed above the dependent iliac crest. The table is angled in the centre. There are objections to the routine use of this position: 1. the assistant surgeon is rarely comfortable and has a restricted view of the operative field; 2. lighting of the wound area may be difficult; 3. haemorrhage control is often more difficult to obtain, as is access to the nerve root canal on the dependent side of the spine

accomplished in comfort and without undue constraints on the duration of the operation.

Jack-Knife or Kneeling Position

In this position, with the use of a simple frame to support the buttocks, excellent operating conditions are provided. Alternatively, the patient may be placed in this position with pillows under the chest so that the abdomen is unsupported. A pillow is placed under the patient's feet and a restraining strap across the legs–though venous obstruction in the lower limbs is then likely to occur. The table is angled. The major objections to the use of this particular posture revolve around the difficulties of setting the patient in position and of dealing with emergencies, which may require the patient to be turned rapidly into a supine position. Particular attention should be paid to the ulnar nerves in this position.

Lateral Position

The use of this position can be recommended in special circumstances, for example, when the patient is extremely obese or when there are special chest problems which may complicate anaesthesia. A pillow should be placed between the patient's legs, a restraining strap crossing the iliac crest, and a sandbag placed above the dependent iliac crest. The table is angled in the centre. There are objections to the routine use of this position: (i) the assistant surgeon is rarely comfortable and has a restricted view of the operation field; (ii) lighting of the wound area may be difficult; (iii) haemorrhage control is often more difficult to obtain as is access to the nerve root canal on the dependent side of the spine.

iv) Instruments (Figs. 3.12, 3.13)

The recommended essential special instruments and disposable supplies are listed below:

1. Self-retaining retractors.
2. Fine sucker.
3. Bayonet forceps.
4. Long-handled carrier for size 11 or 15 blade scalpel.
5. Watson-Cheyne probe.
6. Nerve root retractor, such as a Scaglietti probe (10 inches–25 cm–long).
7. A range of bone rongeurs.
8. A range of pituitary-type rongeurs, straight, angled outwards at 45° and at 90° with cutting tips of varying dimensions.
9. Hammer.
10. Fine osteotomes and chisels.
11. Ring curettes.
12. 6/0 suture material on fine cutting needles with a fine needle holder.
13. Neurosurgical patties and haemostatic gauze or sponge materials.
14. Bone wax.
15. Bi-polar coagulator.

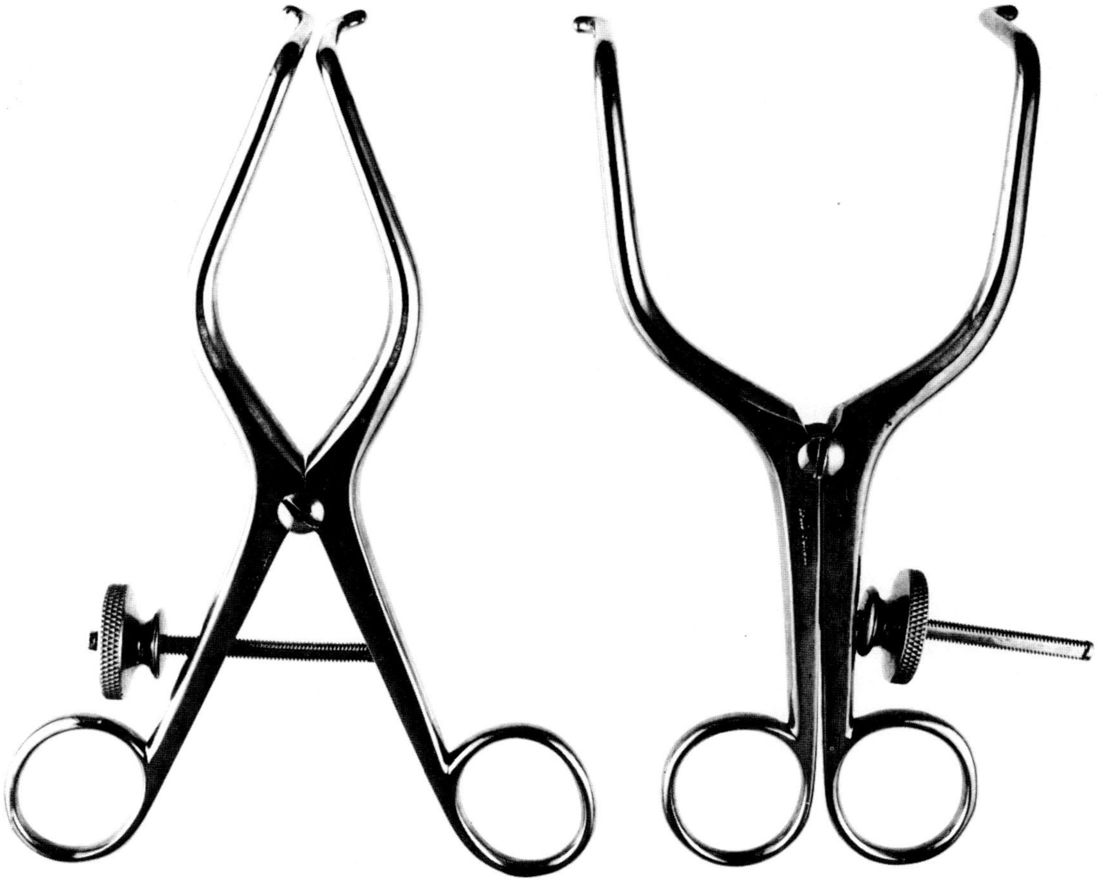

Figure 3.12. A photograph showing the modified Gelpi retractors, which are recommended for use in almost any situation where the spinal canal is to be explored

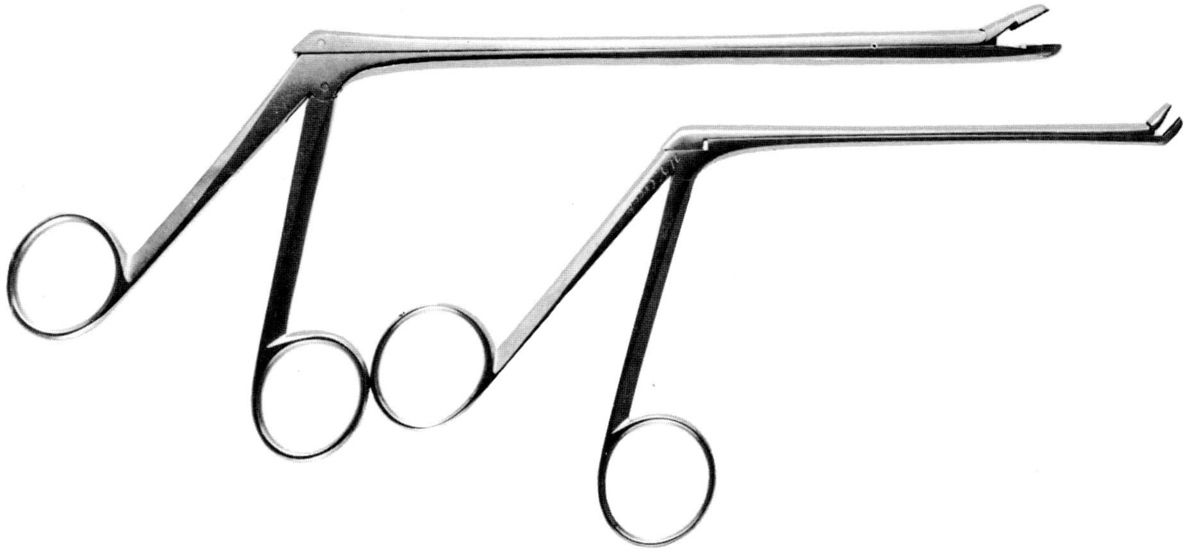

Figure 3.13. A photograph of straight and angled pituitary rongeurs which should be available in various shaft lengths and cup sizes for use in the surgery of disc prolapses

v) Incision

Before the skin incision is made the surgeon should once again inspect the patient's X-rays, paying attention to vertebral anomalies, such as spina bifida occulta and sacralization and noting certain lesions such as spondylolisthesis or isolated disc resorption. The level of the planned exposure of the spine should be noted.

Radiographs of the lumbar spine taken in the operating theatre are often of poor quality and cannot, therefore, be relied upon to identify a particular spinal level.

The skin incision is made in the mid-line or slightly to the right or left of the spinous processes, extending longitudinally a short distance above and below the vertebral interspace to be explored. It is deepened at once through the subcutaneous fat layer to the level of the lumbo-dorsal fascia. In extremely obese patients the depth of the subcutaneous fat layer between the skin and the lumbo-dorsal aponeurosis over the lumbo-sacral area may be 12 cm or more. In such cases this fatty tissue should be carefully handled, avoiding excessive burning with the coagulating diathermy (see "Wound Closure", p. 122).

vi) Separation of Spinal Muscles

An incision is made on one side of the tip of a spinous process, using the cutting current diathermy, passed through a suitable blade-shaped end. The incision continues proximally and distally immediately adjacent to the side of the spinous process *parallel to the adjacent interspinous ligament* and then to the side of the next related spinous process. Bleeding occurs at this stage from posterior branches of the lumbar arteries related to the middle of the side of each spinous process. The muscle mass may be retracted with a closed dissecting forcep placed into the depth of the space, so that the diathermy blade may cut the musculo-tendinous attachments from the inferior surfaces of the spinous processes and from the inter-spinous ligaments near their bases. Throughout this procedure the smoke generated by the diathermy cutting tip may be evacuated with the sucker.

The muscle mass is next separated from the outer surface of each lamina using an appropriate "elevator", such as the Cobb, taking care to preserve the periosteum of the laminae.

Following the use of the muscle elevator which raises the paraspinal muscles laterally to the level of the *apophyseal joint capsules, which should be carefully preserved,* further bleeding may be encountered from posterior branches of the lumbar arteries and veins in the area. This bleeding is readily controlled following the insertion of cotton Raytec swabs (bearing X-ray markers) packed into the depths of the wound along its length (Figs. 3.14–3.16a, b).

The same approach is then repeated on the opposite side of the spinous processes, preserving the interspinous ligaments until the paraspinal muscle mass has been similarly separated from the roof of the spinal canal. Cotton Raytec swabs are again inserted and the self-retaining retractors of the surgeon's choice then prepared for insertion. Some surgeons favour muscle stripping on one side of the spine only (Finneson, 1973).

Unless the technique described is followed carefully, considerable blood loss may occur, even during this preliminary stage of the approach to the disc prolapse.

The cotton Raytec swabs are removed from the lower end of the wound on either side of the S1 spinous process. Hand-held retractors expose the back of the

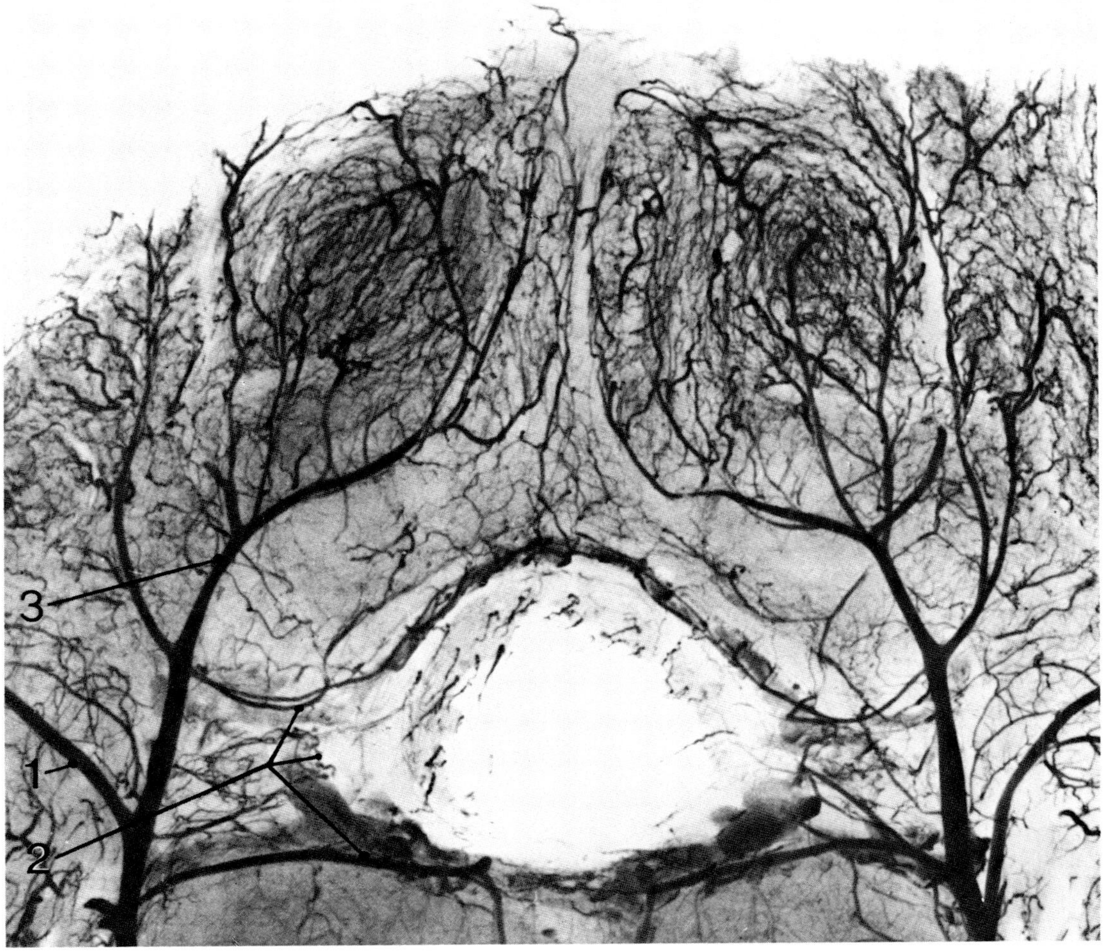

Figure 3.14. A thin transverse section to show details of the arterial distribution in relation to the spinal canal, the vertebral body in front and the lamina and spinous process behind. At the level of the intervertebral foramen, note: **1** the anterior abdominal wall branches; **2** the intermediate or spinal canal branches; and **3** posterior to the intervertebral foramen, the posterior branches in relation to the lamina and spinous process

sacrum allowing the first self-retaining retractor to be inserted and fixed in place. This procedure is repeated at the upper end of the wound and the second self-retaining retractor inserted.

When the self-retaining retractors have been positioned, the surgeon should take note of the time of their application. These instruments obstruct the circulation in the separated paraspinal muscles. At the end of an hour they should be removed for about five minutes to prevent muscle necrosis. During the rest period the wound should be washed out with hydrogen peroxide solution or Ringer's solution.

At this stage, cotton Raytec swabs are again packed firmly along one of the paraspinal gutters while attention is focussed on the opposite side to identify the lumbo-sacral junction. Soft-tissue remnants of muscle fibres and fat are then removed from the interspace which is to be opened. This cleaning-up process can be

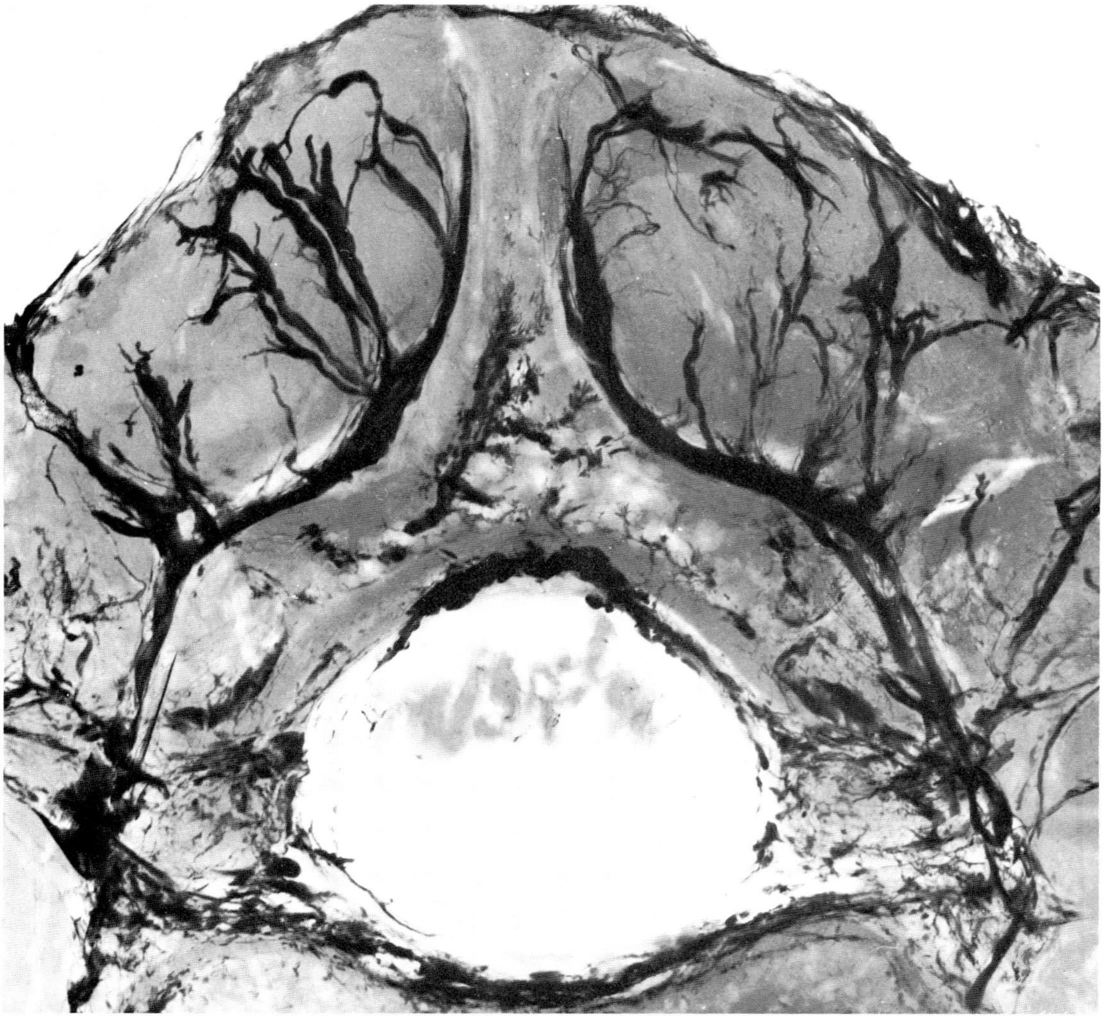

Figure 3.15. A radiograph of a transverse section of a lumbar vertebra from an adult to show the relations of the main stems of the lumbar veins (posterior external vertebral venous plexus) to the spinous process and lamina. [Reproduced by courtesy of J. B. Lippincott & Company from: Clinical Orthopaedics and Related Research, No. 115 (1976)]

Figures 3.16 a and **b.** A photograph of the posterior aspect of the upper lumbar spine of an adult prepared by the Spalteholz method, following injection of the lumbar aorta. The specimen is slightly tilted to the right side to provide a clear view of the posterior spinal branches of three adjacent lumbar arteries. An explanatory diagram is shown alongside, in which the main course of each lumbar artery across the back of the lamina and up the middle of the spinous process is shown with its ascending and descending vertical muscular branches and the arcuate systems formed around the facet joints

Figure 3.17. A radiograph of a thin sagittal section of the lumbar spine, showing the relations of the posterior branches of two lumbar arteries as they course backward behind the intervertebral foramina. These arteries are constant lateral relations of the pars interarticularis of each lamina. In the intervertebral foramen shown on the left, the anterior and posterior spinal canal branches of the lumbar artery can be seen, separated by a clear band, this area being occupied by the nerve root at that level. Note also the branches which encircle the facet joint system and supply it. [Reproduced by courtesy of J. B. Lippincott & Company from: Clinical Orthopaedics and Related Research, No. 115 (1976)]

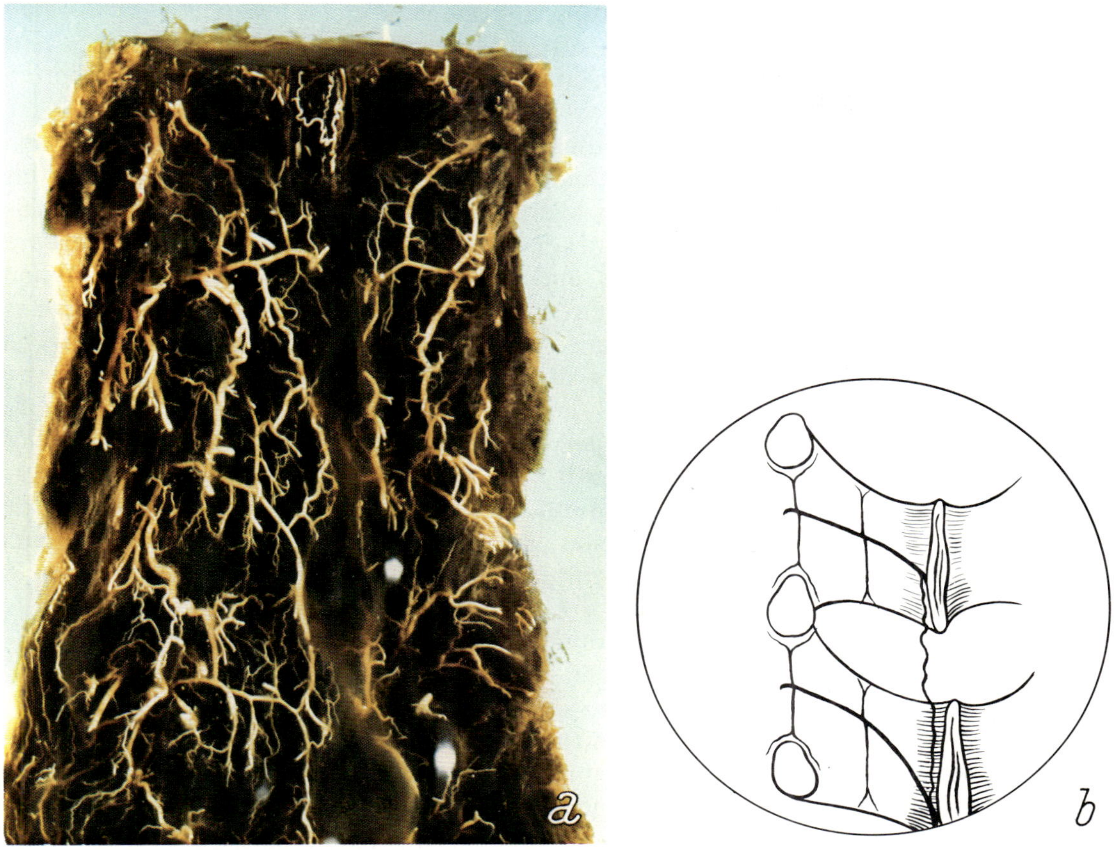

Figures 3.16

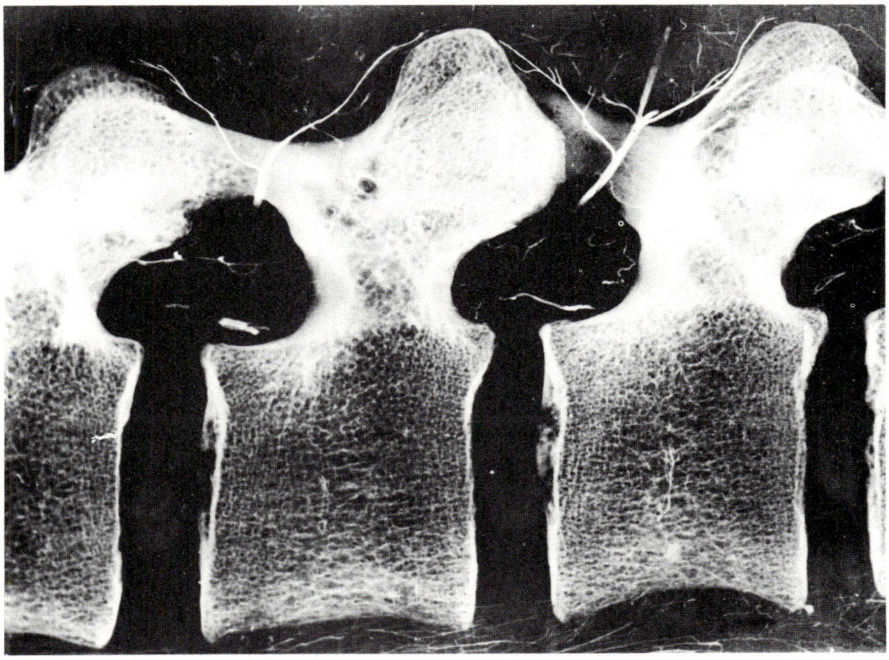

Figure 3.17

accomplished rapidly and neatly by using a straight pituitary rongeur with a 4 mm cup, taking off first the muscle remnants from the interspinous ligament and adjacent lamina and then all the soft tissues from the posterior surface of the ligamentum flavum.

Bleeding is not a problem during these manoeuvres at the lumbo-sacral junction until the extra-synovial fat pad of the apophyseal joint is removed. On avulsing this fat pad, quite brisk arterial and venous haemorrhage will occur. The bleeding vessels are readily identified by the use of a sucker and cotton Raytec swab. The vessels are picked up with the Bayonet forceps and coagulated with the diathermy. When exposure at the L4/5 interspace is required following the initial clearing procedure as described above, the pars interarticularis of the fifth lumbar lamina is exposed. The sucker tip may be used as a dissector at this stage, sucking up remnants of fatty tissue. *The main stem of the posterior branch of the lumbar artery is found constantly at the middle of the outer edge of the pars interarticularis.* From it, arcuate branches pass upwards and downwards towards the capsules of the apophyseal joints (Figs. 3.16a, b, 3.17). Haemorrhage points are easily identified, though care must be taken not to diathermy the main stem far anterior to the anterior margin of the pars interarticularis. Damage to entrant neural arteries at the intervertebral foramen is thereby avoided.

The main stem of the posterior branch of each lumbar artery is accompanied by the corresponding and somewhat larger vein (Crock and Yoshizawa, 1977).

In cases where exposure of both sides of the interspace may be required, the detailed clearing process just described is completed on the opposite side. At this stage, it will be noted that there are some capsular fibres extending medially on to the ligamentum flavum for some distance at its upper margin where it passes beneath

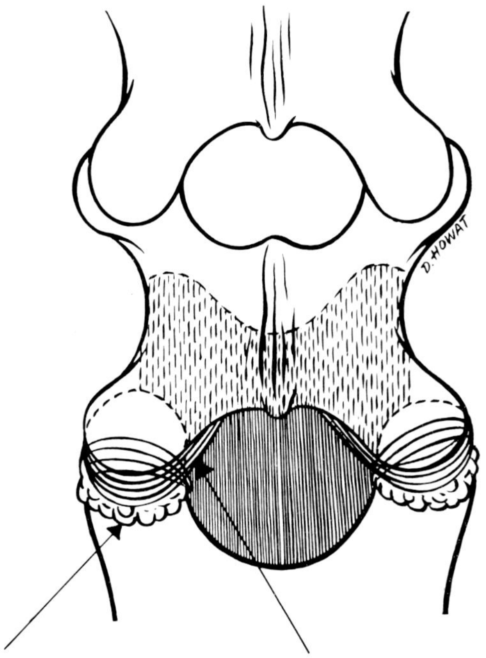

Figure 3.18. A drawing depicting the relations of the ligamentum flavum. The extra-synovial fat pads are shown in exaggerated form. Note the extension of capsular fibres onto the posterior surface of the ligamentum flavum

the inferior margin of the superior lamina of the interspace (Fig. 3.18). These fibres should be removed with a straight pituitary rongeur before opening the ligamentum flavum. Portions of the inferior surface of the superior lamina at the interspace may then need to be excised (using an outward-angled rongeur) and in some cases the interspinous ligament may be removed together with a portion of the inferior surface of the spinous process at the upper level of the interspace (Fig. 3.19). Some surgeons favour the use of chisels or gouges for this particular manoeuvre. Bone wax may be applied to the cut surface of the cancellous bone to control bleeding.

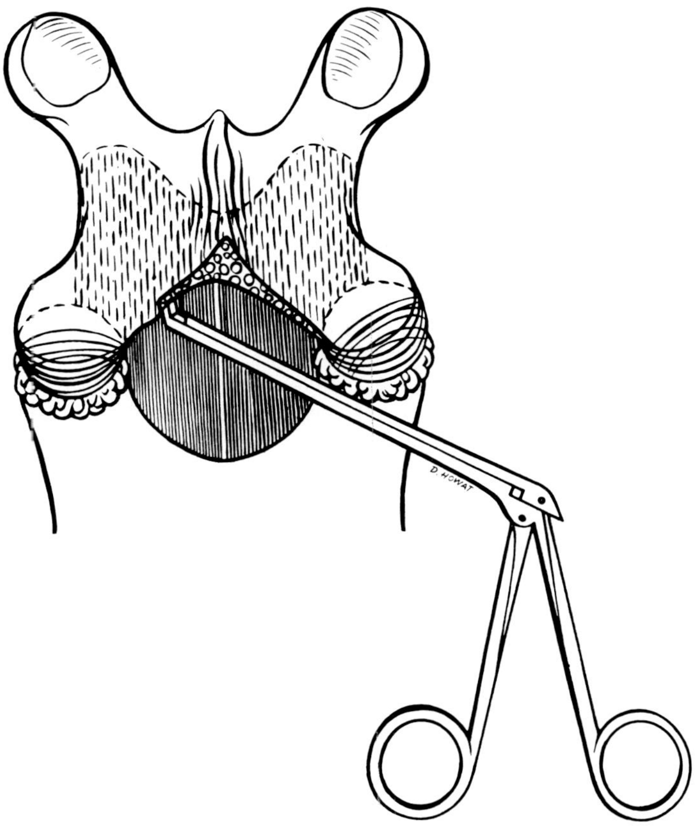

Figure 3.19. A drawing showing the method of removal of portions of the inferior surface of the superior lamina at the interspace, using an outward-angled rongeur. In some cases the interspinous ligament may be removed together with a portion of the inferior surface of the spinous process at the upper level of the interspace

vii) Opening of Spinal Canal

The ligamentum flavum should then be incised vertically in the mid-line using either a No. 11 or 15 blade scalpel. The cut edge of the ligamentum flavum is picked up with a fine-toothed forceps and the incision deepened until either epidural fat or the dura itself is exposed.

The blunt end of the Watson-Cheyne dissector may then be used to widen the opening into the spinal canal. Through the vertical slit in the ligamentum flavum thus created, a small moistened cotton patty is inserted between the ligamentum flavum and the epidural fat, using the curved end of the Watson-Cheyne dissector. The ligamentum flavum is then cut in a lateral direction, first at the lower edge of the interspace, until a flap is raised and turned out laterally.

Even at this early stage of the opening of the spinal canal, the presence of a large prolapse can be suspected when difficulty is experienced during the insertion of the patty or patties, particularly when efforts are made to push them further laterally under the ligamentum flavum as the flap is enlarged.

When the ligamentum flavum has been turned laterally as a flap to the level of the apophyseal joint, a fourth incision is then most commonly made in it, again in a vertical direction to excise the flap.

Following this inital opening into the spinal canal proper, the surgeon must then identify certain landmarks. The Watson-Cheyne probe is invaluable for this purpose. Either the blunt or curved end may be inserted depending on the size of the protrusion at the affected level. If the prolapse is small, then the blunt end may be inserted laterally so that the pedicle on the inferior side of the intervertebral disc space may be palpated. The regional nerve root is then palpated. Moving upwards, the posterior surface of the disc may be felt and the disposition of a prolapse assessed.

viii) Extending Exposure

Wider exposure may be required and this is usually most easily achieved with a 45° outward-angled rongeur. Assuming, for example, that it is necessary to remove more of the outer edge of the ligamentum flavum, then the sucker with a moistened patty on its tip may be used to retract the dura and nerve roots towards the mid-line, while the rongeur is inserted beneath the edge of the ligamentum flavum under direct vision. Depending on the size of the prolapse, it may or may not be possible to insert the angled rongeur. If attempts are made to force the foot-plate of the rongeur between the ligamentum flavum and the nerve root which is being pressed backwards by a large disc prolapse, the root may be bruised or crushed. On occasions, even a thin rongeur cannot be inserted. The interspace will need to be enlarged, either superiorly or inferiorly or in both directions, until sufficient space has been created to allow identification of the nerve root as it traverses the interspace.

When the prolapse is large and sub-rhizal at the L5/S1 level, for example, it may be necessary to enlarge the interspace by removal of part of the superior border of the lamina of S1, commencing initially in the mid-line and passing laterally, and to perform a decompression of the S1 nerve root canal by removing the medial portion of the S1 facet flush with the inner margin of the S1 pedicle. In the operation of nerve root canal decompression, the apex of the facet also needs to be removed (see pp. 23–27).

ix) Management of Venous Haemorrhage

During the more complicated manoeuvres of this type, haemorrhage from the internal vertebral venous plexus surrounding the nerve root and lateral to it may occur. This haemorrhage is usually not troublesome when the patient is in the prone position. On occasions, however, the internal vertebral venous plexus may be distended and brisk venous haemorrhage may occur following damage to some of the radicular branches of this system of veins. The detailed anatomy of the anterior internal vertebral venous plexus in the lumbar region is described on p. 17. Venous haemorrhage is always readily controlled with the gentle use of a patty and sucker as illustrated in Fig. 3.20. Occasionally, bleeding from one of the large venous radicles can be troublesome and it may be necessary to identify this using the sucker and a patty. The bleeding points are grasped with the bayonet forceps and coagulated with low-voltage or bipolar coagulating currents.

At other times, bleeding from several points of the plexiform system of veins can be controlled by light packing with a haemostatic substance held in place with a moistened patty.

Bleeding should be minimal, and good exposure of the field obtained before any attempt is made to retract the nerve root for the final exposure of prolapsed disc material.

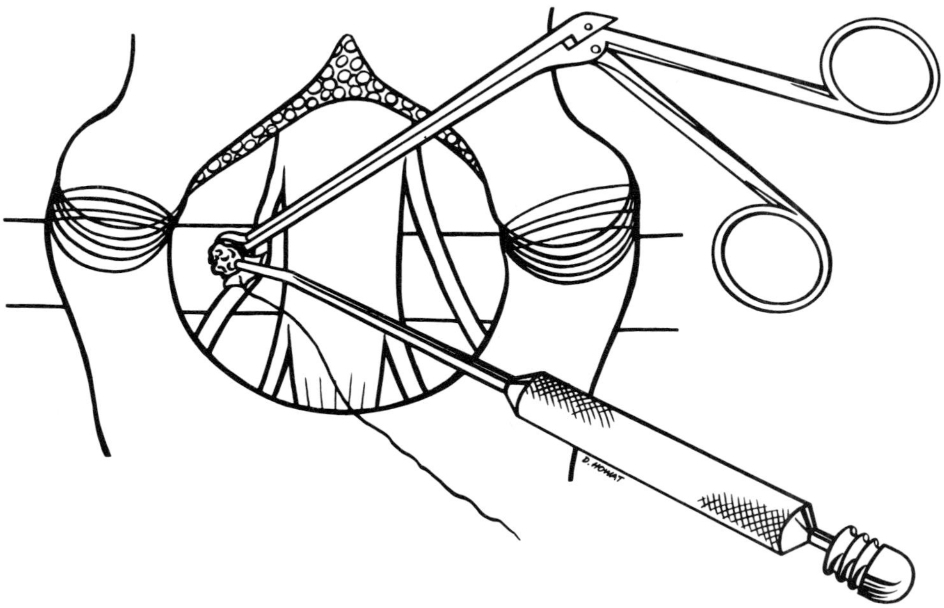

Figure 3.20. A drawing depicting the disposition of the sucker and patty and straight pituitary rongeur at the time of removal of a fragment of prolapsed tissue

x) Excision of Disc Tissue

For the sake of clarity and brevity, special points of technique will be described in relation to individual types of disc prolapse.

Small Sub-Rhizal Prolapse

Partial excision of the ligamentum flavum on one side will afford satisfactory access to the canal. Initially, identification of the landmarks of pedicle, disc and affected nerve root is made using the sucker and patty as a medial retractor and the blunt end of the Watson-Cheyne dissector in the lateral part of the canal.

Blunt dissection will separate the epidural fat, and the nerve root can usually be easily retracted medially. The discrete rounded prolapse with intact annular fibres is then outlined and a suitable root retractor inserted. The surgeon may use the sucker with a moist patty on its tip as a retractor laterally in the interspace while the assistant holds the nerve root medially. In a dry field it should then be possible to incise the annular fibres over the prolapse in a cruciate fashion using a No. 11 or 15 blade scalpel. The prolapsed tissue then begins to emerge spontaneously and it may be picked out with a straight pituitary rongeur of appropriate dimension varying from 1 to 4 mm bite.

Only a small volume of disc tissue can be removed in such cases and curettage of the interspace is not recommended.

Large Sub-Rhizal Prolapse

In such cases, adequate exposure on the side of the prolapse is essential. Technical details for the enlargement both superiorly and inferiorly have been outlined above. Identification of the affected root may be a problem, because in such circumstances the root is often flattened and its lateral margin not easily identified, being of the

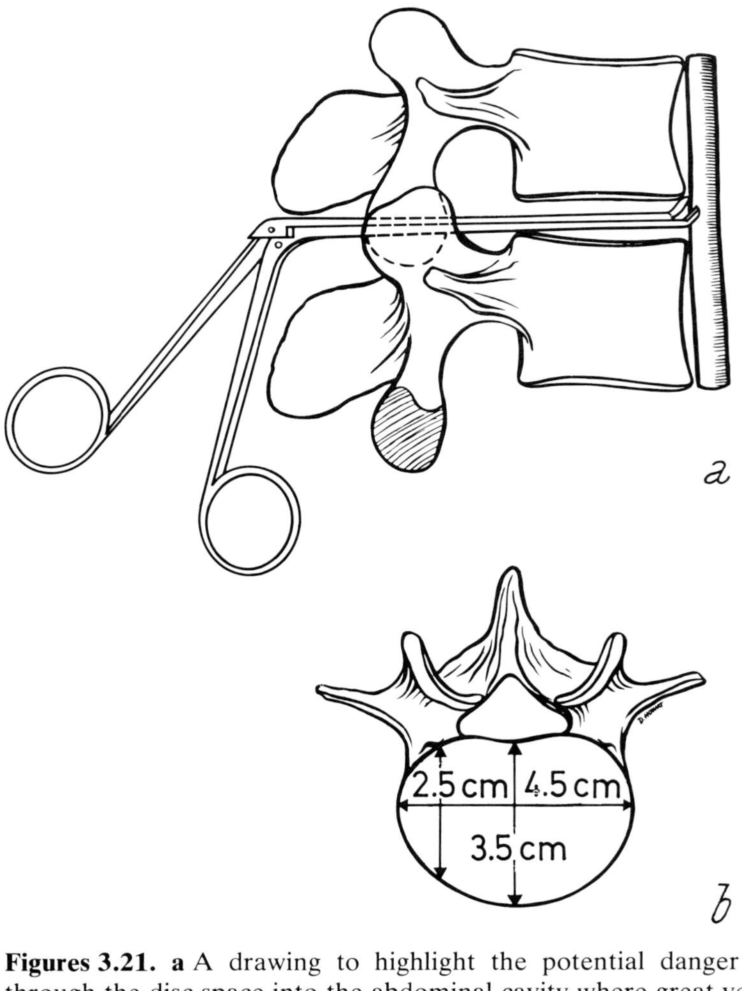

Figures 3.21. **a** A drawing to highlight the potential danger of penetration of a rongeur through the disc space into the abdominal cavity where great vessels or other intra-abdominal structures may be injured. **b** A drawing to illustrate the dimensions of a lumbar vertebral body in an adult of average size

same colour as the disc prolapse beneath it. Use of an operating loop may be helpful, as it is essential under such circumstances to identify the nerve root sleeve at its junction with the dura above or to identify the main stem of the nerve root at the level of the inferior pedicle. By either method, with the use of an appropriate nerve root dissector, the outer edge of the nerve root can be identified and retracted medially. Very fine straight and curved pituitary rongeurs will be required in such a case to remove the first of the fragments of prolapsed tissue, possibly through a minute incision in intact annular fibres. Only after the initial removal of fragments with small instruments will it become possible to complete the dissection and retraction of the nerve root medially from the bulk of the prolapse.

As the tension on the nerve root is released, retraction becomes easier. The opening in the annular fibres may be enlarged under vision and rongeurs of increasing cup size inserted for removal of free disc fragments from the interspace. The sucker with a patty on the end of it may be used as a retractor held by the surgeon in his left hand, while, with the rongeur in his right hand, the fragments are lifted out from the interspace (Fig. 3.20). In such cases, quite large amounts of the disc material may be removed, but the risk of penetration of rongeurs deep into the interspace with the possibility of damage to intra-abdominal structures is high (Fig. 3.21). The use of ring curettes is recommended in such cases for curettage of loose disc fragments and vertebral end-plate material. When large amounts of disc material have been removed, of the order of several grams of tissue, then it is wise to perform a nerve root canal decompression on both sides of the interspace, completing removal of ligamentum flavum far laterally and removing the inner margin of the superior articular facet of the inferior vertebra at the interspace on each side. In addition, with angled rongeurs it may be necessary to remove the apices of both the superior facets on the inferior side of the interspace. Excision of the whole facet joint in the course of this operation should be avoided.

The Management of Sequestrated Disc Fragments

The finding of free fragments of disc tissue in the spinal canal may pose specific problems at operation. These problems relate, more than anything else, to the site of origin of the disc tissue. If, for example, free fragments of disc tissue are found at the lumbo-sacral level, yet the posterior annular fibres of the L5/S1 disc space are found to be normal, then exploration of the higher interspace is essential. In these circumstances careful palpation of the L5/S1 disc with the blunt end of the Watson-Cheyne dissector, beneath the dural sac towards the mid-line, will be necessary before it can be safely assumed that the disc tissue has not prolapsed from that interspace. If, on the other hand, the L4/5 interspace has been exposed and a rather adherent nerve root retracted from the back of the disc to reveal a circumscribed rounded defect in the annulus, then free sequestrated disc material may be found at the lower interspace.

Central Disc Prolapse

The presence of a central disc prolapse is usually, though not always, suspected in the early stages of opening of the spinal canal. For example, it may be opened on one side and the nerve root which comes into view cannot be retracted towards the mid-line, though the disc beneath and lateral to it appears normal. In such a case, *digital palpation of the dural sac is essential* and will lead the surgeon to establish this diagnosis. Wide exposure is then required even involving excision of the whole of the spinous process and central part of the arch of the lamina on the superior side of the interspace.

Trans-Dural Approach

Having determined to remove the fragments by a trans-dural approach, then the special instruments listed above must be available, especially the fine sutures and needle holders which will be required to repair the dural opening. In addition long lintine strips with attached threads should be available, as these may need to be placed along each edge of the dural sac to prevent seepage of blood into the sub-arachnoid space after the dura has been opened.

The dural vessels in the mid-line may be coagulated over the length of the proposed dural incision, using low voltage coagulating current. This done, the dura is incised with a No. 15 blade scalpel and a protective probe introduced near the top of the incision. This is followed downwards progressively as the full length of the dural incision is made.

Cerebrospinal fluid is allowed to escape. It should be aspirated from the wound, but *at all times the sucker should now be covered with a patty.* An inexperienced surgeon or an inexperienced assistant may, from any point onwards in this operation, inflict irreversible damage on filaments of the cauda equina. Remembering that the vessels of the cauda equina are minute, only smooth rounded instruments should be used to retract the filaments from the mid-line laterally on each side (Fig. 3.22). At no stage should an unguarded sucker be placed within the dural sac itself as a nerve root may be avulsed up the sucker.

Bearing these hazards in mind, the actual process of removal of disc tissue is easily and rapidly accomplished by the trans-dural route following separate incision of the dura and the posterior longitudinal ligament over the disc space. It is likely, however, that the prolapse will have emerged on one side of this ligament.

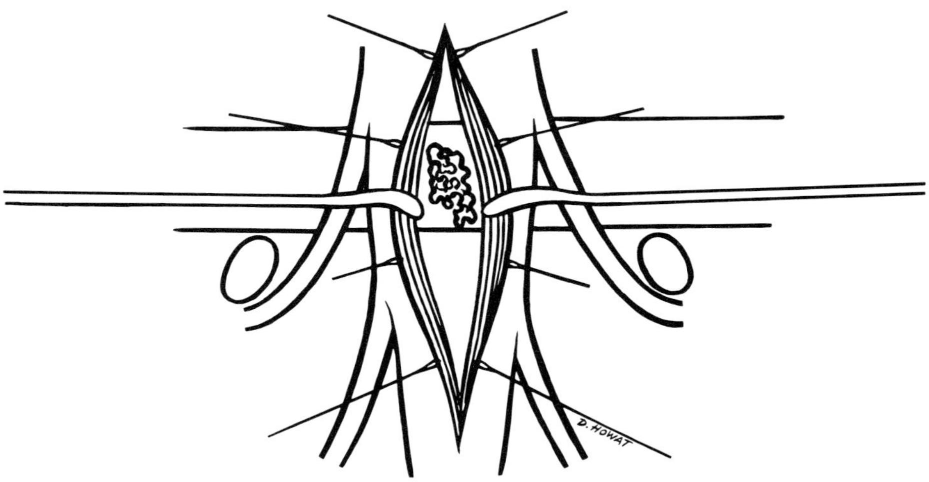

Figure 3.22. A drawing to illustrate exposure of a central disc prolapse trans-durally filaments of the cauda equina being retracted from the mid-line laterally on each side with smooth rounded instruments

Depending on the volume of disc material that can be removed with straight or angled pituitary rongeurs of varying sizes, so the question of curettage of the disc space may arise. If large quantities of disc material can be removed easily, it is wise to use a ring curette to clear other remnants, recalling once again the risk of instruments penetrating into the abdominal cavity.

Although some authors recommend closure of the anterior layer of the dural sac following this procedure, this is not always necessary. However, careful closure of the posterior layer should be effected using a continuous 6/0 dural stitch. The retaining sutures which were earlier inserted, are used to retract the dura in the final stages of closure and care is taken at all times to avoid transfixion of any of the cauda equina filaments in the closing suture.

In cases of this type, especially when many fragments of intervertebral disc tissue have been removed from the interspace, it is wise to perform bilateral nerve root canal decompression to complete the procedure, to prevent recurrence of sciatica later following reduction in height of the disc space.

xi) Disc Prolapses Associated With Other Special Problems

Spinal Canal Stenosis

This situation should be recognized pre-operatively in most instances, especially if myelography has been performed. The disc prolapses found in these cases are often small. It is essential to perform an adequate spinal or nerve root canal decompression on both sides in such cases.

Nerve Root and Other Anomalies

The recognition of nerve root and vascular anomalies requires excellent technique during the exposure. A lower lumbar nerve root sometimes arises from the dural sac at right angles, passing directly laterally through the intervertebral foramen across the posterior surface of the disc. Mistaken easily for a prolapse at operation, it may be incised, excised or avulsed in error.

Isolated Disc Resorption

Unilateral sciatica in cases of isolated disc resorption is not common (Crock, 1976). The most important part of the surgery for this condition is the nerve root canal decompression and "foraminotomy" which can usually be performed with preservation of the relevant laminal arch. The "disc prolapse" in such instances usually consists of a small fragment of vertebral end-plate cartilage, which may be adherent to the under-surface of the nerve root. Careful dissection is then required to remove it, as the root may be flattened in these circumstances.

Spondylolisthesis

Disc prolapse may occur at the level of a spondylolisthesis or above it. Excision of the prolapsed disc fragments is essential, but questions of complete spinal canal and nerve root canal decompression including removal of the loose lamina, together with decisions on the use of spinal fusion techniques then arise.

xii) Upper Lumbar Disc Prolapse

Upper lumber disc prolapses may occur in the L 1/2, L 2/3 area in association with the conus medullaris in some cases. Operations in this area carry hazards of spinal cord injury, and retraction of the dural sac must be performed with great care at all times. Similarly, the introduction of large-jawed pituitary rongeurs or large ring curettes may be hazardous. Extra-peritoneal approaches to these prolapses can be recommended with confidence.

xiii) Preserving the Bony Canal

In the past it has been common practice to remove either one half side of a lamina or to cut a narrow channel in it between the two ligamenta flava related to it, while seeking an elusive disc prolapse. This interference with the roofing apparatus of the spinal canal is to be avoided, particularly in cases with spinal canal or nerve root canal stenosis, because it may lead to the development of stenosis of the canal following growth of new bone into the area of the laminal defect (see Chapter 9, p. 253).

Exploration of an intervertebral disc space can be accurately and competently performed through a limited inter-laminar exposure, carried out along the lines recommended above (p. 116). If no lesion is found at one level, due to error, then it is better to look at the next level upwards or downwards from the primary exploration without disturbing the integrity of the lamina.

xiv) Wound Closure

The use of suction drainage is recommended routinely, except in cases where the dura has been breached.

Undue haste, poor haemorrhage control and careless handling of rongeurs or root retractors may lead to serious dural injuries. Indeed, dural tears may be inflicted even before the ligamentum flavum has been opened if rongeurs "slip" into the spinal canal.

Dural tears are most likely to occur in complicated cases, for example, where there is associated spinal canal stenosis and opening of the canal proves difficult, or again, in the course of separating an adherent root from a disc prolapse. These defects should be identified carefully and repaired with fine sutures.

Careful attention to wound closure is important. Deep sutures may be placed in the muscle layer, but these should be tied only to the point of approximation of the muscle masses in the mid-line. Most attention should be focussed on tight closure of the lumbo-dorsal fascia with interrupted sutures.

In extremely obese patients with thick layers of subcutaneous fat, the use of multiple sutures in this tissue should be avoided. Excessive use of diathermy in the fatty layer and rough handling of this tissue will result in the leakage of liquified fat from the wound. Infection in this layer may subsequently become troublesome. These problems may be prevented by using three or four heavy grade nylon sutures passed through the skin and full depth of the fatty layers beneath it and tied as "mattress" stitches. When these "tension sutures" have been tied, the skin edges may be approximated with fine interrupted sutures.

4

Intervertebral Disc Calcification

4.1. *Introduction*

Although calcification of the nucleus pulposus is not a common pathological finding in intervertebral discs, it warrants discussion for a number of reasons.

4.2. *Complications*

First of all, it is one of the few causes of *acute excruciating spinal pain,* the most common being pathological fractures, acute inflammatory lesions, some tumours and the vascular catastrophe of dissecting aortic aneurysm.

Secondly, paraplegia of sudden onset may complicate prolapse of calcified nuclear material into the thoracic spinal canal. This cause of paraplegia may go unrecognized if the calcified nuclear material is dispersed into the spinal canal where it may be difficult to see on plain X-rays. An erroneous diagnosis, such as acute ascending polyneuritis or vascular accident to the cord may then be made.

Thirdly, while Kohler and Zimmer (1968) have stated that it is relatively common in adults, the belief is widespread that it is of little clinical significance. Indeed, Nachemson (1976) included intervertebral disc calcification in a list of radiological findings in the lumbar spine which, in his view, have no significance as causes of low back pain.

Surgeons in consultant practice should beware of generalizations about disease processes which may lead them to think that certain pathological changes cannot be related to a patient's symptoms.

While it is clear that nucleus pulposus calcification may be associated with localized spinal pain of moderate severity and that the pain usually responds to simple conservative methods of treatment, it is equally clear that this disc disorder may have serious consequences for individual patients and that surgical operations may be required in the course of treatment.

4.3. Patterns in Children

Clinical syndromes associated with nucleus pulposus calcification in children are well recognized, though rare. Bouts of acute painful wry neck or severe spinal pain of sudden onset, with fever, moderate elevation of the erythrocyte sedimentation rate and occasional increase in white cell counts, subside rapidly with rest. Typically, widespread calcification of variable density outlines the area of one or more of the

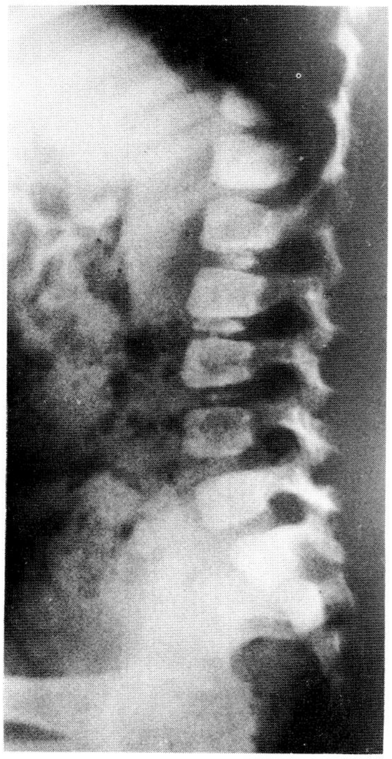

Figure 4.1. A lateral X-ray of the thoraco-lumbar spine in a child aged 11, showing nucleus pulposus calcification at multiple levels. Note the straight lumbar spine due to muscle spasm

Table 4.1

Age	Sex	Site
54	F	L3/4
46	M	T10/11
42	F	T11/12
46	F	L3/4
45	F	L5/S1
51	F	T9/10, T10/11
33	F	T12/L1
38	F	L1/2
57	F	L4/5, L5/S1
47	F	L1/2
56	M	L1/2
60	F	T8/9

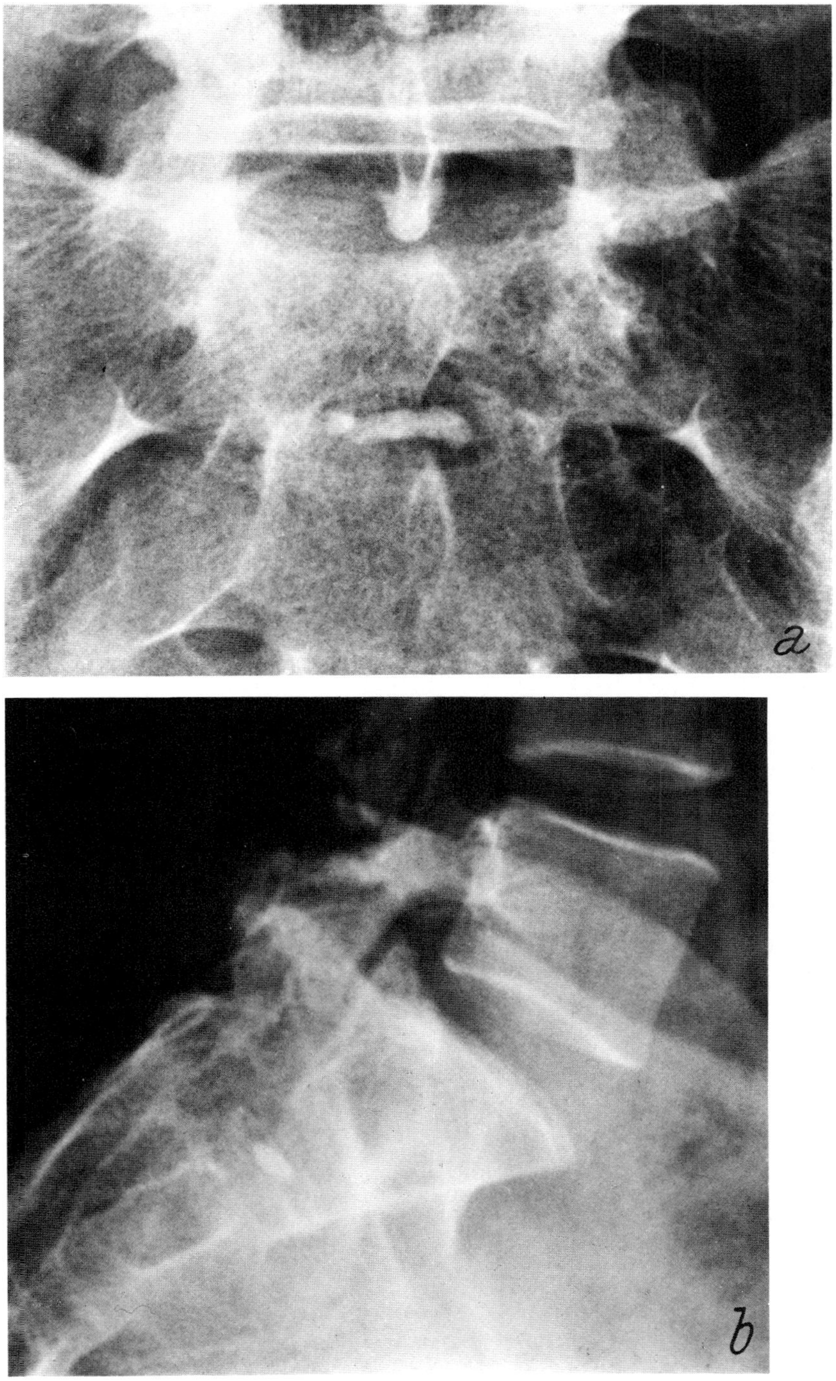

Figures 4.2. Antero-posterior (**a**) and lateral views (**b**) of the sacrum in a female aged 36, showing nucleus pulposus calcification in a rudimentary sacral intervertebral disc

nuclei pulposi. This calcification usually disappears within a few weeks of its first recognition on the X-ray examination of the spine (Fig. 4.1).

The natural history of symptomatic paediatric intervertebral disc calcification has been defined recently by Sonnabend *et al.* (1982), following a review of 35 papers on the subject. Most of these cases occur in the cervical discs. Trauma seems to play a part, at least as a precipitating factor. In children, the disorder is usually asymptomatic in the thoracic spine.

In this review of 89 children with symptoms attributed to the lesion, the sex ratio boys:girls was 1.5:1, but in 19 children who were asymptomatic, it was 0.5:1.

Crock (1982) reported twelve cases of intervertebral disc calcification in adults, ten of whom required surgical treatment for the relief of severe intractable pain, not responsive to conservative measures of treatment. Only two of these patients were males.

The sites of disc calcification also differed markedly from that seen in children (Table 4.1).

In dogs with disc calcification, involvement of the sacral *intervertebral* discs occurs in about 4 or 5%. Apparently not previously reported in man, I have observed a female patient with the condition in the first sacral intervertebral disc, where it has caused troublesome sacral pain for a number of years (Figs. 4.2a, b).

4.4. Patterns in Adults

The radiological appearances of calcific deposits in this series of twelve cases were classified into four groups.

1. Small discrete irregularly opaque shadows within the nucleus pulposus lying nearer the posterior than the anterior boundary (Figs. 4.3a, b, 4.4).
2. Widespread calcification of variable density giving the nucleus pulposus a fluffy outline (Figs. 4.5, 4.6).
3. Small discretely outlined zones of calcification lying adjacent to one vertebral end-plate but peripherally located in the nucleus pulposus (Figs. 4.7a, b).
4. Discrete aggregates of densely calcified material confined to the area of the nucleus pulposus (Figs. 4.8a, b, 4.9, 4.10).

Computerised tomography may provide valuable information on the spatial distribution of calcified disc tissue with particular reference to its relation to the spinal canal and its neural contents (Fig. 4.11).

a) Clinical Features

Examples of type 1 nucleus pulposus calcification are illustrated in Figs. 4.3a, b, 4.4. These patients, one female (Figs. 4.3a, b) and the other male (Fig. 4.4), presented

Figures 4.3a and **b.** Antero-posterior and lateral X-rays of the mid-dorsal spine in a female patient aged 60 showing *type 1* nucleus pulposus calcification

Figure 4.4. Lateral X-ray of the thoraco-lumbar junction in a male aged 56 years showing *type 1* nucleus pulposus calcification. This X-ray appearance remained unchanged in eight years

Figure 4.5. Lateral X-ray of the thoracic spine showing *type 2* nucleus pulposus calcification at the T11/12 intervertebral disc space in a female patient aged 42

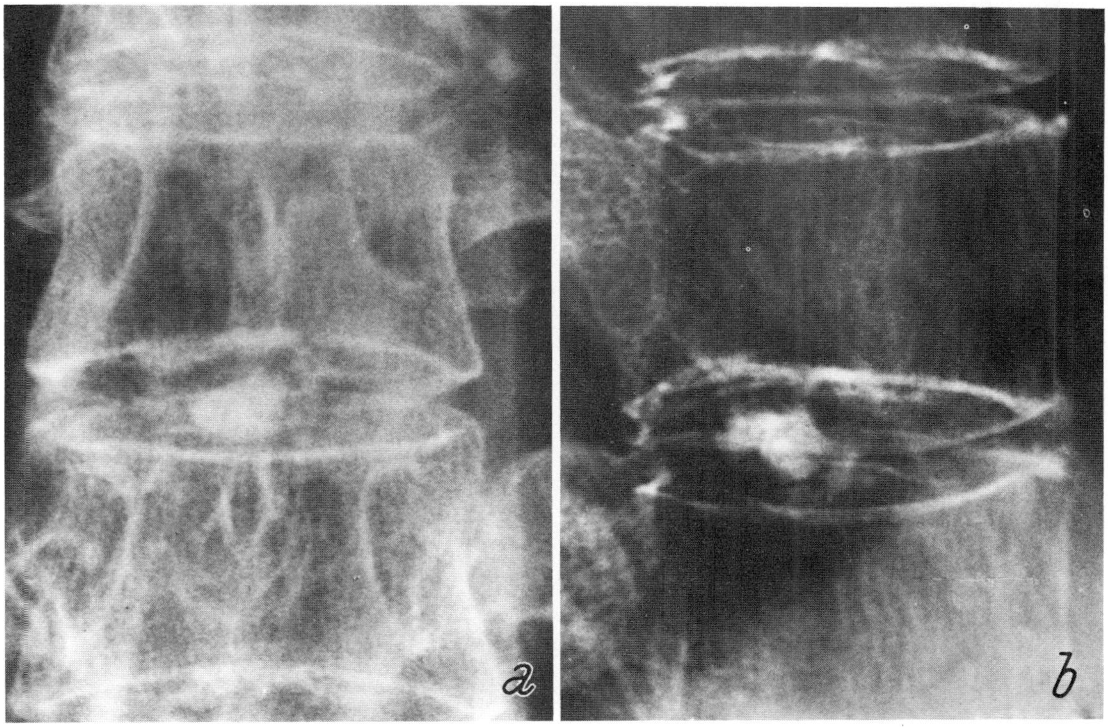

Figures 4.3

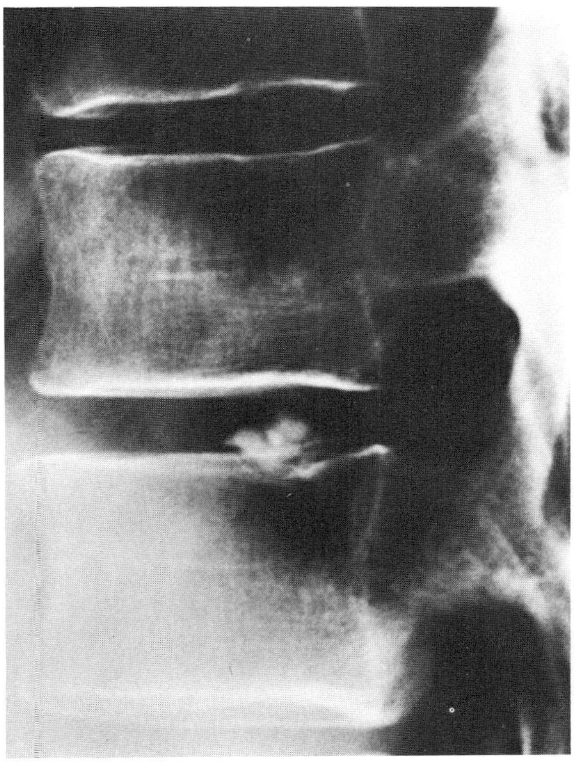

Figure 4.4

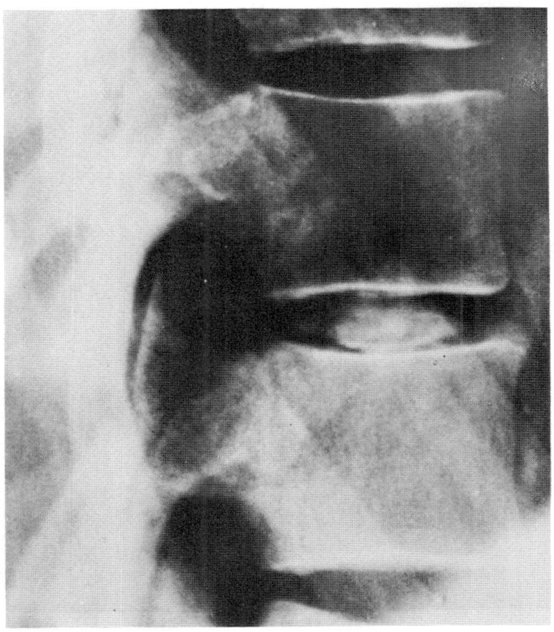

Figure 4.5

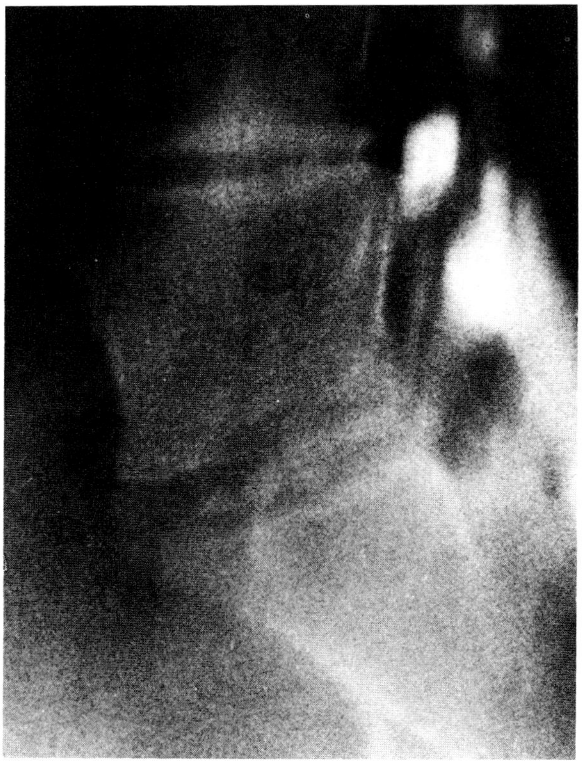

Figure 4.6

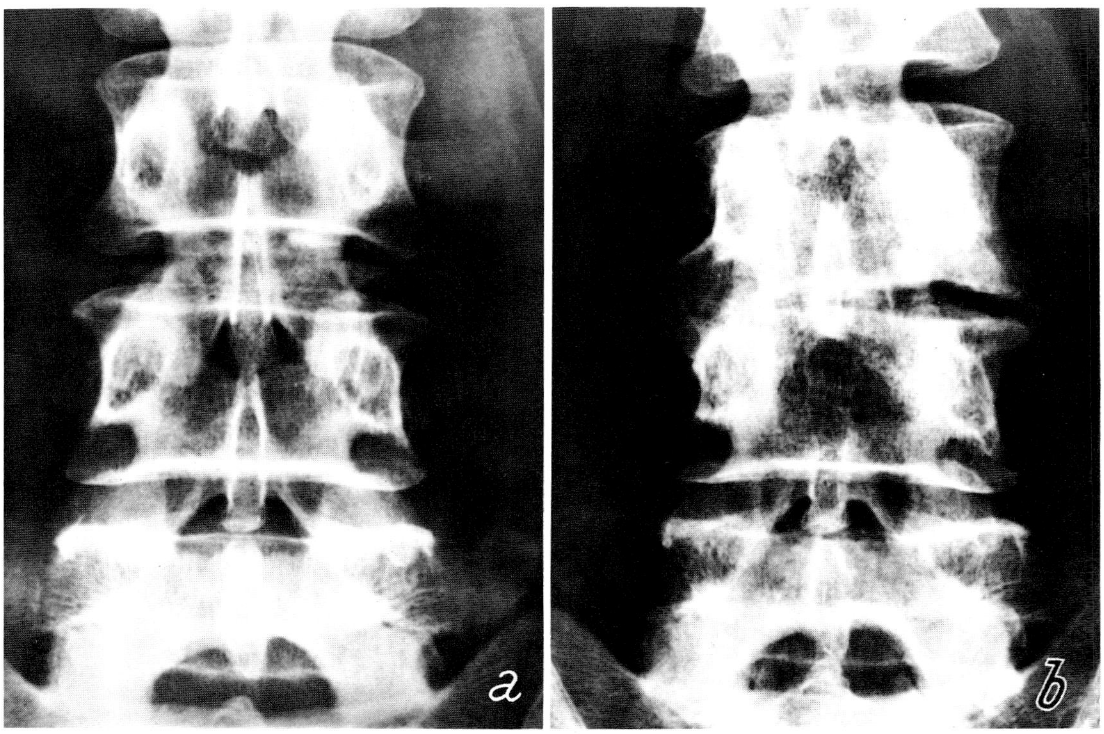

Figures 4.7

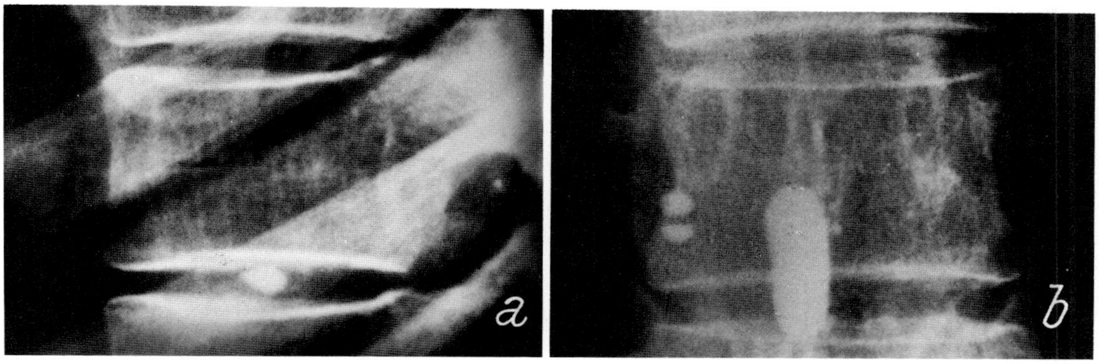

Figures 4.8 a and b. Lateral and antero-posterior radiographs of the thoracic spine in a female patient aged 47 years showing *type 4* nucleus pulposus calcification at the T8/9 intervertebral disc level. The middle lobe of the right lung was adherent to this disc in the paravertebral gutter, the remainder of the pleural cavity being free of adhesions

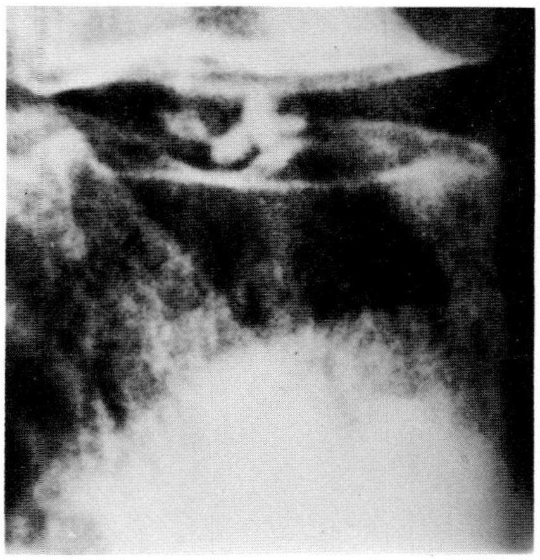

Figure 4.9

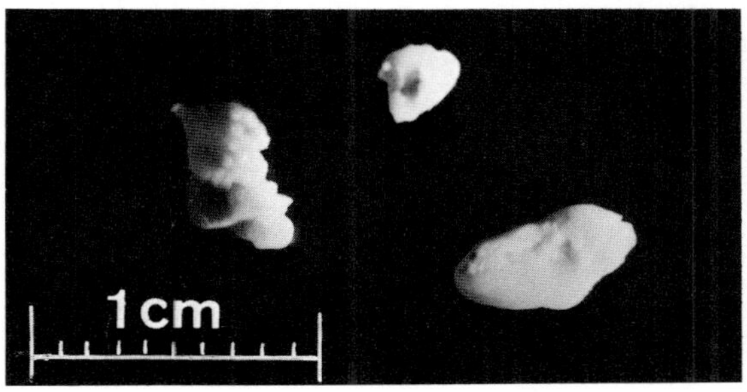

Figure 4.10

Figure 4.9. A lateral radiograph of the thoracic spine showing *type 4* nucleus pulposus calcification at the T10/11 intervertebral disc space in a male patient aged 46

Figure 4.10. A photograph of the calcium calculi removed at operation from the disc shown in Fig. 4.9

Figure 4.6. Lateral tomogram of the L4/5 and L5/S1 area of the spine in a female patient aged 45 years showing *type 2* nucleus pulposus calcification at L5/S1

Figures 4.7. a Antero-posterior view of the lumbar spine in a female patient aged 54 years showing *type 3* nucleus pulposus calcification at the L3/4 level on the right side of the photograph. **b** Antero-posterior photograph of the lumbar spine showing spontaneous interbody fusion at the L3/4 level six years after partial disc excision

Table 4.2. Protocols

	Case 1	Case 2	Case 3
Sex	Female	Male	Female
Age	54	46	42
Occupation	Home duties	Workman	Home duties and nurse
X-ray	L 3/4	T 10/11	T11/12
Type of lesion	3	4	2
Date of presentation	May, 1970	February, 1971	October, 1973
Date of operation	October, 1970	1976	September, 1974
Trauma	None	Heavy blow to trunk	Heavy lifting
Major symptoms	Excruciating lumbar back pain with referred leg pain	Lower thoracic pain, weakness of legs	Severe low thoracic spinal pain, radiating around lower ribs
Intra-disc hydro-cortisone injection	Not administered	Not administered	Not administered
Previous surgery	None	Lumbar spine fusion – 8 years earlier for tuberculous disease, T11 to L1	Nil
Type of operation	Trans-lumbar canal partial disc excision	Interbody fusion	Interbody fusion
Result	Improved. Spontaneous interbody fusion observed in X-rays several years after operation	Improved	Improved
	Case 4	**Case 5**	**Case 6**
Sex	Female	Female	Female
Age	46	45	51
Occupation	Home duties and factory worker	Home duties	Home duties and telephonist
X-ray	L 3/4	L 5/S1	T9/10, T10/11
Type of lesion	3	2	3
Date of presentation	August, 1975	1976	1977
Date of operation	September, 1975	1976	1977
Trauma	Lifting	None	None
Major symptoms	Excruciating mid-lumbar pain, (R) hip flexed	Severe low back pain – marked lumbar spasm	Severe thoraco-lumbar junction pain
Intra-disc hydro-cortisone injection	No help	No help	No help
Previous surgery	None	Lumbar spinal fusion – 20 years earlier L 4/5 for degenerative disc disease	Multiple operations including lumbar fusion for lumbar spondylosis and degenerative spondylolisthesis at L4/5 level
Type of operation	Trans-lumbar canal partial disc excision	Interbody fusion	Extra pleural partial disc excisions
Result	Improved	Fair	Fair

	Case 7	Case 8	Case 9
Sex	Female	Female	Female
Age	33	38	57
Occupation	Home duties and nurse	Home duties and nurse	Home duties
X-ray	T12/L1	L1/2	L4/5, L5/S1
Type of lesion	3	3	2
Date of presentation	December, 1976	1973	1978
Date of operation	March, 1978	1978	March, 1979
Trauma	None	Heavy lifting	Back pain persisted following motor vehicle accident
Major Symptoms	Severe mid- to upper lumbar pain, occasional (L) thigh pain	Severe upper lumbar back pain	Severe lumbar back pain, buttock pain. Marked muscle spasm
Intra-disc hydrocortisone injection	No help	No help	No help
Previous surgery	Cervical fusion	Intercostal neurectomy	Lumbar laminectomy
Type of operation	Extra-pleural interbody fusion	Extra-peritoneal disc excision	Extra-peritoneal partial disc excisions
Result	Fair	Improved	Improved

	Case 10	Case 11	Case 12
Sex	Female	Male	Female
Age	47	56	60
Occupation	Home duties and factory worker	School teacher	Home duties
X-ray	T8/9	L1/2	T8/9
Type of lesion	4	1	1
Date of presentation	July, 1979	February, 1972	1976
Date of operation	October, 1979	No operation	No operation
Trauma	Lifting and twisting	Digging	None
Major symptoms	Severe thoracic pain, aggravated by deep breathing, radiating around chest wall	Upper lumbar back pain	Mid-thoracic back pain
Intra-disc hydrocortisone injection	Not administered	Not administered	Not administered
Previous surgery	Lumbar laminectomy	None	None
Type of operation	Trans-pleural disc excision	No operation	No operation
Result	Improved	Improved with brace and analgesics	Improved with brace and analgesics

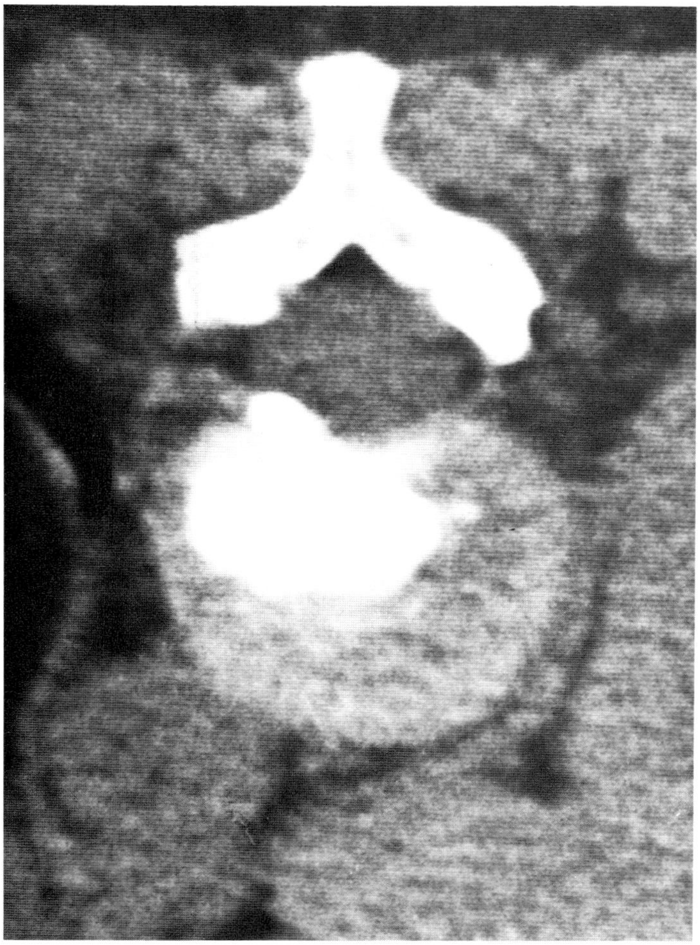

Figure 4.11. A computerised tomograph showing the pattern of calcification of disc tissues at the disc between the vertebrae T11/12, in a female, aged 49 years. The calcification (type 2) is shown extending postero-laterally into the spinal canal where it is related to the antero-lateral aspect of the spinal cord on the left side

with spinal pain of sudden onset, localized respectively to the mid-thoracic spine and to the upper lumbar zone. In both, symptoms were controlled promptly with simple measures including the use of spinal supports for some months. The radiological appearance of the calcification shown in Fig. 4.4 remained unchanged in X-rays taken at follow-up eight years later. There were no outstanding clinical features characterizing these cases.

By contrast, more serious problems were seen in the ten patients whose details are shown in Table 4.2. Eventually all were treated surgically.

In four of the patients in the surgical group, nucleus pulposus calcification was found in the mid- and low lumbar discs. These patients presented with severe low back pain and paraspinal muscle spasm. One had a unilateral psoas muscle spasm preventing hip extension. The severity of the pain was such that family members complained bitterly that conservative treatment was ineffective, and they insisted that their relative should be admitted to hospital.

Table 4.3. Patterns of nucleus pulposus calcification

	Female	Male
Type 1	1	1
Type 2	3	–
Type 3	5	–
Type 4	1	1

In the other six patients in the surgical group, nucleus pulposus calcifications were localized in the upper lumbar and lower thoracic discs. Again, *the pain of which they complained was intense in character,* localized in the upper lumbar and upper abdominal regions, and in the thoracic spine and radiating to one or both sides of the thoracic cage. Deep breathing, coughing and sneezing aggravated the pain. Paraspinal muscle spasm was also marked. One patient, the only male in the series, presented with low thoracic pain and weakness of his legs. There were no specific abnormal neurological findings in any of these patients.

b) Pathological Findings

There were two striking observations made at operation. One concerned the local inflammatory response apparently induced by the nucleus pulposus calcification in the region of affected discs. The other related to the appearance and texture of the calcified material removed.

Within the spinal canal, in the retro-peritoneal space and between the parietal and visceral pleura, adhesions were found related to the affected discs. The most remarkable evidence of this pathology was seen in the right hemi-thorax (case 10) where well-formed filmy adhesions had to be divided between the visceral pleura of the middle lobe of the lung in the paravertebral gutter and the antero-lateral surface of the disc between T8 and T9, immediately adjacent to the nucleus pulposus calcification (Figs. 4.8a, b) on the right side of the disc space.

The calcified material removed from the intervertebral discs at operation was either white in appearance, with the consistency of soft paste, or in the shape of irregular calculi, slightly yellowish in colour.

Histological examination was carried out on tissue removed in five cases. In each case degenerative fibro-cartilage was found associated with calcification. Chemical analysis confirmed the presence of calcium in the tissues. No abnormal cartilaginous proliferation was found in any case, nor was there any evidence of specific inflammation.

c) Surgical Treatment

The types of operation carried out in the ten patients reported by Crock (1982), are set out in Table 4.2.

Summary

While calcification of the nucleus pulposus is a rare disorder of thoracic and lumbar discs in adults, it seems reasonable to draw attention to a number of observations made in this series of ten patients who underwent surgical operations for this problem.

Nine out of ten of the patients were female and in eight out of the ten there was some history of trauma.

Six of the patients had had some form of spinal surgery performed prior to the onset of their nucleus pulposus calcification.

While the pathological changes induced within the disc itself include some features of non-specific inflammation, it is interesting to note the capacity of this lesion to induce non-specific inflammatory changes at the surface of an affected disc.

Observations of retro-peritoneal fibrosis, perineural fibrosis in the spinal canal and localized pleural reactions have been reported in this series.

The pain in certain cases of nucleus pulposus calcification is acute in onset, intense in character and frequently unrelieved by conservative measures. In particular, intra-disc injections of hydrocortisone appear to be ineffective, whereas in cases of acute supraspinatus tendonitis they often relieve patients of pain.

Analysis of the findings in the ten patients presented in this chapter suggests that acute nucleus pulposus calcification deserves more serious consideration in clinical practice than is normally accorded to it.

5

Spondylolisthesis

5.1. *Planning of Treatment*

Spondylolisthesis is a condition in which one vertebral body slips forward on the one below it. Associated with the forward displacement of the vertebral body there is either a laminal defect or degenerative arthritis of the inferior laminal facet joints.

The most common type of spondylolisthesis requiring surgical treatment is that seen with pseudarthroses in the lamina, so-called *spondylolytic spondylolisthesis*. Pseudarthroses occur in the pars interarticularis on each side. These take the form of asymmetrical false joints with false capsules and synovial linings in which osseous loose bodies may be found.

In *degenerative spondylolisthesis* the slip of the vertebral body is associated with degenerative arthritis of the inferior facet joints of the lamina; this condition is seen most commonly in women after the menopause.

Spondylolisthesis usually occurs at one level in the lumbar region, though rarely two or more adjacent levels may be involved (Fig. 5.1). Spondylolisthesis is one of the academic subjects that has appealed to orthopaedic surgeons for many years. It has been classified in various ways, five clinical groups being widely recognized: congenital, isthmic, degenerative, traumatic, and pathological.

In this chapter, conservative treatment will not be discussed, beyond pointing out that many patients with this condition who present for the first time with symptoms will respond to a variety of conservative measures.

Likewise, the academic aspects of this subject will not be dealt with in depth. Readers may refer to the published work of Newman, Wiltse, McNab, and Louis, listed in the short bibliography which is found at the end of this book.

a) History

Patients may develop a wide range of symptoms and signs, including: back pain, referred leg pain, a combination of back and leg pain, or in severe cases, evidence of lower cauda equina dysfunction with impairment of bladder function and impotence. In the extreme example of vertebral body slip, described as *spondyloptosis,* the pelvic

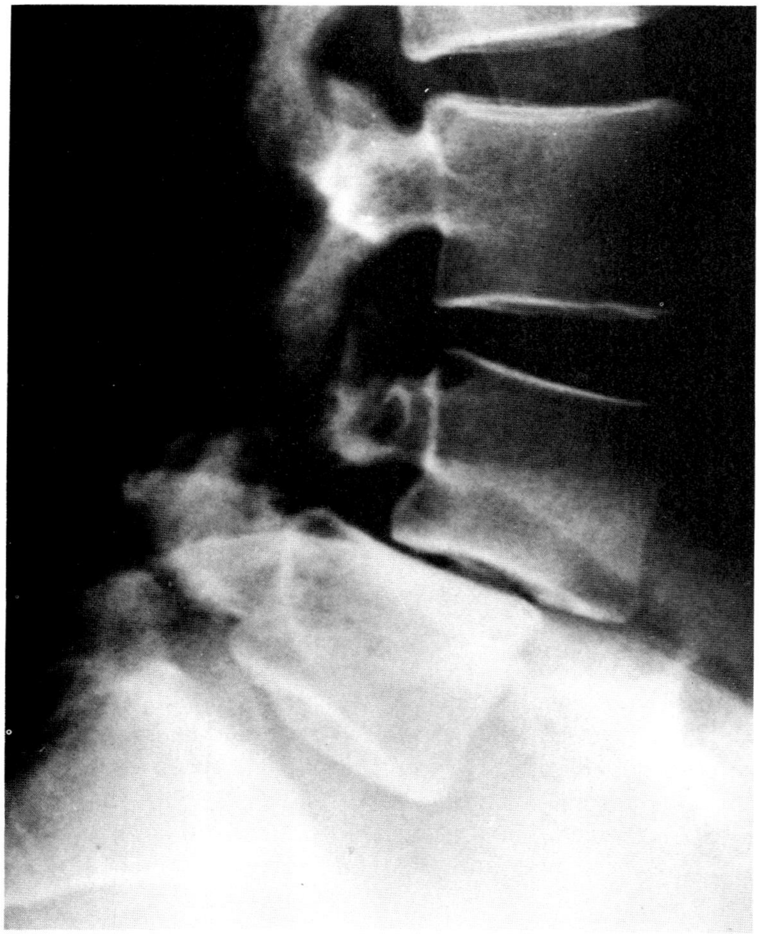

Figure 5.1. A lateral radiograph of the lumbar spine of a woman aged 45 years showing spondylolytic spondylolisthesis, Grade 1, at L5/S1 with a normal intervertebral disc, and Grade 2 at L4/5 with disc resorption at that level. *This patient only required conservative treatment* for low back pain

outlet may become obstructed during labour, rendering Caesarean section essential (Fig. 5.2).

In practice, no single operation will necessarily produce a cure in patients with spondylolisthesis. Hence it is necessary to make a careful analysis of each case, attempting to introduce some rationale to the planning of treatment.

In assessing individual patients with a view to selecting a particular type of operation for use in treatment, one must first take account of the outstanding features in the clinical history. Careful analysis of individual symptom patterns may indicate, for example, that decompression of the spinal canal alone may be the operation of choice. This will be the case where the patient's dominant symptoms are bilateral buttock and leg pain.

Where the symptom pattern combines the complaints of back and leg pain, then both decompression of the spinal canal and combined spinal fusion may be indicated. For the treatment of back pain alone, spinal fusion may be indicated.

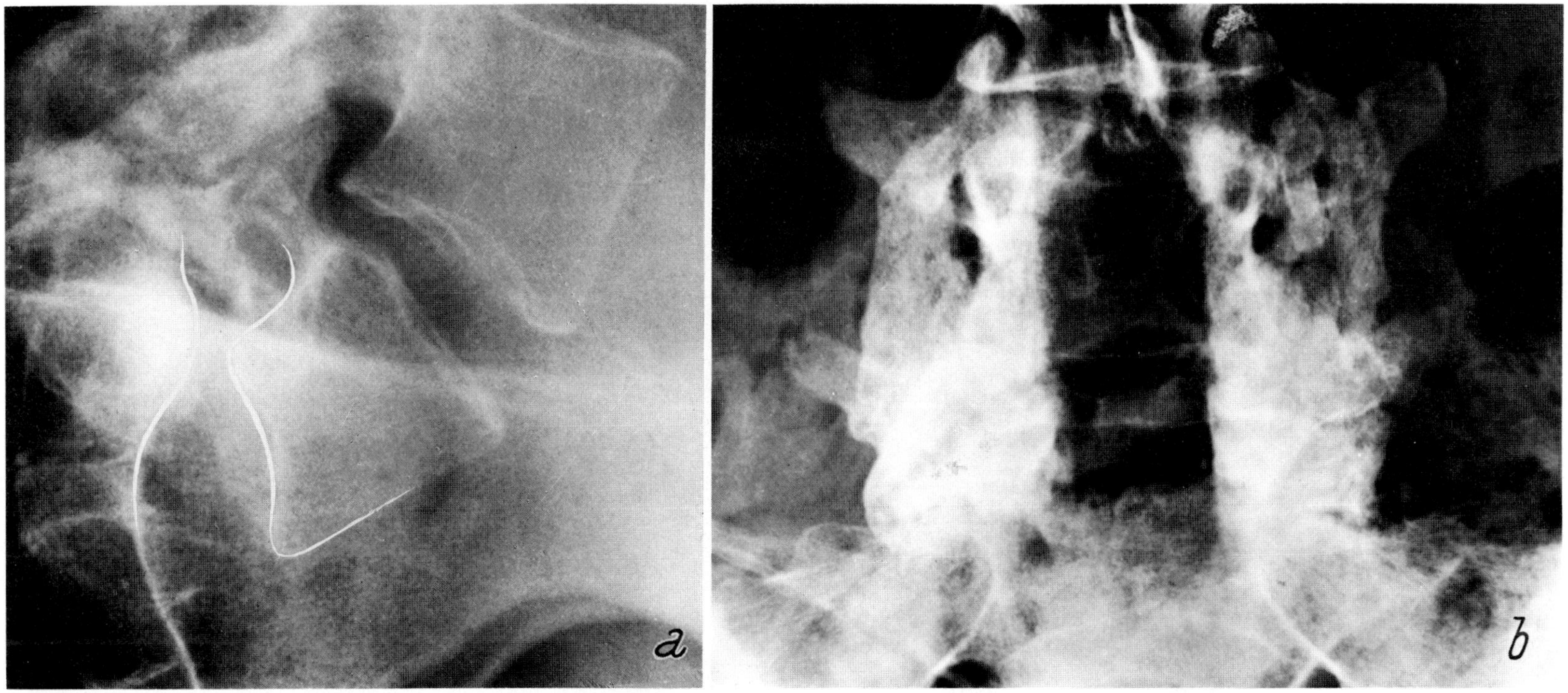

Figures 5.2. **a** A lateral radiograph of the lower lumbar spine showing spondyloptosis of L5, with the vertebral body slipped forward and rotated, lying anterior to the 2nd sacral vertebra. **b** An antero-posterior view showing multi-level intertransverse fusion with spinal canal decompression

b) Physical Parameters

Having considered the history, four physical parameters should be analyzed in each case before the definitive decision can be taken on the type of surgical procedure required.

i) Role of Laminal Pseudarthroses in Symptom Production

The first of these is the role of the laminal pseudarthroses in symptom production. The structure of the pseudarthroses varies considerably. Defects in the pars inter-

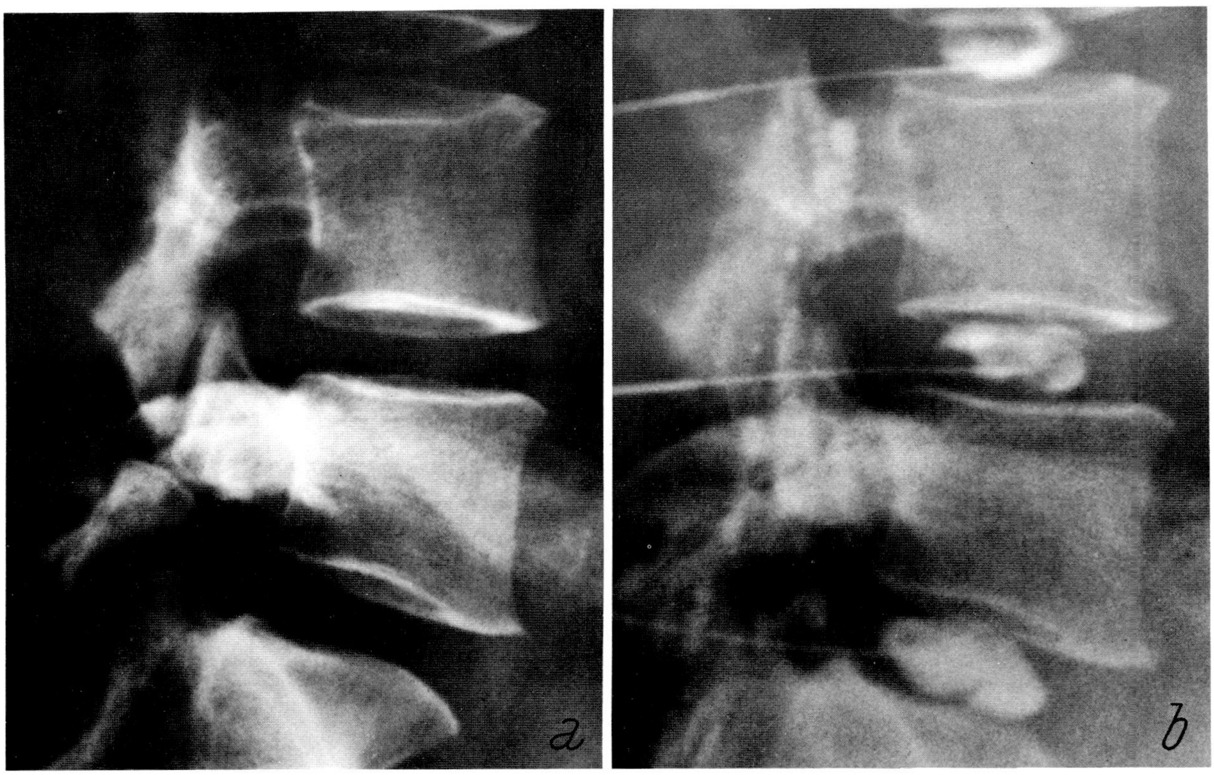

Figures 5.3. a A lateral radiograph of the lower lumbar spine showing a spondylolytic defect in the lamina of L5. **b** Normal discograms at L3/4, L4/5 and L5/S1 in this case

Figures 5.4. a A drawing to illustrate a spondylolytic defect in the lower of two laminae which are viewed obliquely. **b** An oblique radiograph of the lower lumbar spine showing a normal lamina with the pars interarticularis outlined in the middle of the photograph and the spondylolytic defect involving the lowest lamina shown on the film. Loose bodies in the pseudarthrosis are clearly visible

Figures 5.5 a–d. Photographs of loose laminae ("rattlers") removed at operations from patients with spondylolytic spondylolisthesis. The specimens have been photographed from above except for **b,** which is a lateral photograph. In **a,** note the complex nature of the pseudarthroses with the loose body on the right side of the photograph. In **b,** the large pseudarthrosis is visible in profile and the inferior facet of the lamina is visible on the bottom right of the photograph. The views of the specimens in **c** and **d** show the asymmetric nature of the pseudarthroses on either side of the lamina

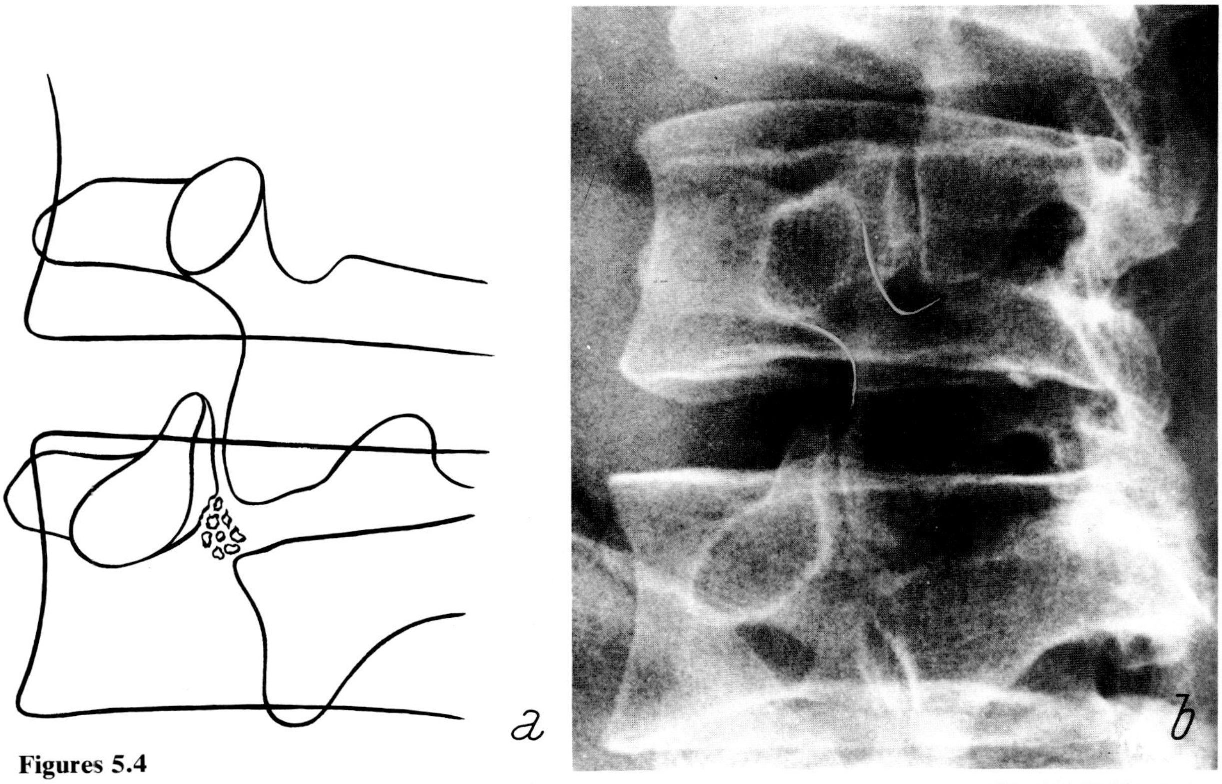

Figures 5.4

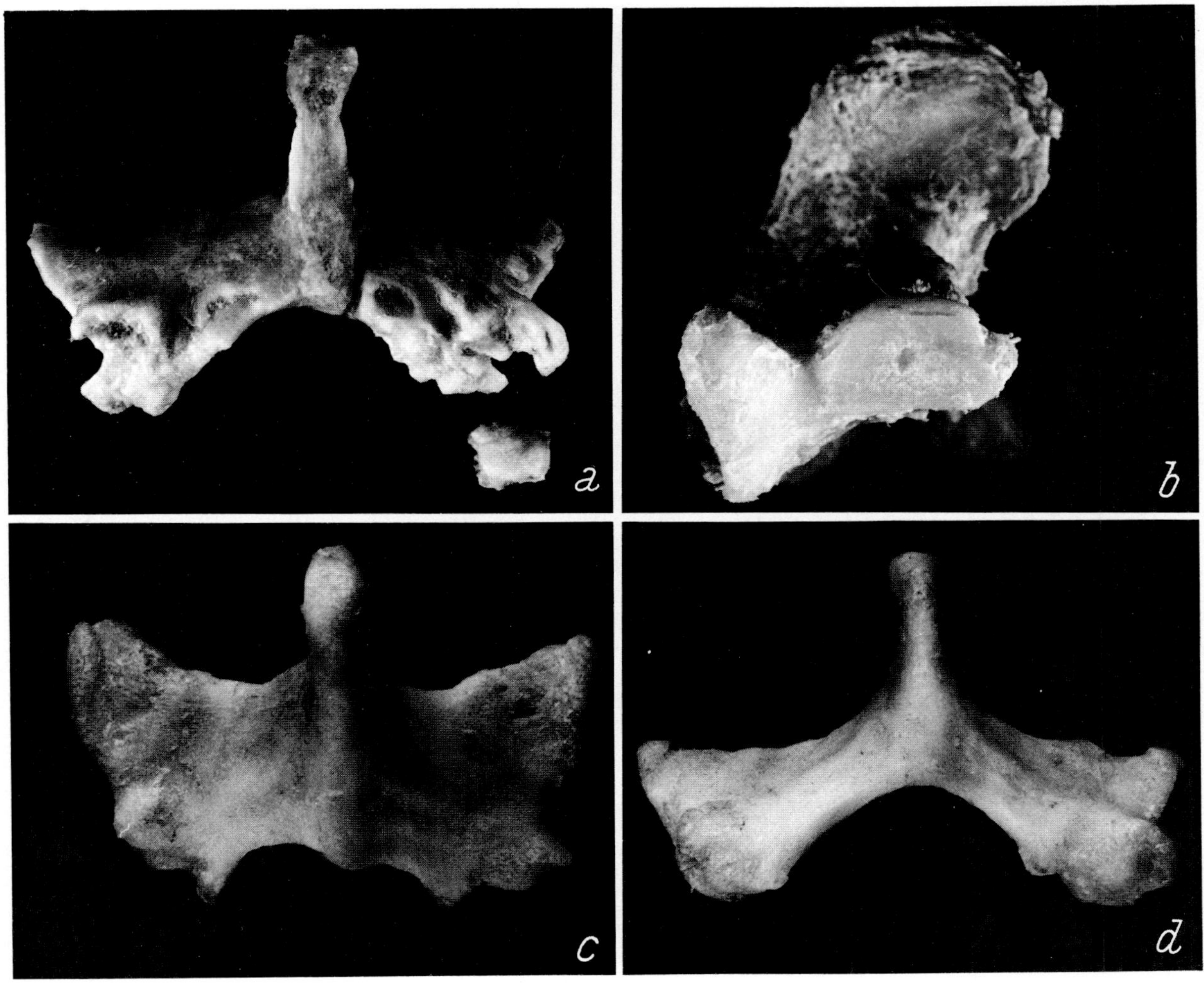

Figures 5.5

articularis are usually bilateral, though rarely symmetrical. They are often associated with bulky false joints from which recognizable synovial tissue may be extracted and in which a number of loose bodies may be found. These pseudarthroses are immediate posterior relations of the emerging nerve roots at the intervertebral foramina on both sides. Their obtrusions into the intervertebral foramina and nerve root canals may be the sole cause of referred leg pain in patients with spondylolytic spondylolisthesis, or in rare cases of spondylolysis (Figs. 5.3a, b). In the usual case with bilateral laminal defects, the spinous process, lamina and the inferior articular processes remain as a single unit which is loose in the vertebral column. When the spinous process is grasped with an instrument during operation, this whole unit can be moved freely. It has been described as the "rattler". Removal of the "rattler" is said to relieve nerve root pressure. However, if only the "rattler" is removed, the proximal portions of the pseudarthroses which remain attached to the pars interarticularis on each side, leading up to the superior articular facets, remain in the spine. The related nerve roots cannot be seen throughout their courses unless these proximal segments of the pseudarthroses are also removed, thereby completing the nerve root decompressions. *Simple removal of the "rattler", therefore, is always inadequate* (Figs. 5.4a, b, 5.5a–d, 5.6).

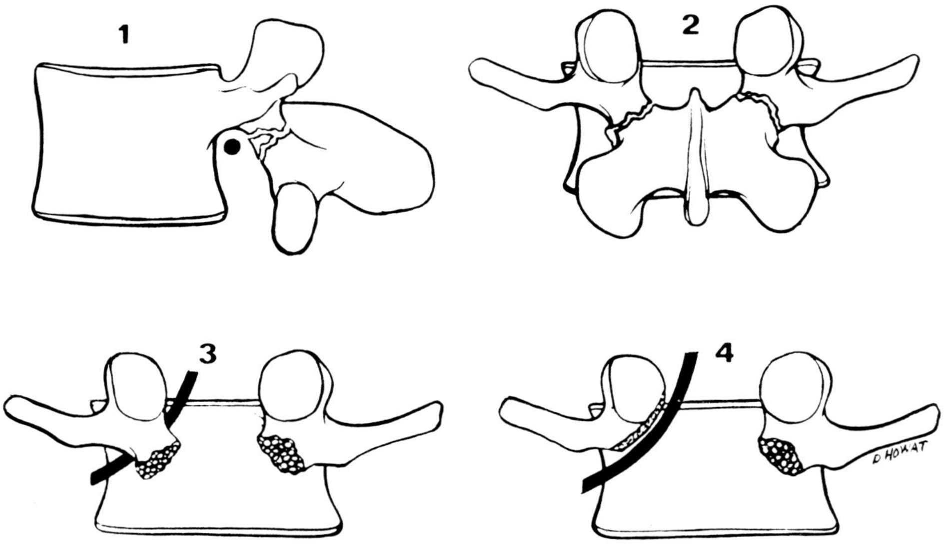

Figure 5.6. **1** and **2** show the relationship of the laminal pseudarthroses to the spinal nerves. The soft tissues such as ligamentum flavum, false capsule and synovium are not depicted. **3** and **4** show the nerve root relations after removal of the "rattler" of spondylolysis, and the correct method of decompression **(4)** of the root canal and intervertebral foramen on the left side of the drawing

ii) State of Discs Adjacent to Slip

The second parameter to be considered concerns the state of discs adjacent to the vertebral slip, both above and below it. *Discography* may be an essential special investigation where the symptom pattern is characterized by a mixture of back and leg pain. For example, in the case of spondylolisthesis at L4/5, if the discograms at L3/4 and L5/S1 are normal, then operative treatment should be restricted to the L4/5 segment alone (Figs. 5.7a, b). In other circumstances, the presence of

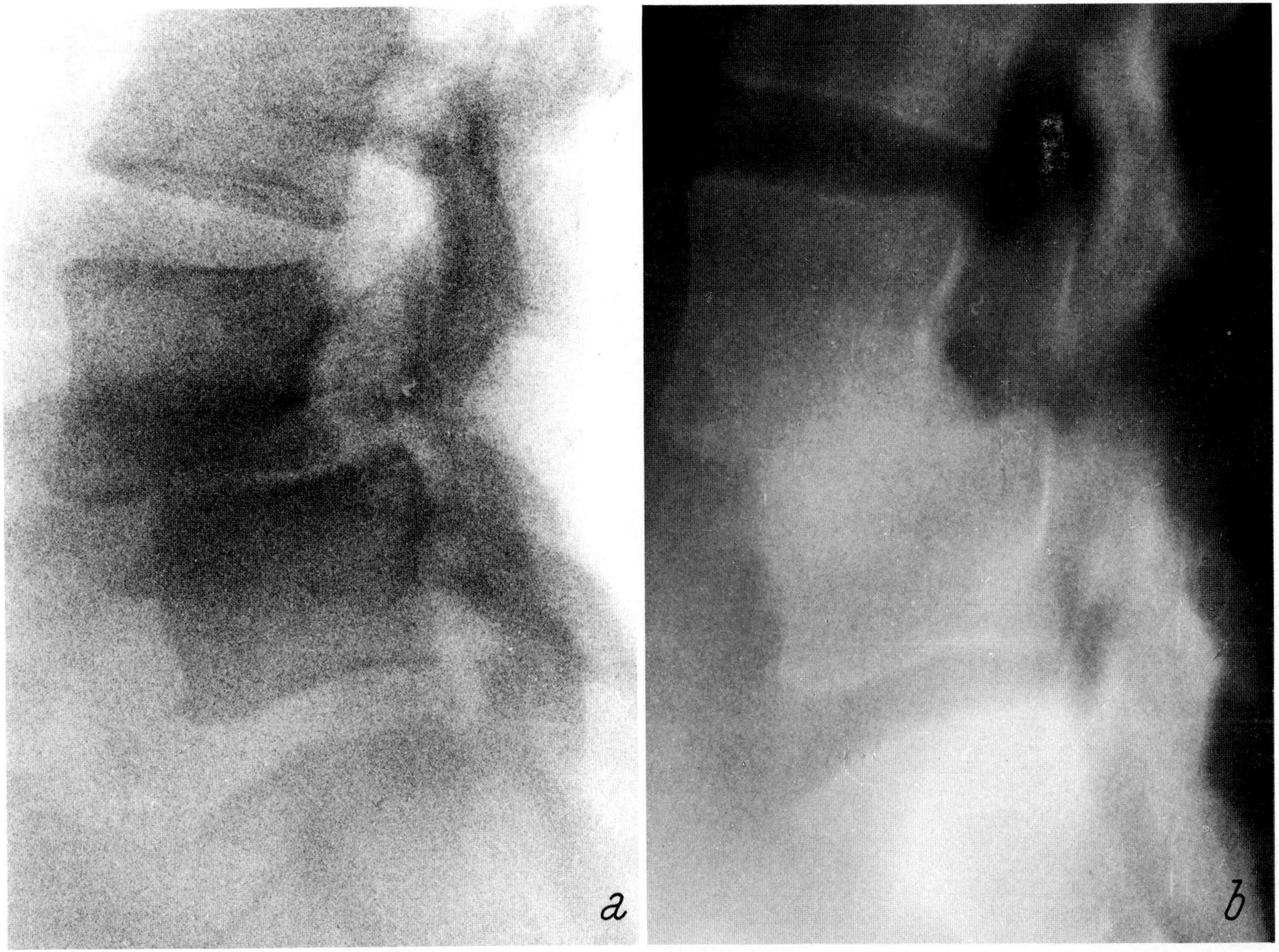

Figures 5.7. **a** A lateral radiograph of the lumbar spine in a 45 year-old man showing Grade 2 spondylolisthesis at L 4/5. **b** Interbody grafts have been inserted transversely. The tomogram shows the appearance one year after operation

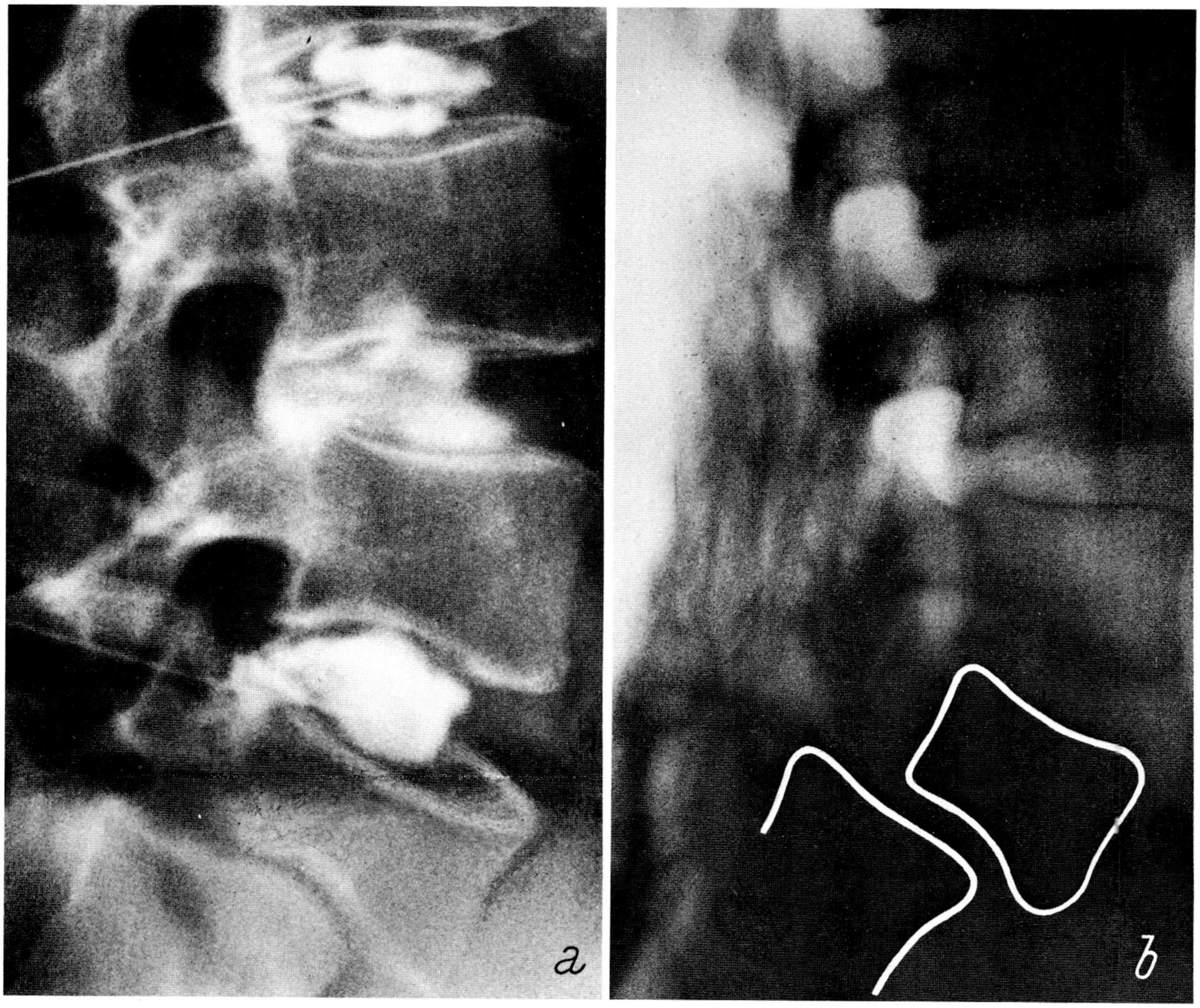

Figures 5.8. a A lateral radiograph of the lumbar spine of a man aged 45, showing Grade 2 spondylolisthesis at L5/S1, with discograms at L2/3, L3/4 and L4/5. Post-traumatic disc disruptions are shown at each level, causing severe back pain. The patient had fallen from a height of 25 feet (8 metres). **b** A lateral tomogram of the same patient's spine taken 9 months after an extensive multi-level posterior spinal fusion, which was planned after the discography shown in Fig. 5.8a

disruptive disc lesions demonstrated by discography above the level of the spondylolisthesis may help in planning the extent of a spinal fusion procedure (Figs. 5.8a, b).

Finally, in assessing the state of the discs in cases of spondylolisthesis where unilateral sciatica is a problem, *lumbar myelography* is essential to exclude the diagnosis of disc prolapse, either at the level of the vertebral slip, or at some adjacent disc space.

iii) Shape of Spinal Canal

The third parameter to be considered is the shape of the spinal canal. When a patient with spondylolisthesis is found to have laminal abnormalities, then again,

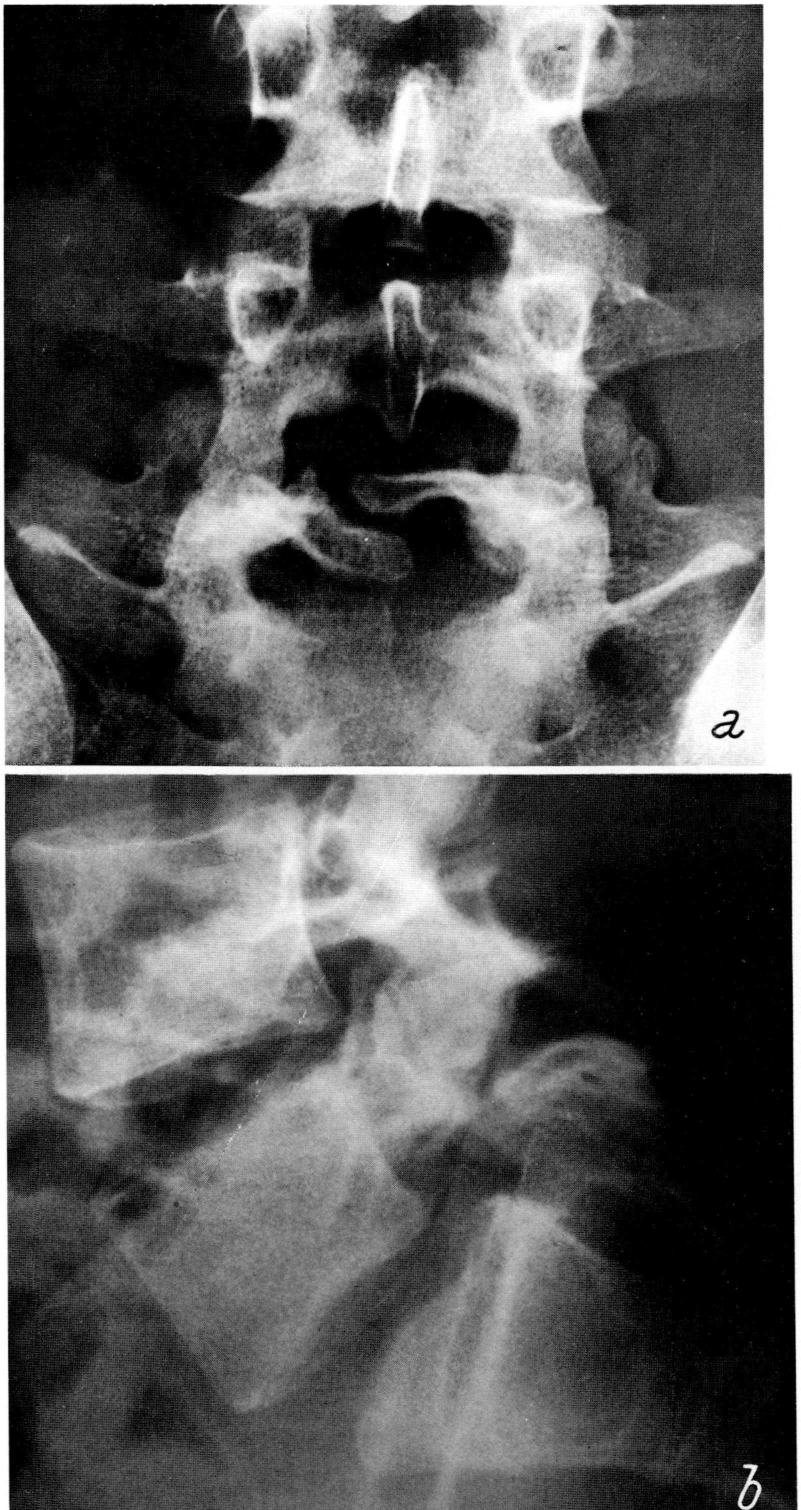

Figures 5.9 a and **b.** Antero-posterior and lateral radiographs of the lower lumbar spine in a 21 year-old male with Grade 1 spondylolisthesis. Spondylolytic defects are visible at L5/S1 but the lamina is grossly abnormal with spina bifida occulta. In such patients, if surgery is contemplated, myelography is essential

myelography is essential if the symptoms include referred leg pain (Figs. 5.9a, b). In such cases, associated spinal canal stenosis may be found. Spinal fusion alone may then be contraindicated, concomitant decompression of the spinal canal being necessary.

iv) Degree of Vertebral Slip

The fourth parameter for consideration is the degree of vertebral slip. Increase in the degree of slip usually occurs gradually over a number of years, often in association with progressive narrowing of the related intervertebral disc (Figs. 5.10a, b). In the

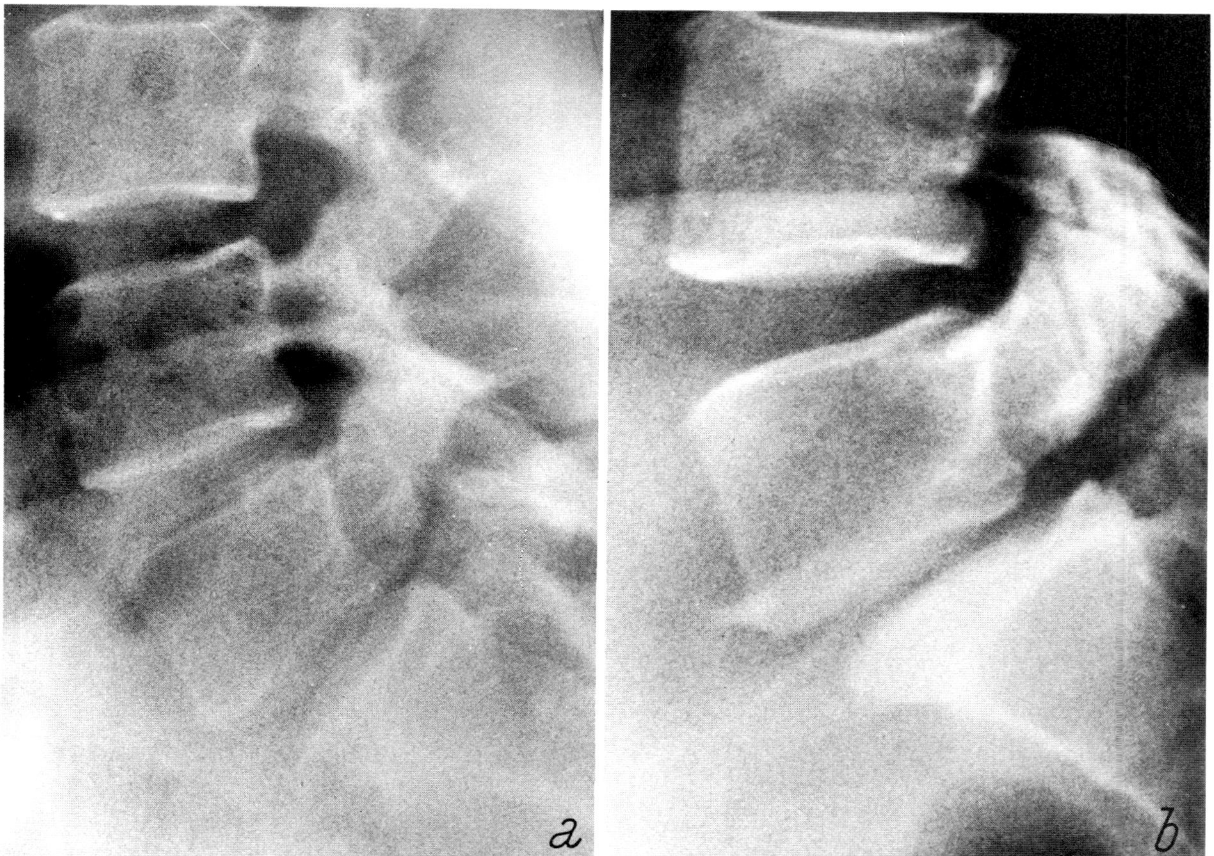

Figures 5.10a and **b.** Lateral radiographs of the lumbar spine in an adult showing in **(a)** spondylolytic spondylolisthesis Grade 1 at L5/S1 with a normal intervertebral disc. The same spine five years later **(b)** showing disc resorption and increase in slip to Grade 2

presence of grade one or grade two spondylolisthesis, anterior interbody fusion may be satisfactory. However, this method should be reserved for thin patients who have had neither previous abdominal surgery, nor antecedent history of venous thrombosis. For cases with higher grades of slip, in which spinal fusion is being considered, standard methods of posterior fusion or inter-transverse-alar fusion may be considered. Freebody (1971) has described a method for anterior lumbar interbody fusion applicable even in advanced grades of spondylolisthesis. This

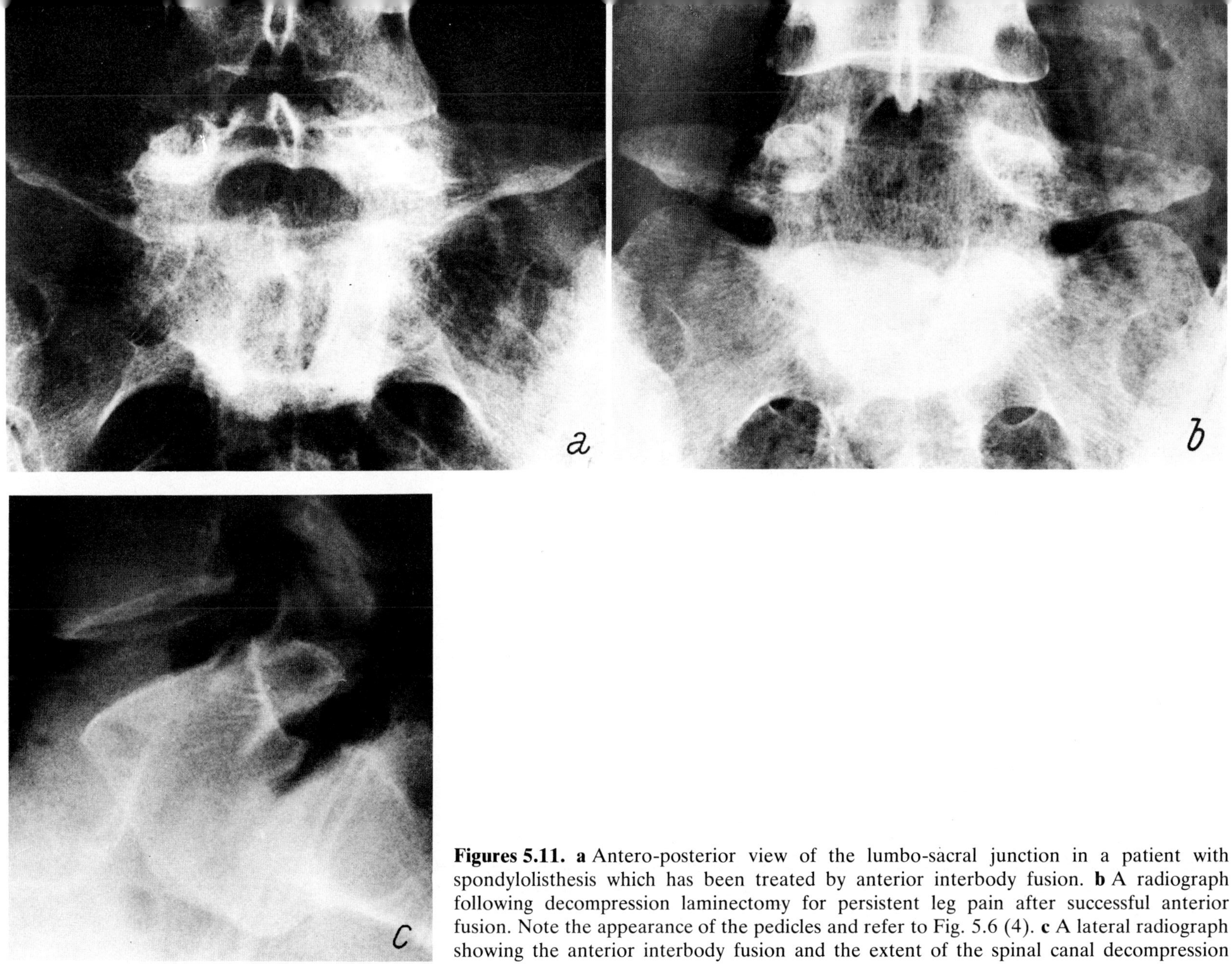

Figures 5.11. **a** Antero-posterior view of the lumbo-sacral junction in a patient with spondylolisthesis which has been treated by anterior interbody fusion. **b** A radiograph following decompression laminectomy for persistent leg pain after successful anterior fusion. Note the appearance of the pedicles and refer to Fig. 5.6 (4). **c** A lateral radiograph showing the anterior interbody fusion and the extent of the spinal canal decompression

method calls for special training and even then its success rests on the surgeon having above-average skill.

In recent years, attempts have been made to reduce higher grades of slip, either by manipulation under anaesthesia or by the use of femoral traction. Once reduced, anterior interbody fusion may be used, supplemented by one of a variety of devices now available for fixation, such as the plate and screws designed by Professor Louis of Marseilles, France. These manoeuvres are mentioned for the sake of completing the record of surgical measures in current use. If they are to be used at all, then *the considerable attendant risk of these heroic efforts must be thoroughly appreciated,* with particular reference to cauda equina injuries.

By contrast Bohlman and Cook (1982) have reported success by combining spinal canal decompression and in-situ posterior interbody fusion, using fibular grafts in two cases of spondyloptosis.

In children, symptomatic spondylolisthesis may require surgical treatment and this should be undertaken early if there is any fear of increase in the degree of vertebral slip. Bilateral inter-transverse-alar fusion is usually effective.

The operation for the removal of the "rattler" and decompression of the nerve root canals recommended by Gill and White (1965) can be recommended for use in adults whose symptoms are predominantly those of referred leg pain, which is usually bilateral. Following the Gill and White operation, some increase in vertebral slip may occur in a few patients. However, if back pain persists as a major problem, then spinal fusion may be required. The choice of method, be it inter-transverse-alar or anterior interbody fusion, will depend on the particular skills and preferences of the surgeon, bearing in mind that either method applied to this particular problem requires special training.

While theoretically it may be desirable to perform spinal fusion and spinal canal and foraminal decompression operations simultaneously, this is not always possible. Furthermore, if the cases have been selected for surgical procedures according to the recommendations set out above, the results are usually good and the combined operations are then unnecessary.

There will be a few patients who may continue to complain of referred leg pain after successful spinal fusion and, conversely, a few who will complain of back pain after relief of their leg pain (following spinal canal and foraminal decompression). These patients will require relevant secondary operations (Figs. 5.11a–c).

The choice of treatment in patients with symptomatic degenerative spondylolisthesis follows the same general lines outlined above. However, in this condition, spinal fusion alone is usually the operation of choice.

5.2. Technique of Postero-Lateral Inter-Transverse-Alar Spinal Fusion

a) Indications

This operation has virtually replaced the older methods of posterior spinal fusion introduced by Hibbs and Albee earlier this century, along with many variants such as "H" grafts and screw fixation with facet grafts.

When the transverse processes are sturdy this method of spinal fusion can be recommended for the treatment of:

1. spondylolisthesis, especially in children;
2. lumbar spondylosis causing back pain;
3. failed anterior interbody fusions.

b) Preliminary Preparation

Blood loss is often considerable so that transfusion facilities with three or four litres of blood must be available.

The patient's spinal X-rays must be displayed in the operating room.

c) Positioning

Patients should be placed prone on a suitable frame to avoid compression of the abdominal cavity (see pp. 106–107).

d) Incisions

In children a long mid-line incision is recommended, extending from L2 to the lower sacrum.

In adults, the laterally placed, parallel vertical incisions advocated by Wiltse (1978) are recommended (Figs. 5.12a–c).

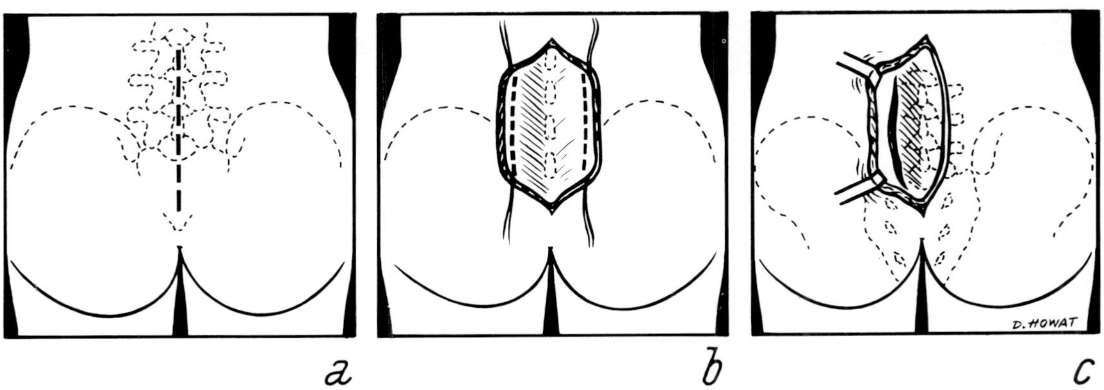

Figures 5.12a–c. Drawings to illustrate the mid-line skin incision and the laterally placed incisions in the lumbo-dorsal fascia for the paraspinal sacro-spinalis splitting approach recommended by Wiltse

e) Exposure of the Graft Bed

If the mid-line incision is used, the paraspinal muscles are separated as described on pp. 110–113. Their dissection is carried laterally beyond the facet joints until the posterior surfaces of the transverse processes and the alae of the sacrum on both sides can be palpated. The bulky paraspinal muscle mass is then retracted backwards and laterally to the level of the tips of the transverse processes. Blood loss is

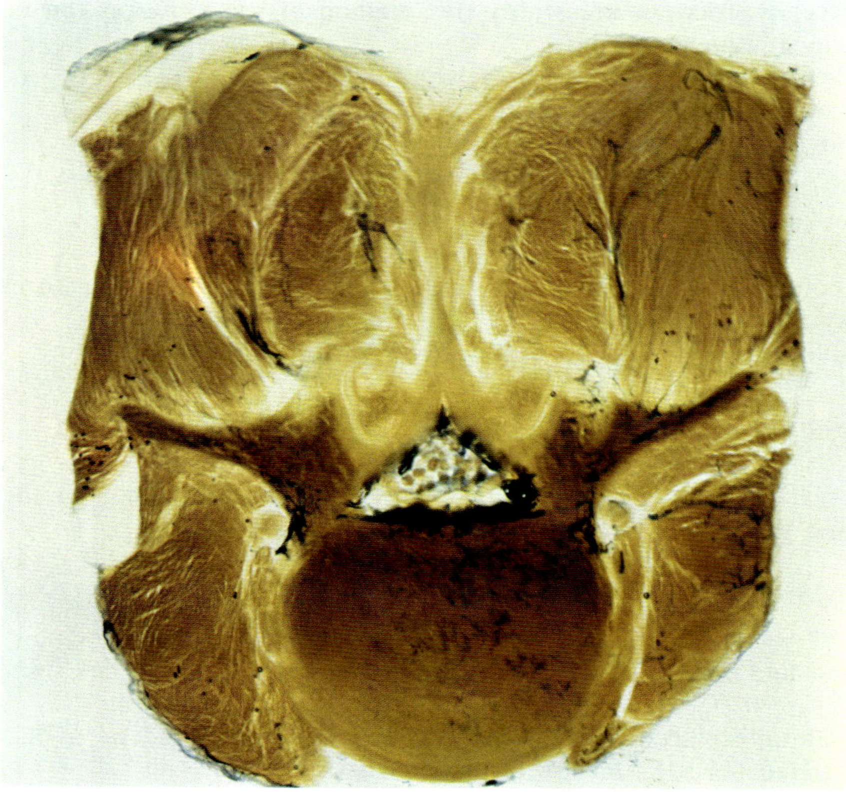

Figure 5.13. A photograph of a transverse section of a mid-lumbar vertebra, with the paraspinal muscles intact. The specimen has been cleared by the Spalteholz technique. Note the arrangements of the paraspinal muscles posteriorly, with a plane of cleavage clearly visible between the muscle bundles related to the posterior aspects of the transverse processes at their junctions with the superior articular facets. This is the plane of cleavage recommended for use in inter-transverse-alar fusions by Dr. L. Wiltse of Long Beach, California

considerable during this stage of the operation and it is often difficult to see the transverse processes of L5 in the depth of the wound unless the paraspinal muscles have been separated from as high as the lamina of L2.

Using the lateral paraspinal muscle splitting incision of Wiltse (1978), less extensive longitudinal dissection of these muscles is required to gain good exposure of the bony structures to be "fused". Modified Gelpi retractors inserted between the separated muscle fibres aid in obtaining a clear view (Fig. 5.13).

Figures 5.14. a A drawing of the lower lumbar spine seen from behind to show the intertransverse ligaments between L4, L5 and S1. On the right side note the preparation of the graft bed for an inter-transverse-alar fusion. The arrow indicates an upturned segment of bone cut from the ala of the sacrum and turned up towards the transverse process of L5. **b** A drawing to depict the preparation of the graft bed for an inter-transverse-alar fusion. Note the use of a curette to roughen the surface of the outer aspect of the superior facet of L5, leaving intact the capsule of the joint at that level. A chisel is shown turning up the flap of cortico-cancellous bone from the ala of the sacrum towards the transverse process of L5. **c** A photograph of a dissection of the lumbar spine viewed from the side, to show the siting of intertransverse grafts in relation to the spine as a whole (see arrows)

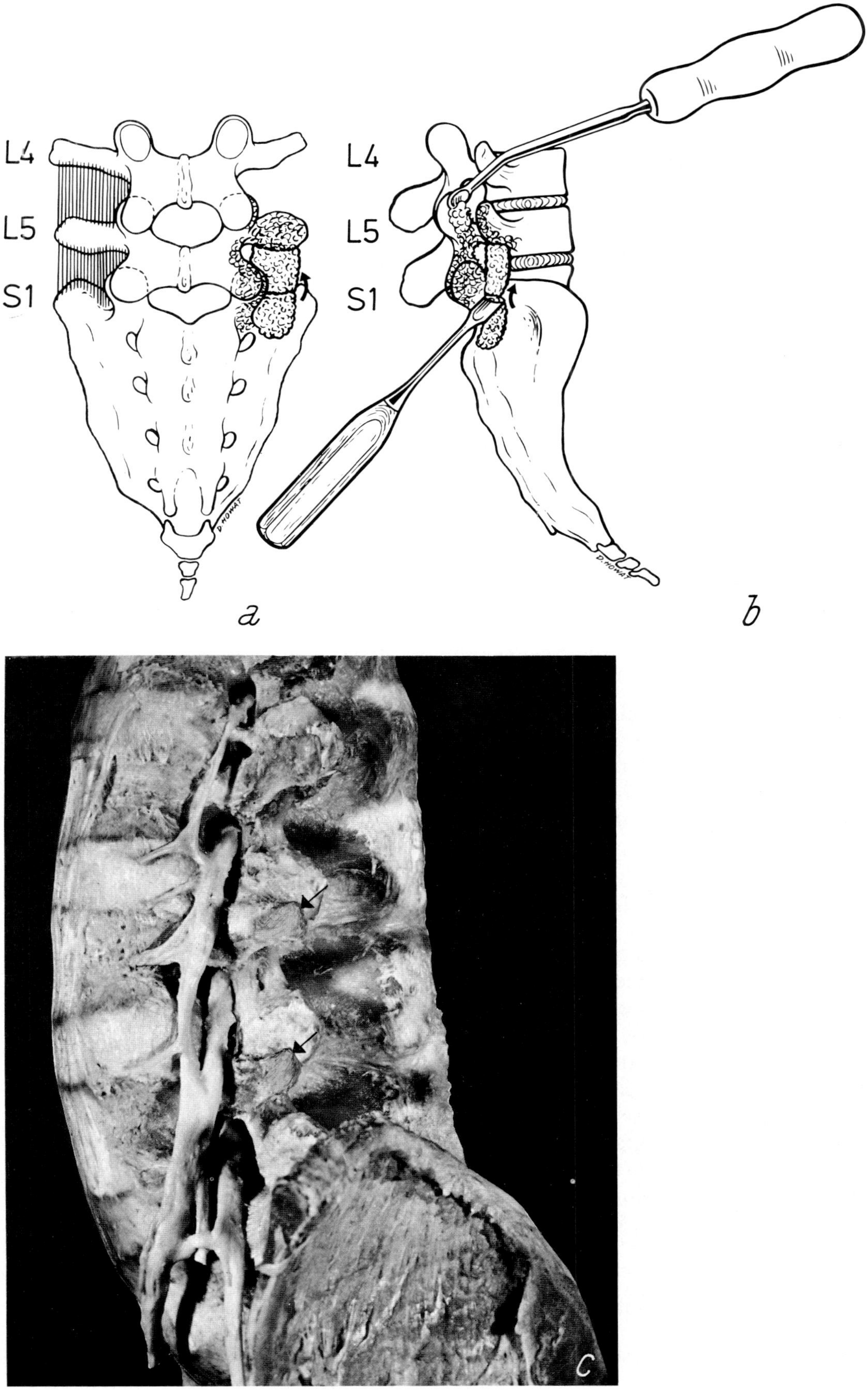

Figures 5.14

Preparation of the bed for the graft requires meticulous attention to detail. The intertransverse ligaments and muscles should be preserved. *For fusions at L5/S1 level* the capsules of the lumbo-sacral facet joints should be excised allowing access to the joint surfaces for excision of their articular cartilages and sub-chondral bone plates. The facet joint capsules between the superior facets of L5 and the inferior facets of L4 should be preserved intact. All remnants of soft tissues must be removed from the sacral alae, from the inferior facets of L5, from the lateral aspects of the partes interarticulares on both sides cephalad to the outer aspects of the superior facets of L5, from the outer aspects of the pedicles of L5 and the posterior surfaces of the transverse processes of L5.

The exposed surfaces of the transverse processes of L5 should then be decorticated carefully, using a gouge and hammer or Leksell type rongeur. Then, with a stout curved curette the cortical bone on the outer sides of the L5 pedicles and superior facets of L5 should be broached to expose bleeding cancellous bone. The lateral aspect of the pars interarticularis of L5 lamina on both sides should also be roughened (Figs. 5.14a–c).

Cortico-cancellous flaps cut from the postero-superior surface of the alae of the sacrum on both sides should be turned upwards to lie on the intertransverse ligaments, adjacent to the transverse processes of L5.

f) Preparation of Graft Bone

Autogenous grafts should be cut from the postero-lateral aspect of the iliac crest, access to this being obtained usually by undercutting the tissues between the lumbo-dorsal fascia and the iliac crest on one side.

Thin strips of cortico-cancellous bone, with other slivers of cancellous bone can be obtained usually in sufficient bulk from one side of the pelvis.

g) Placement of the Grafts

Thin strips of cancellous graft should be packed into the facet joints of L5/S1–then other strips should be placed *accurately* along the length of the spine extending from the upper edges of the decorticated transverse processes, but below the level of the intertransverse ligaments, at the space immediately above the level to be "fused".

Cortico-cancellous strips–with the cortical surfaces directed outwards to lie facing the paraspinal muscles–should be packed in carefully at the conclusion of this stage of the operation (Figs. 5.15, 5.16).

After placing the graft chips with equal care on both sides of the spine, the wounds should be closed with suction drainage. Where multi-level fusions have been performed, some surgeons have used screw fixation of the facet joints to aid in stability until fusion has occurred (Fig. 5.17).

Figure 5.15. A drawing depicting the inter-transverse-alar graft mass on the left side

Figure 5.16. An antero-posterior tomogram showing satisfactory intertransverse grafts at L4/5 in a patient with sacralization of the last lumbar vertebra. (Mr. Chris Haw's case)

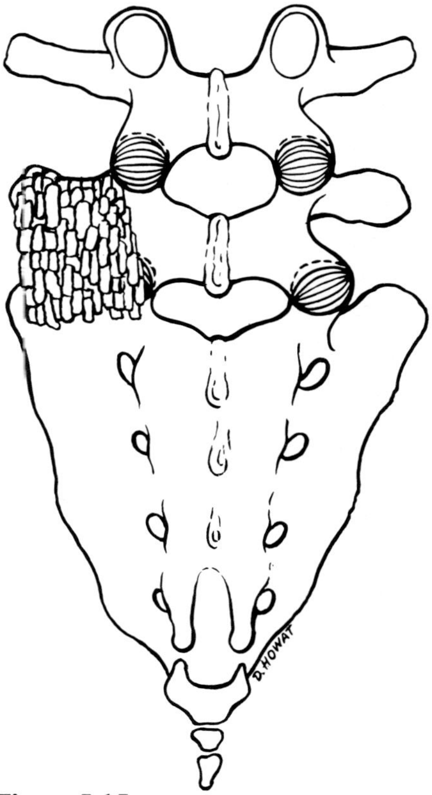

Figure 5.15

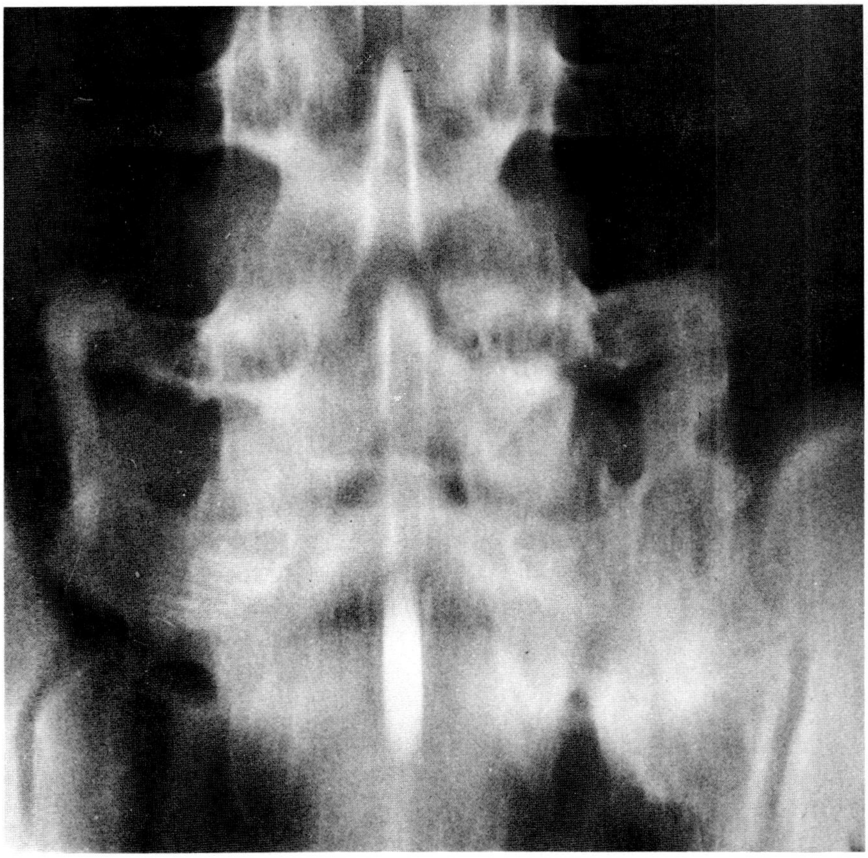

Figure 5.16

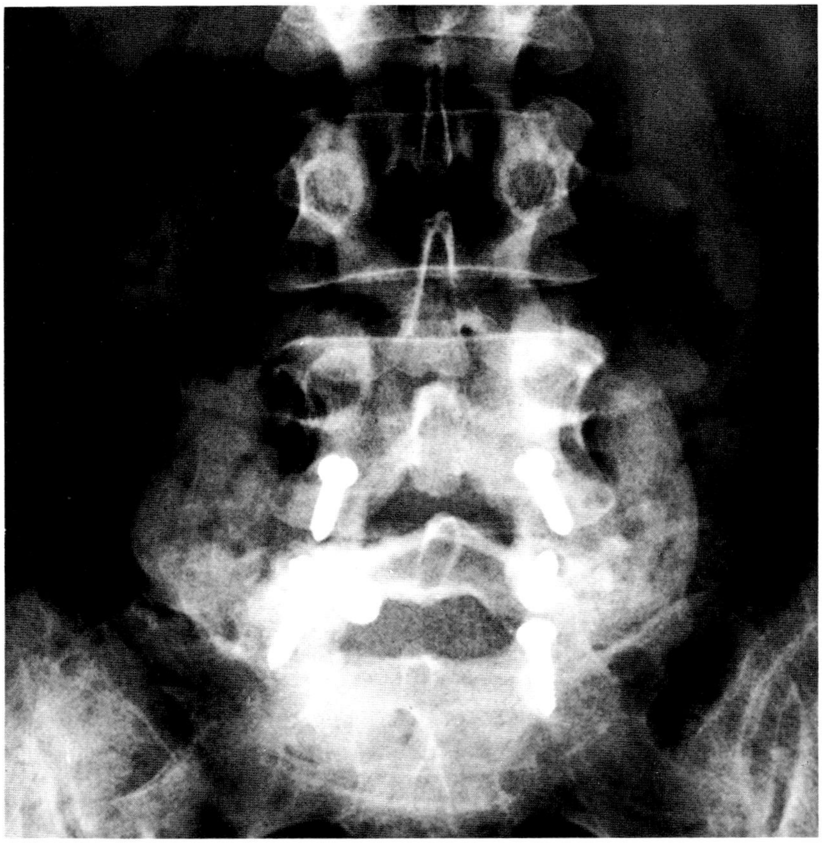

Figure 5.17. An antero-posterior radiograph of the lower lumbar spine showing a multi-level inter-transverse-alar fusion with supplementary screw fixation of the facets in the fused area. (Mr. John Cloke's case)

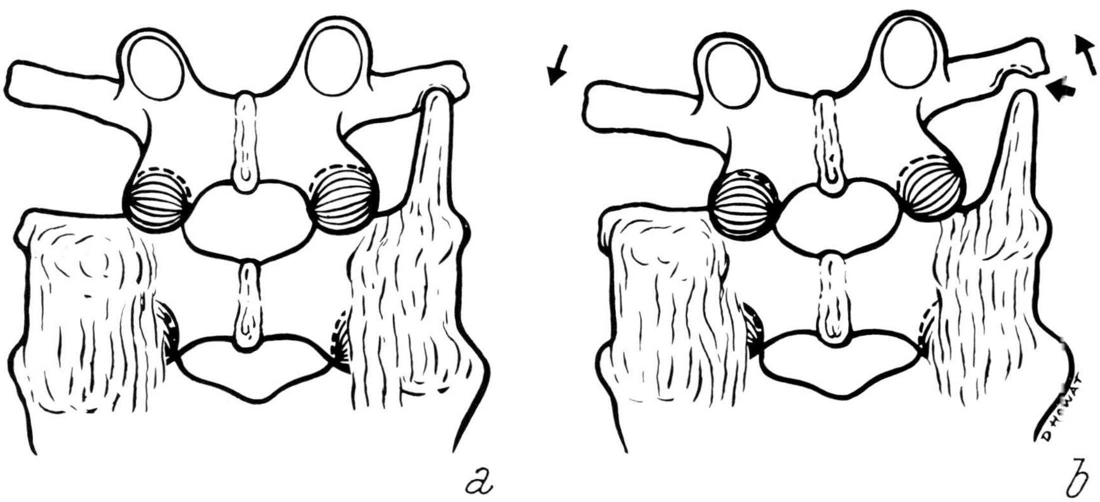

Figures 5.18 a and **b.** A drawing showing inter-transverse-alar grafts with an "unwanted segment" of graft extending up on the right side producing a pseudarthrosis between the tip of the grafted bone and the transverse process, visible when the patient flexes to the side. This is a cause of local chronic back pain easily relieved by excision of the "unwanted segment" of graft

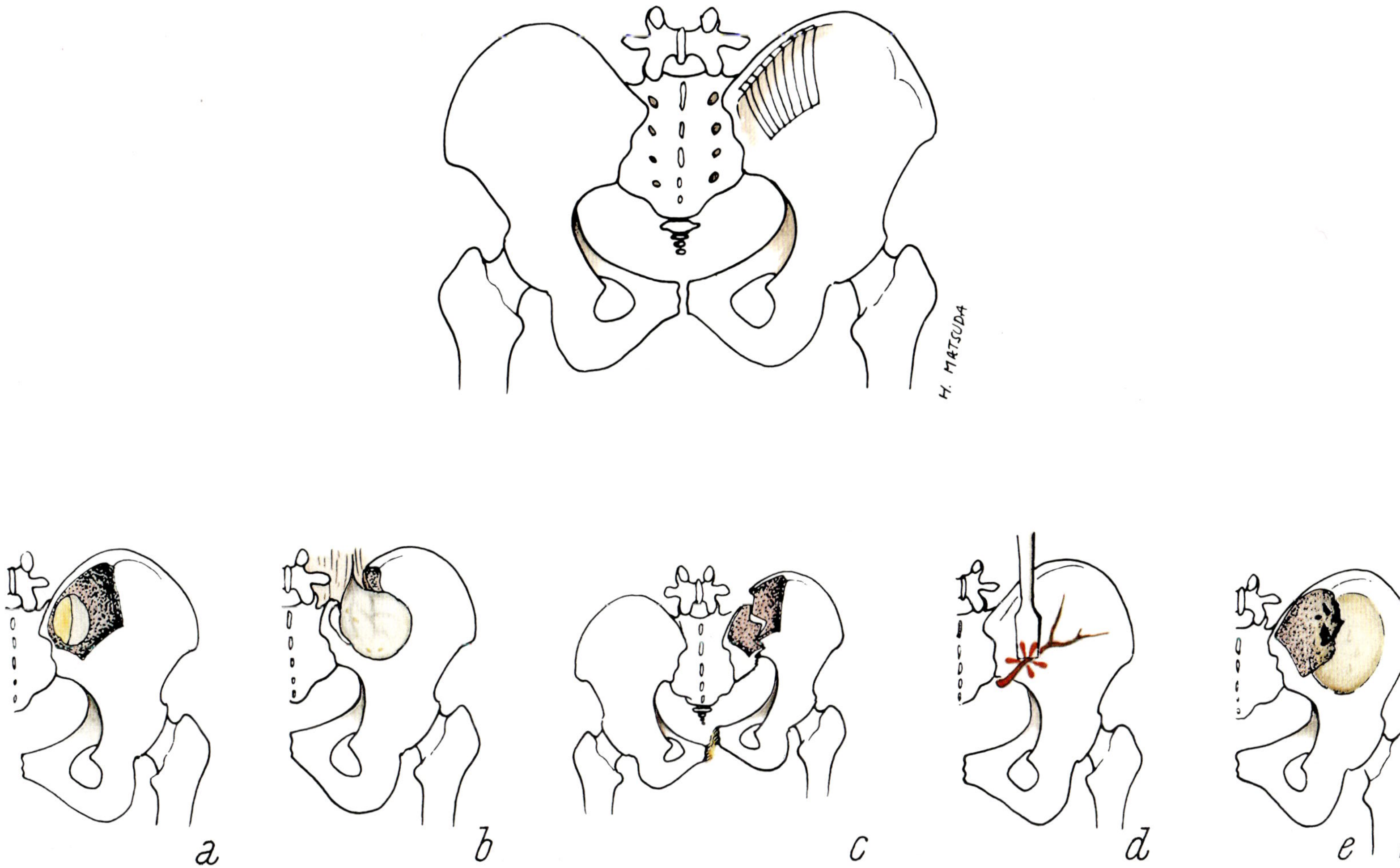

Figures 5.19 a – e. Drawings depicting the potential hazards at the donor site after removing cortico-cancellous grafts from the posterior third of the iliac crest. **a** Shows penetration of the sacro-iliac joint. **b** Lumbar hernia. **c** Dislocation of the sacro-iliac joint and symphysis pubis. **d** Potential for haemorrhage from the superior gluteal artery. **e** Gross local sepsis

h) Post-Operative Care

Retention of urine is common and it should be managed as recommended on p. 82. The use of catheters is best avoided.

Following multi-level spinal fusions, wearing of surgical corsets or braces is recommended. Patients are encouraged to get out of bed early and to walk short distances within a few days of their operation.

i) Complications

Unless this operation is performed with the attention to detail outlined above, failure rates from non-union will be high. In cases of failure, when examining X-rays taken months after operation, it is often difficult to identify any grafted bone on one or other side of the spine. Conversely, in some cases, segments of "unwanted graft" may impinge on adjacent mobile segments of the posterior elements of the spine–often far removed from the site of the primary pathology, causing chronic back pain (Figs. 5.18a, b).

If grafted bone breaches the intertransverse muscles and ligaments, it may hypertrophy, producing nerve root irritation and foraminal stenosis. This problem has been recognized by Kirkaldy-Willis (1980) in C.T. Scans of the lumbar spine taken after inter-transverse-alar fusion operations.

j) Infections

See pp. 240, 241.

k) Graft Site Problems

Wiltse (1978) has warned of the risk of damaging cuneal nerves as they cross the posterior iliac crest, leading to chronic pain at the donor site.

Major complications may occur during or after the removal of large quantities of bone from the region of the posterior ilium. Attention should be focussed on the potential problems of severe haemorrhage during graft removal, sacro-iliac joint injury, lumbar hernia formation, pelvic dislocation and deep-seated infection of the pelvic bones (Figs. 5.19a–e).

5.3. Spinal Canal and Nerve Root Canal Decompression With Foraminal Enlargement

After the initial exposure of the affected area of the spine (pp. 110–113), the interspinous ligaments should be excised from the superior and inferior aspects of the spinous process of the "rattler"–that hyper-mobile segment of the roof of the spinal canal found in spondylolysis and spondylolytic spondylolisthesis which consists of the spinous process, the inferior articular facets and the lamina, split across its pars interarticularis on both sides and carrying the two distal surfaces of the pseudarthroses. The false joint capsules of these pseudarthroses, along with any loose bodies from within them, should then be removed with straight pituitary rongeurs. If the pseudarthroses have complex bulky opposing bony surfaces, it will not be possible to remove the "rattler" intact after excising the ligamentum flavum from both its superior margin and anterior surface. In such cases, the lamina is best divided along one side of the spinous process with a forward-angled rongeur. The spinous process is then grasped with a large bone nibbler and with the dura under constant vision, one half of the "rattler" may be rotated carefully and twisted slowly until it separates from the deep soft tissues which bind it to the proximal portion of the pseudarthrosis. The opposite segment of the "rattler" is then removed in like manner. This done, assuming that it is the L5 lamina which has been removed, the L5 nerve roots on both sides remain obstructed by the proximal portions of the laminal pseudarthroses and their soft tissue coverings. Removal of all these tissues on both sides is necessary to leave the pedicles of L5 clearly defined, the L5 nerve roots decompressed and the joints between the superior facets of L5 and the inferior facets of L4 essentially intact (Figs. 5.6, 3, 4).

5.4. Direct Repair of the Bony Defects in Spondylolysis and Spondylolisthesis

While the Gill and White procedure just described has been shown to give good long-term relief of leg pains in adults, there is a place for the conservation of the "rattler" in young patients in whom spinal fusion may be deemed unnecessary. Direct bone grafting of the laminal pseudarthroses, with internal fixation using screws, has been described by Buck (1979).

6

The Surgical Management of Spinal Canal Stenosis

6.1. Lumbar Canal Stenosis

The causes of spinal stenosis may be classified as follows:

1. Congenital Causes
   a) Achondroplasia and other forms of dwarfism.
   b) Congenital small spinal canal, with short vertebral pedicles.
   c) Hemi-vertebrae with lumbar scoliosis.
   d) Congenital cysts arising from the dura or arachnoid, in an otherwise normal spinal canal.

2. Acquired Causes
   a) Degenerative spondylosis, including degenerative spondylolisthesis.
   b) Vertebral fractures, post-traumatic or pathological.
   c) Spinal infections.
   d) Paget's disease.
   e) Following some spinal operations.

Radiographs have been chosen to illustrate some of the differences between cases of spinal stenosis of congenital and acquired origin (Figs. 6.1–6.5).

The experience of individual surgeons in treating cases of spinal canal stenosis due to different causes will vary, especially among those working in large cities where special units may be found, such as:

a centre for spinal injuries;
a cancer institute;
an unit for the study of dwarfism.

Since 1961, working in the orthopaedic department of a university teaching hospital with only a small children's section, my experience in treating cases with spinal stenosis of different causes has been as follows:

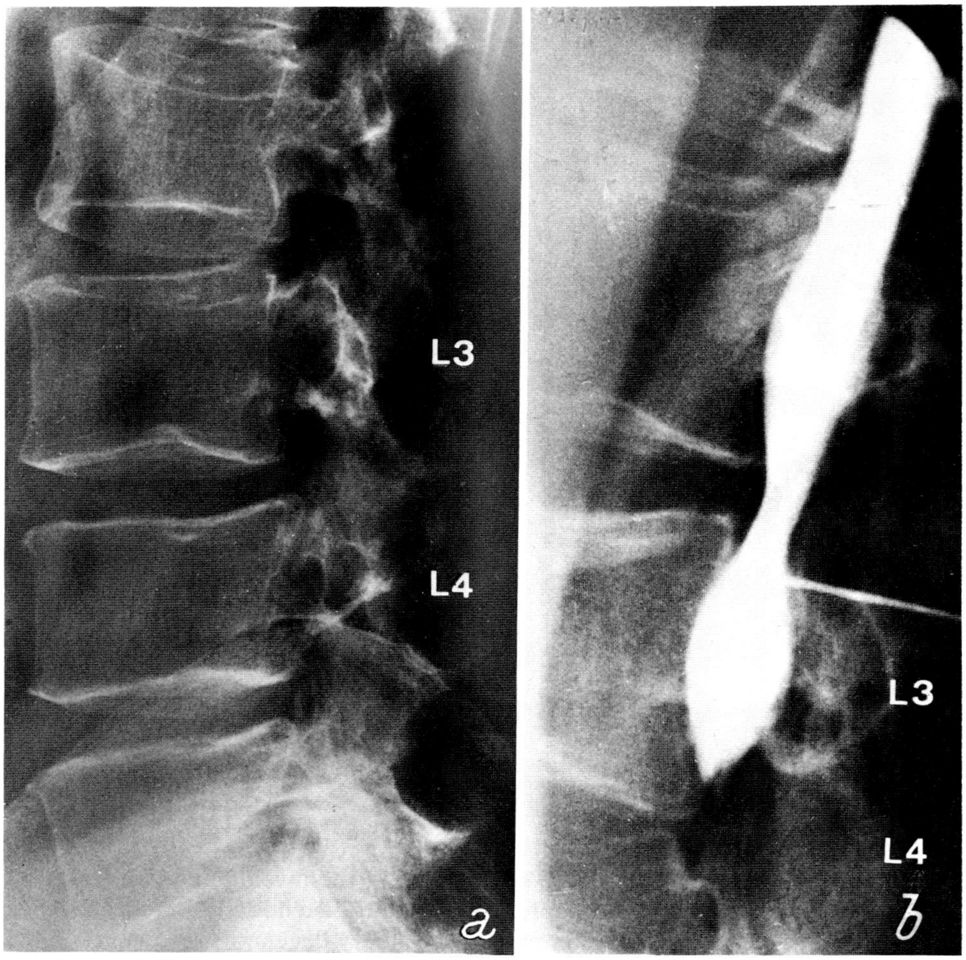

Figures 6.4. **a** A lateral radiograph of the lumbar spine of a male patient aged 58 years. Note the preservation of the disc spaces and there is no evidence of degenerative spondylosis. *The pedicles of L3 and L4 appear short.* **b** A lateral radiograph of the same spine showing a myelogram with complete spindling and obstruction of the column at the L3/4 level. This appearance is typical of spinal canal stenosis at a single level

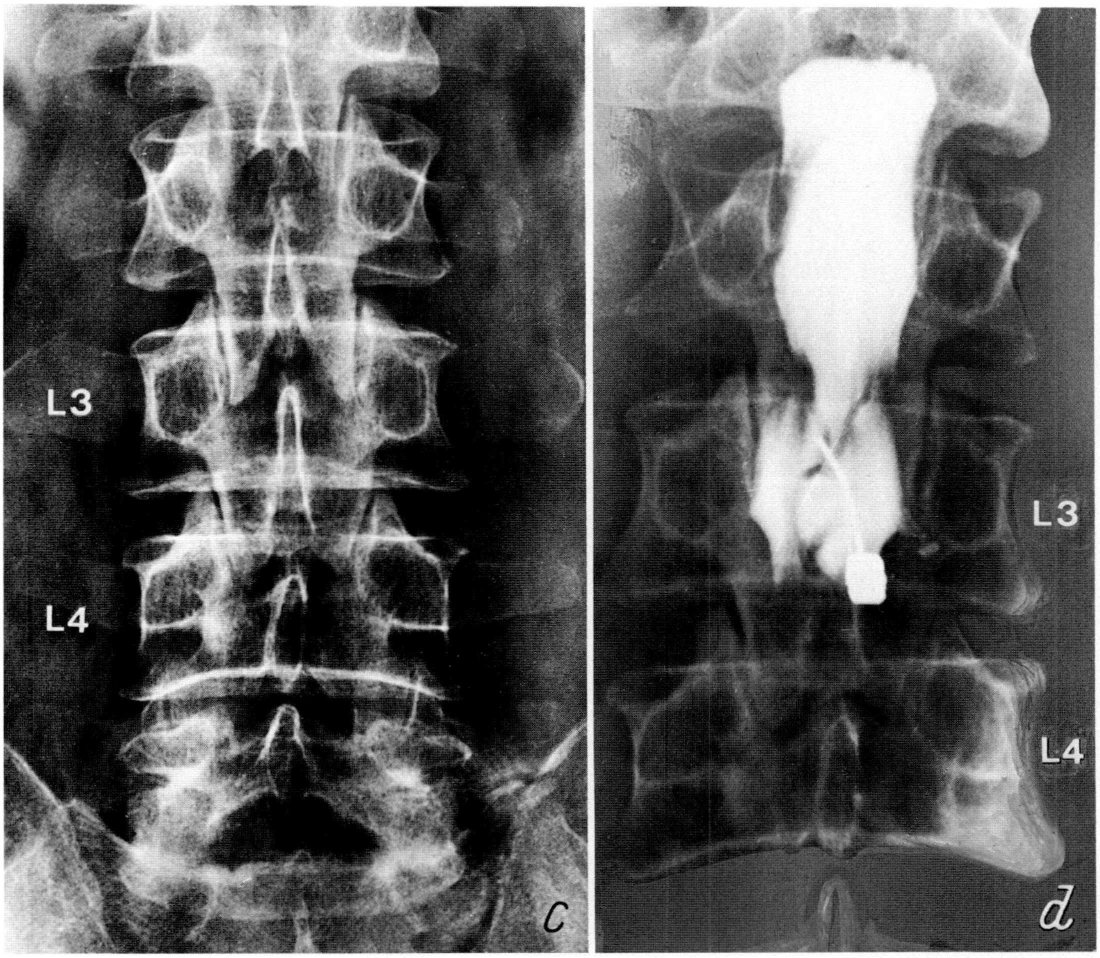

Figures 6.4. c An antero-posterior radiograph of the same spine. Note the orientation of the facets of L3/4. These are vertically orientated so that the medial margins of the inferior facets of the L3 lamina approach the mid-line in contrast to the normal anatomical arrangements seen in Fig. 6.9. **d** An antero-posterior radiograph showing the myelographic appearance in this patient with complete obstruction to the flow of Myodil at the L3/4 level. This patient presented with the classic clinical features of cauda equina claudication with pain and numbness in the legs and a sense of weakness after walking short distances

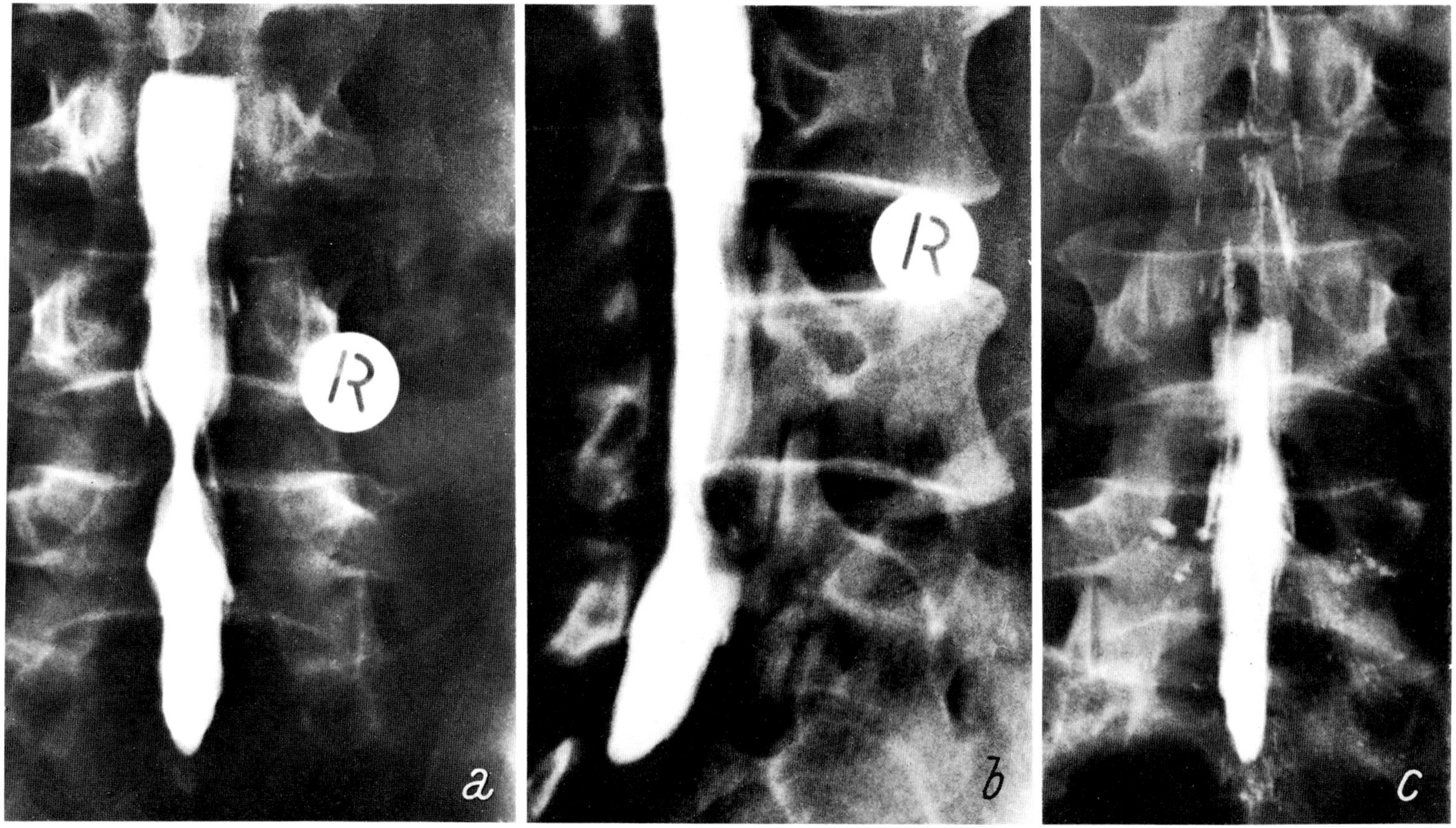

Figures 6.5. **a** An A-P radiograph of the lower lumbar spine of a man aged 55 years who presented with bilateral buttock and leg pain aggravated by walking and standing. The myelogram shows the classic appearance of spinal stenosis at the L4/5 level, the hour-glass deformity being due to *facet intrusions* on both sides, contributed to in part by a bulky ligamentum flavum. **b** An oblique view of the same spine showing the myelographic defect at L4/5 with the intimate relation of the inferior facet of the 4th lumbar lamina to the myelographic defect. Note that in both views of this patient's spine the intervertebral disc spaces are of normal height. **c** An antero-posterior radiograph of the same spine showing the post-operative appearance after a single level spinal canal and nerve root canal decompression. Residual myodil is present showing that the spindling defect is no longer present. The patient's symptoms were relieved and at follow-up ten years later he was symptom free

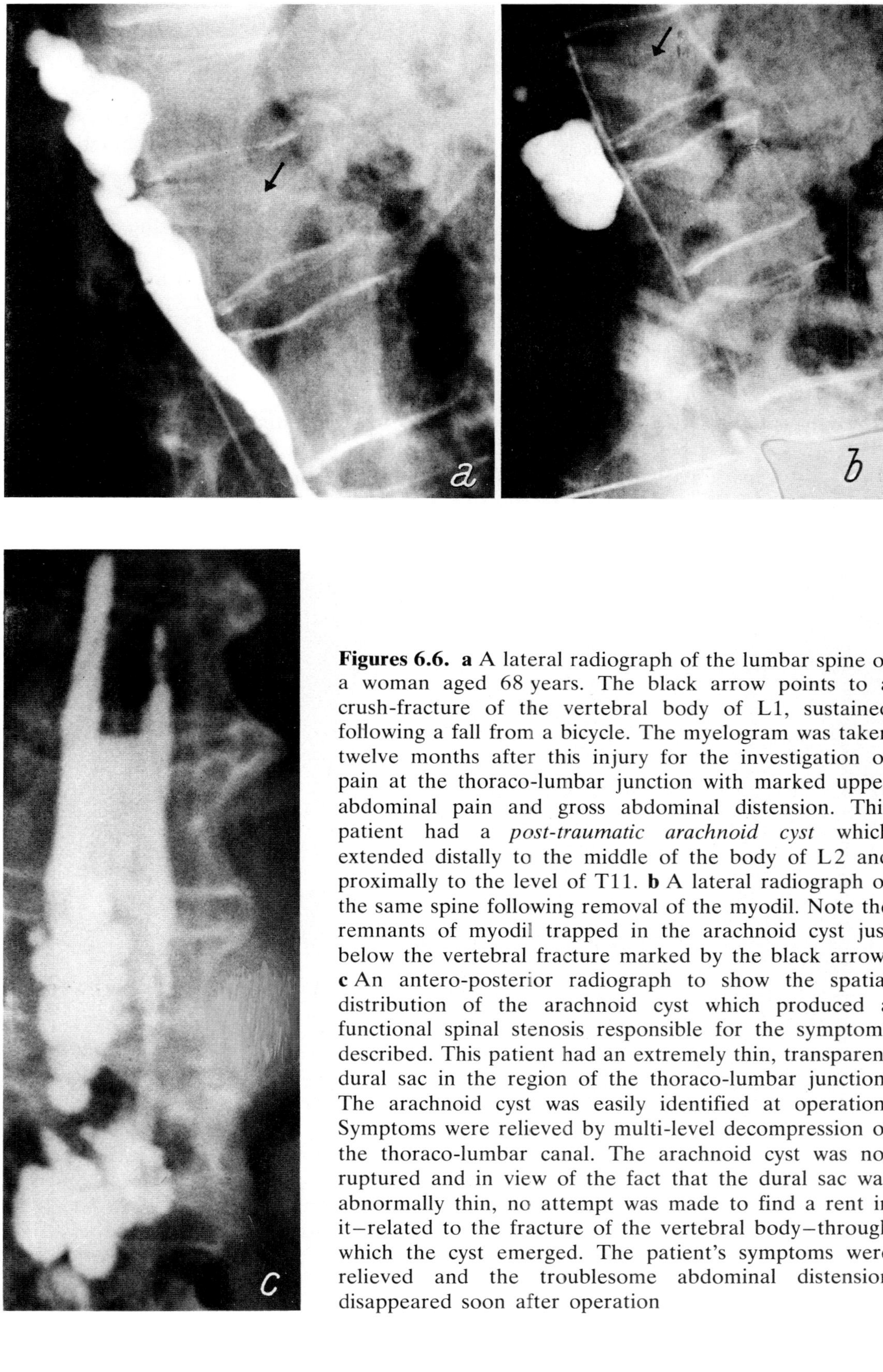

Figures 6.6. a A lateral radiograph of the lumbar spine of a woman aged 68 years. The black arrow points to a crush-fracture of the vertebral body of L1, sustained following a fall from a bicycle. The myelogram was taken twelve months after this injury for the investigation of pain at the thoraco-lumbar junction with marked upper abdominal pain and gross abdominal distension. This patient had a *post-traumatic arachnoid cyst* which extended distally to the middle of the body of L2 and proximally to the level of T11. **b** A lateral radiograph of the same spine following removal of the myodil. Note the remnants of myodil trapped in the arachnoid cyst just below the vertebral fracture marked by the black arrow. **c** An antero-posterior radiograph to show the spatial distribution of the arachnoid cyst which produced a functional spinal stenosis responsible for the symptoms described. This patient had an extremely thin, transparent dural sac in the region of the thoraco-lumbar junction. The arachnoid cyst was easily identified at operation. Symptoms were relieved by multi-level decompression of the thoraco-lumbar canal. The arachnoid cyst was not ruptured and in view of the fact that the dural sac was abnormally thin, no attempt was made to find a rent in it–related to the fracture of the vertebral body–through which the cyst emerged. The patient's symptoms were relieved and the troublesome abdominal distension disappeared soon after operation

a) Congenital

a) Two patients with dwarfism complained of symptoms suggestive of spinal stenosis. In one of these, an achondroplastic dwarf with a small lumbar canal, myelography was performed with only 1.5 mls. of myodil. Multi-level canal stenosis was demonstrated in the lumbar spine. The patient's symptoms subsided with rest. Neither of these patients required surgical treatment.

b) Ten adult patients. One presented with paraparesis.

c) Three adult patients, two of whom were elderly women. One man aged 34 years presented with cauda equina claudication and paraparesis.

d) Three adult patients; in one the cause of the arachnoid cyst may have been traumatic (Figs. 6.6a–c).

b) Acquired

a) Many patients, with wide-ranging symptoms of spinal stenosis were in this group. Their ages ranged between 55 and 75 years.

b) Five patients with stenosis following vertebral fractures. Two patients with stenosis following pathological fractures (Figs. 6.7a, b).

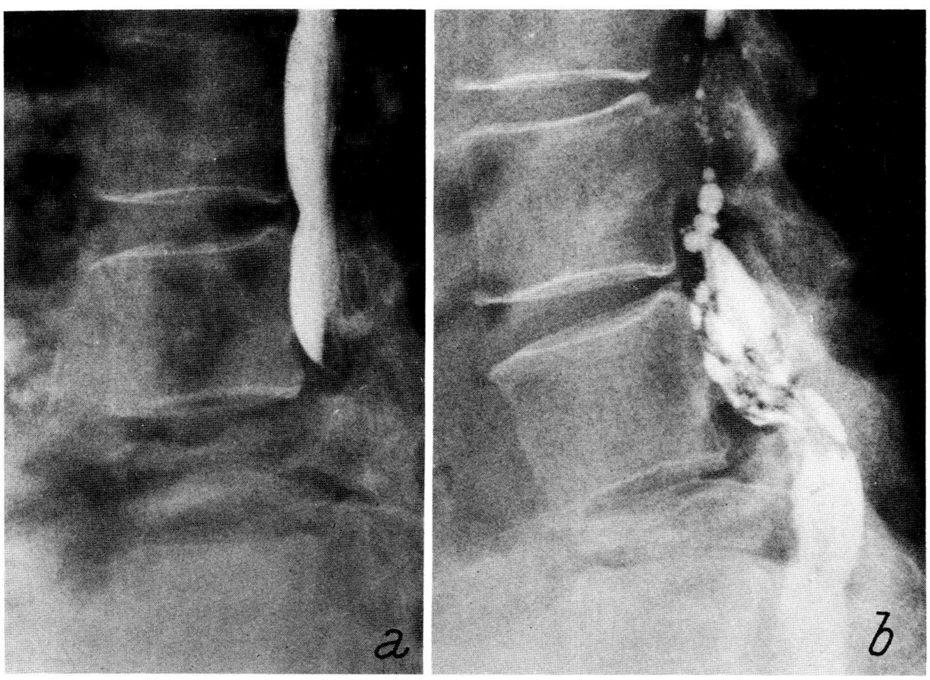

Figures 6.7. a A lateral radiograph of the lower lumbar spine of a woman aged 59 years showing complete obstruction to the flow of myodil in a myelogram at the level of L4, the site of a pathological fracture of the vertebral body due to a primary tumour of bone. **b** Following decompression of the lumbar spinal canal, note the restoration of the flow of myodil. The patient's symptoms of referred leg pain were relieved and she lived for approximately nine months after this film was taken, dying with secondary pulmonary tumours. The primary lesion was sarcomatous

c) Ten patients.

d) Although Paget's disease is common in Australia, I have never seen a case of spinal canal stenosis which resulted from it and required surgical treatment.

e) Many patients (see Chapter 9).

Although Sarpenyer described congenital stricture of the spinal canal in 1945, Verbiest (1954) deserves much of the credit for focussing attention on the various clinical syndromes associated with stenosis of the spinal canal. He, along with other members of the International Society for the Study of the Lumbar Spine: Kirkaldy-Willis, Paine, Cauchoix, and McIvor (1974), Verbiest (1976), Weinstein, Ehni, and Wilson (1977) has made scholarly contributions to medical literature on this subject.

6.2. Clinical Features

a) Symptoms

Most patients describe a variety of symptoms which may include:

a) Back pain,	often aggravated by standing or walking.
b) Leg pain,	of variable distribution, unilateral or bilateral, fluctuating.
c) Paraesthesiae,	ranging from feelings of numbness and heaviness, sometimes with an associated burning pain, sometimes with a feeling of coldness.
d) Weakness in the legs,	ranging from unilateral loss of power resulting in sudden falls to paraparesis, related to walking and relieved by rest.
e) Restless legs,	uncontrolled leg movements experienced especially at night in bed.
f) Disturbances of bladder function,	frequency or incontinence after walking.

Despite wide-ranging descriptions of symptoms, all of these patients complain of claudication, related either to their pain, paraesthesia, weakness or, occasionally, to all three symptoms together.

Intermittent claudication of vascular origin can usually be distinguished from cauda equina or nerve root claudication on clinical grounds. Pain in the legs of vascular origin is cramp-like and centres on the calf or buttock muscles. Impairment of arterial circulation is indicated by:

loss of hair on the legs;
absent peripheral pulses;
bruits along the course of the main arteries in the lower abdomen or at the groins.

b) Physical Signs

There are no characteristic findings. Signs vary depending on the underlying pathological condition causing the stenosis.

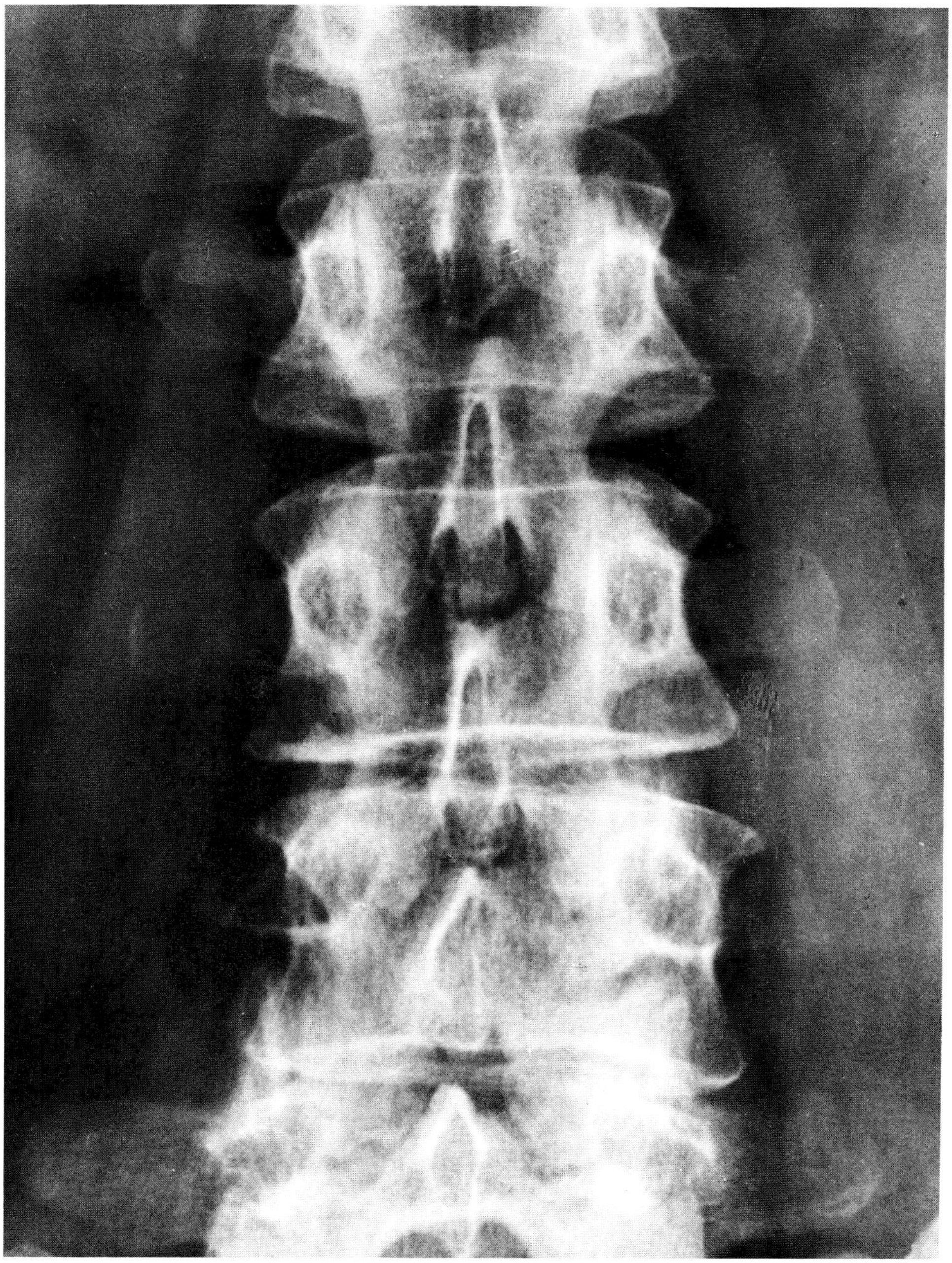

Figure 6.8. An antero-posterior radiograph of the lumbar spine in an adult in whom gross pathology is noted, particularly in the roof of the spinal canal. Although there is evidence of spondylosis at L3/4 with asymmetrical narrowing of the disc space, the major changes are in the laminal structures where facet hypertrophy, laminal thickening and spinous process interdigitation have reduced the interlaminar spaces at L2/3 and L3/4 to minute porportions

6.3. Radiological Investigations

a) Plain X-Rays

In congenital lumbar canal stenosis, certain findings can be important:

vertebral anomalies, with scoliosis;
narrowing of the diameter of the spinal canal, with short vertebral pedicles;
alterations in the pattern of orientation of facet joints.

In canal stenosis of degenerative origin the following findings can be important:

gross lumbar scoliosis, due to asymmetrical narrowing of the disc spaces or to acute necrosis of the vertebral end plate;
facet joint hypertrophy;
reduction in inter-laminar spaces and overriding of adjacent laminae (Figs. 6.8–6.10).

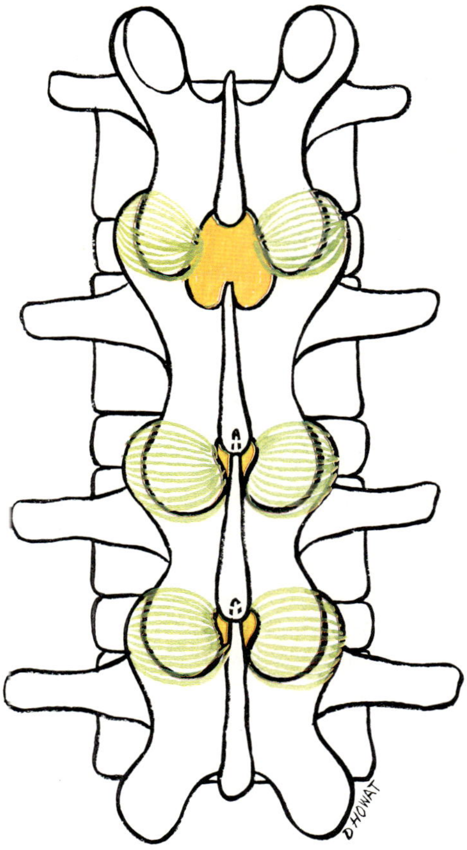

Figure 6.9. A drawing based on the X-ray shown in Fig. 6.8 to highlight the pathological changes which may occur in the roofing structures of the spinal canal leading to the development of multi-level canal stenosis. At the top of the drawing the ligamentum flavum is of normal proportions and there is wide separation between the medial margins of the capsules of the facet joints. In addition, the interspinous space is clearly defined. By contrast, at the lower two levels, note the interdigitation of the spinous processes, the hypertrophic changes in the facets and the almost complete occlusion from view of the ligamentum flavum at both these levels

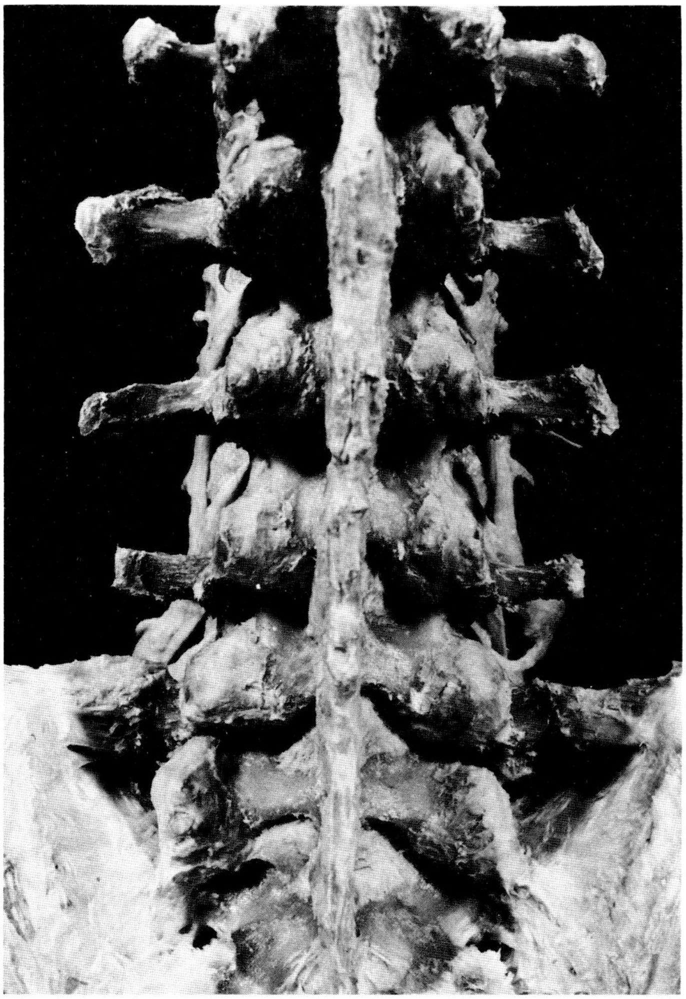

Figure 6.10. A photograph of a dissection of a normal lumbar spine viewed from behind. Note the orientation of the facet joints at L3/4, L4/5 and L5/S1. These are separated widely from the mid-line, so that the ligamentum flavum can be seen clearly at each level. Shadows are cast on the ligamentum flavum by the lower margins of the laminae, highlighting the anatomical feature of the superior attachment of the ligamentum flavum to the anterior surface of the superior lamina at a particular interspace. (Dissected by Dr. M. C. Crock)

Figures 6.11. **a** A lateral radiograph of the lumbar spine of a man aged 47 years presenting with classical symptoms of cauda equina claudication. Note the myelographic defect and the normal disc height at L4/5 and L5/S1. *This is an example of incomplete obstruction* and in such cases it is necessary to posture the patient at the time of myelography so that adequate studies of the flow of the dye can be obtained. What appears to be a complete obstruction may turn out to be incomplete if the patient is postured in the vertical or head down position. **b** An antero-posterior radiograph of the same spine showing the single level canal stenosis due to pathology in the roof of the spinal canal

Figures 6.12. **a** A lateral radiograph of the lumbar spine of a man aged 47 years showing the classical myelographic appearance of arachnoiditis of the cauda equina. **b** An antero-posterior radiograph of the same myelogram showing typical features of distortion of the column of dye due to arachnoiditis of the cauda equina (see Figs. 6.15a–c)

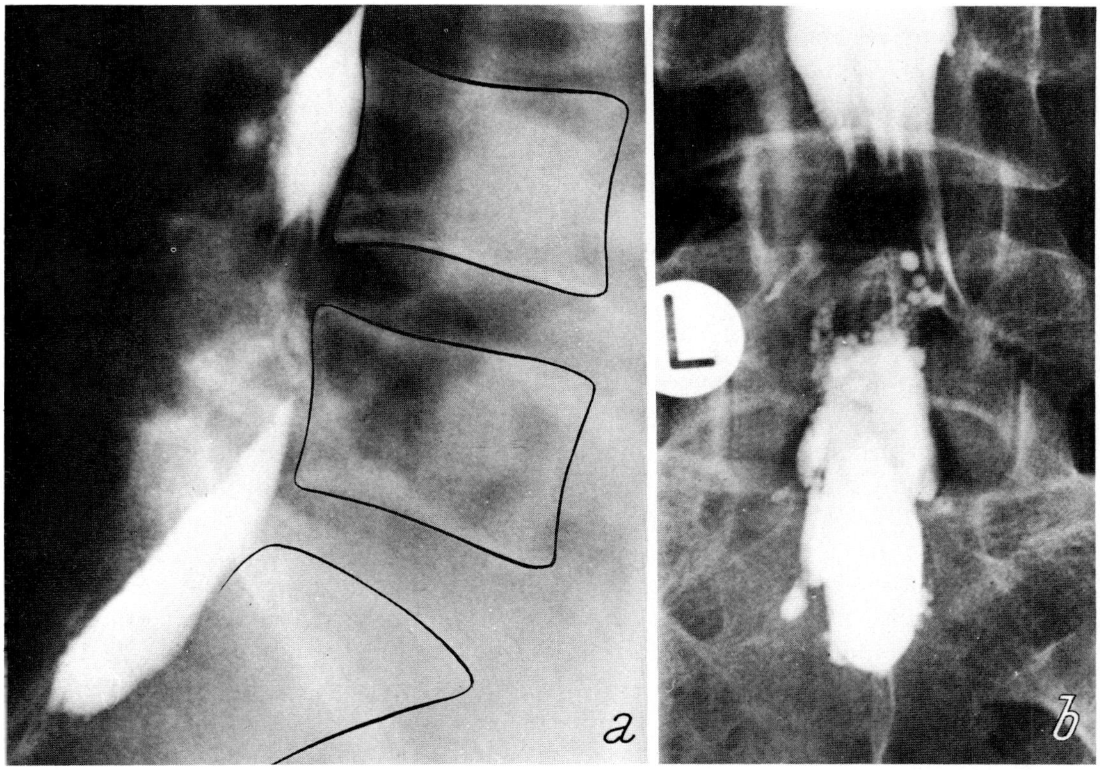

Figures 6.11

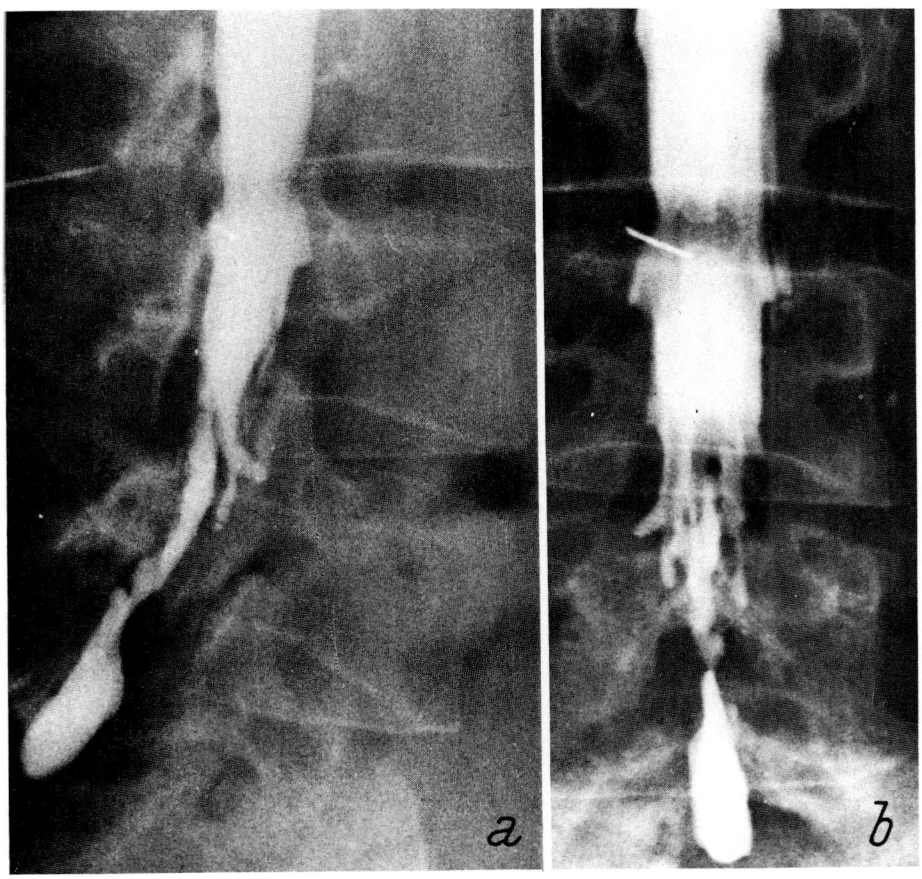

Figures 6.12

b) Computerized Axial Tomography

Although this investigation has revolutionized the investigation of spinal stenosis in the past few years, it has not superseded the use of either plain X-rays or myelograms (Lancourt *et al.*, 1979).

c) Lumbar Myelography

This investigation is the cornerstone for planning surgical treatment, being the most reliable method by which multi-level stenoses can be demonstrated. In addition, it can provide information about the nature and severity of pathological changes at or below the site of obstruction, providing the movement of dye in the spinal canal is studied carefully during myelography. For example, by tilting the patient into head-down or erect vertical positions, observing the flow of the dye with these changes in posture, distinctions can be drawn between complete and partial blockages, areas of arachnoiditis in the cauda equina can be identified and obstructions at multiple levels in the canal can be recognized (Figs. 6.11a, b, 6.12a, b).

6.4. Conservative Treatment

Conservative measures must always be tried. Many patients with disabling symptoms will improve following the use of spinal supports. Epidural injection of hydrocortisone may be useful, though if the patient's symptoms are made worse, this might indicate that the stenosis requires decompression.

6.5. Surgical Treatment

Elderly patients tolerate multi-level spinal canal decompressions satisfactorily. However, special care should be exercised in operating on older patients. Cardiac monitoring should be used during surgery. Blood loss can be considerable, up to 1,200 ml in cases requiring decompression over three or more segments. When anaesthetized, they should be turned slowly and with great care for positioning on the operating table.

a) Positioning

Use of the prone position on the operating table is essential, the chest and pelvis being supported on a suitable frame. Exaggerated postures should be avoided. The head and trunk should be kept almost horizontal, but the legs can be flexed slightly at the hips and knees (see Chapter 3, Figs. 3.8–3.11). Mental confusion due to cerebral oedema may occur in the post-operative period in elderly patients following operations performed under general anaesthesia in the prone position, if the table has been tilted towards the head-down position.

b) Surgical Pathology

In the *congenital group,* problems may arise simply because the spinal canal is too narrow, the structure and tissues of the vertebral column being otherwise normal. However, even in this group, the major complication of severe spinal stenosis may be found–arachnoiditis of the cauda equina.

In the *acquired group,* many pathological lesions will be found. The largest sub-group–(a)–provides the widest range of pathology, followed closely by patients in sub-group (e), many of whom may have been operated on in error, the underlying primary diagnosis of spinal stenosis having been overlooked.

Vertebral osteoporosis is often marked, the soft laminal bone being very vascular. *Laminar thickness* varies between 2.5–5.0 mm in the normal lumbar vertebrae. It may be increased to as much as 25.0 mm in some cases.

The normal *ligamentum flavum* is highly elastic, varying in thickness between 1.0 and 2.5 mms. Sometimes it is greatly thickened, retaining its elasticity. In other cases, while thicker than normal, it becomes inelastic and friable, with visible patches of ectopic calcification. Following spinal injuries, it may ossify.

Changes in the *facet joints* are common, with gangliform degeneration of joint capsules, hypertrophy of individual facets, osteophyte formation and intra-articular loose bodies.

Within the spinal canal, epidural fat may be absent in the stenotic area. The dural sac and contents show important changes; the dura may be thickened and opaque, or thin and extremely friable.

Arachnoiditis of the cauda equina may occur, identified on digital palpation of the dural sac at operation by loss of the normal soft balloon-like consistency, the affected segment being firm and rubbery to touch, like a par-boiled sausage.

Changes in the anterior wall of the spinal canal can be related to pathology of the intervertebral discs with herniation or sequestration of fragments. Osteophytes may arise from the vertebral bodies.

c) Technique

i) Exposure

Exposure of the affected vertebral segments is obtained using the techniques described on pp. 110–117. Identification of the affected level or levels should be confirmed by examinating the patient's X-rays. X-ray control is not usually necessary, providing the lumbo-sacral junction is identified as a routine.

In patients with anomalous fused lumbo-sacral articulations, the first mobile segment of the lumbar spine should be identified.

At each level, after self-retaining retractors have been inserted, the laminal interspaces should be cleared of remnants of muscle fibres and fatty tissues. When the inter-laminal spaces are obstructed by hypertrophic facets, and the laminae override each other, it may be difficult to gain access to the spinal canal. The partes interarticulares of the laminae on both sides should be clearly exposed. Particular care should be taken in these cases to avoid damaging the arteries that supply the cauda equina. These vessels arise from branches of the posterior portions of each lumbar artery, anterior to the partes interarticulares of each lamina on both sides of the spine. Use of diathermy to coagulate bleeding vessels should be avoided near the origins of these branches.

ii) Enlargement of Bony Canal

Adjacent spinous processes should be excised flush with the laminae. Next, the edge of the inferior margin of the superior lamina at the laminal interspace should be excised, using a rongeur of suitable shape. When the medial margins of the inferior facets meet near the mid-line, removal of this laminal edge may be difficult. Attention should then focus on the facet joints, their infero-medial margins being exposed and any associated degenerate capsular tissues or ganglia removed.

The most effective technique for enlarging the laminal interspace, to expose the underlying ligamentum flavum, is to excise the medial aspects of these facets, using a fine osteotome, directed laterally and caudally. The cutting edge of the osteotome will emerge from the facet to strike the inferior lamina and the "non-articular" inner segment of the subjacent superior facet. If the lamina is osteoporotic, this manoeuvre can be carried out with a straight, short pituitary rongeur.

When the ligamentun flavum has been widely exposed, it may be thinned with a rongeur and then removed in the usual manner to expose the spinal canal.

Using a Watson-Cheyne probe, the pedicles should be palpated above and below, separating the dura carefully from the walls of the spinal canal. Having identified the medial margin of the inferior pedicle at the interspace, the medial edge of the superior facet related to this pedicle should be excised flush with the inner margin of the pedicle. The line of this cut in the facet, where it merges with the lamina, should mark the lateral extent of removal of bone when the central segment of the lamina is removed. In this way, the partes interarticulares will be preserved at each vertebral level on both sides of the canal. Removal of the facets in toto should be avoided, as this will lead to serious vertebral instability in some patients.

Bleeding from the cut surfaces of the laminae should be controlled by the application of bone wax regularly as the decompression is proceeding. This will help to reduce blood loss significantly in elderly patients with osteoporosis.

Once the canal has been exposed on both sides, the dural sac should be inspected carefully and palpated (Fig. 6.13).

iii) Haemostasis

Haemorrhage from the internal vertebral venous plexus on either side of the dural sac should be controlled by packing strips of a suitable haemostatic agent–such as gelfoam–along the antero-lateral margins of the spinal canal. The gelfoam should be covered with moistened linteen strips until the posterior surface of the dura is outlined on either side by these strips and the field should, by then, be bloodless.

iv) Dural Opening

Arachnoiditis of the cauda equina should be suspected if the dura is opaque and non-pulsatile. Digital palpation will confirm the suspicion when the firm texture, described above, is felt. If this condition is diagnosed, the surgeon should first complete the decompression over the planned length of the spine. The dural sac

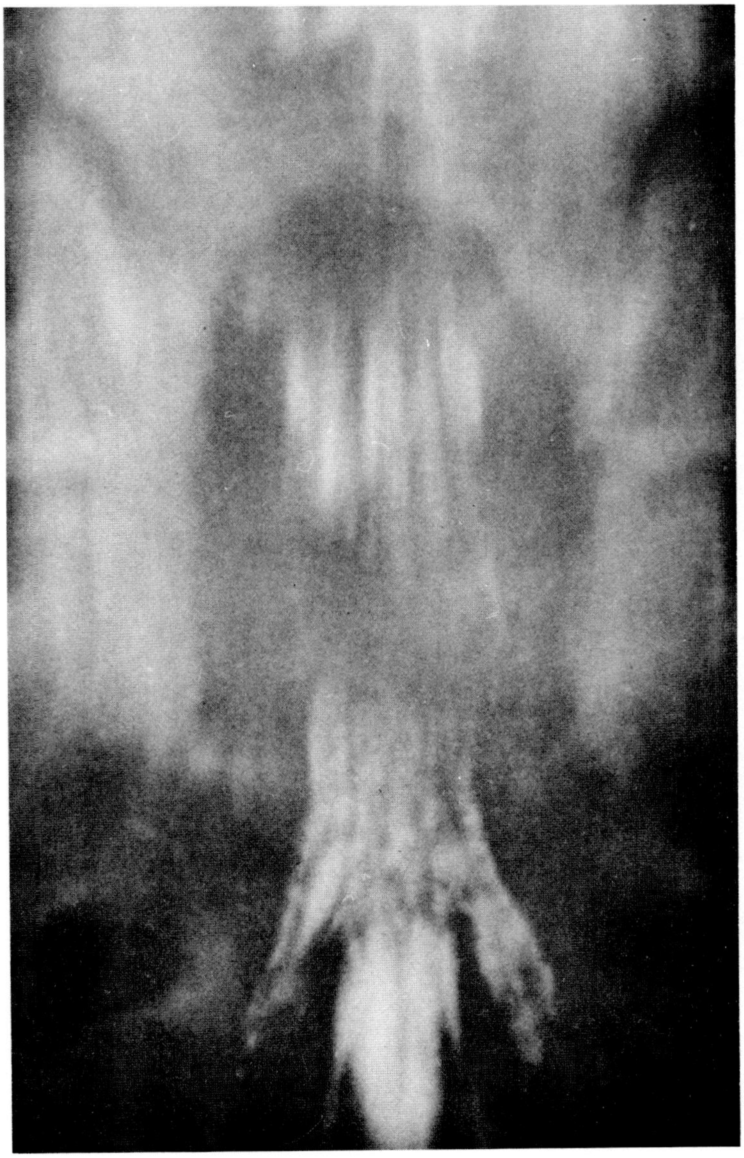

Figure 6.13. An antero-posterior tomogram of the lower lumbar spine taken following decompression of the spinal canal to show restoration of the normal contours of the dural sac following treatment for single level canal stenosis at L4/5. Note the smooth margins to the laminae on both sides of the vertebral column. The technique of spinal canal decompression should be such that the post-operative films have this appearance, with preservation of the partes interarticulares and greater portions of the facet joints on both sides. The lateral extent of laminal dissections should not proceed beyond the medial margins of the pedicles at each level. Multi-level decompressions of the lumbar canal may be carried out in this manner without fear of causing vertebral instability

should then be opened carefully in the mid-line over a segment firm to the touch of the surgeon's finger. The dura will be quite thick, but its cut edges will be distinct from the underlying greyish-pink thick arachnoid. The filaments of the cauda equina will not be visible, as they are ensheathed by the inflamed arachnoid membrane.

The aim in exposing the inflamed arachnoid membrane is to leave the dural sac widely open. Dissection should continue proximaly either to the level where the dural sac pulsates or to a point where cerebrospinal fluid can be seen contained by transparent arachnoid membrane.

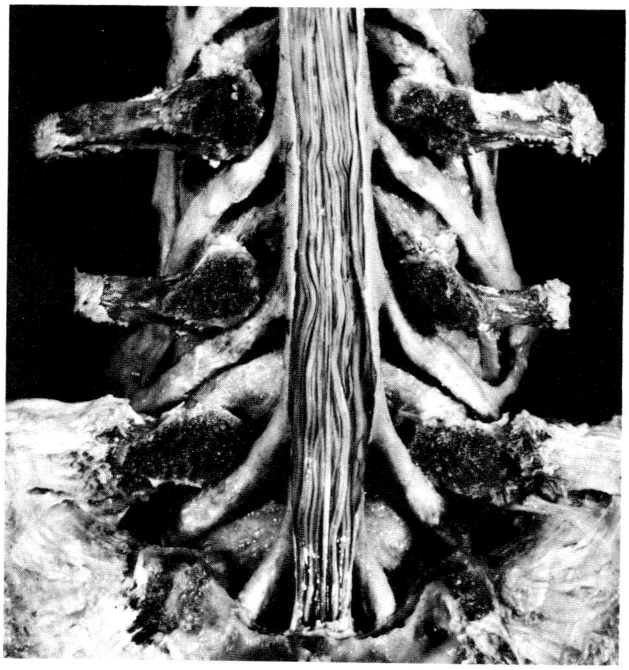

Figure 6.14. A photograph of a dissection of the lumbar spine of a woman aged 46 years. The posterior part of the dural sac has been removed to show the cauda equina which is still ensheathed in transparent arachnoid membrane. During explorations of the lower lumbar spine the dural sac is usually transparent and filaments of the cauda equina can be seen floating in the cerebrospinal fluid. (Dissected by Dr. M. C. Crock)

The margins of the opened dura should be fixed with a few interrupted silk sutures to the muscles along the lateral edge of the bony margins of the spinal canal, over the area of the decompression (Figs. 6.14, 6.15a–c).

Assuming that no other lesions, such as prolapsed disc fragments, have been found during the operation, the wound may now be closed, without drainage. Particular care should be taken to ensure that the lumbo-dorsal fascial layer is sealed.

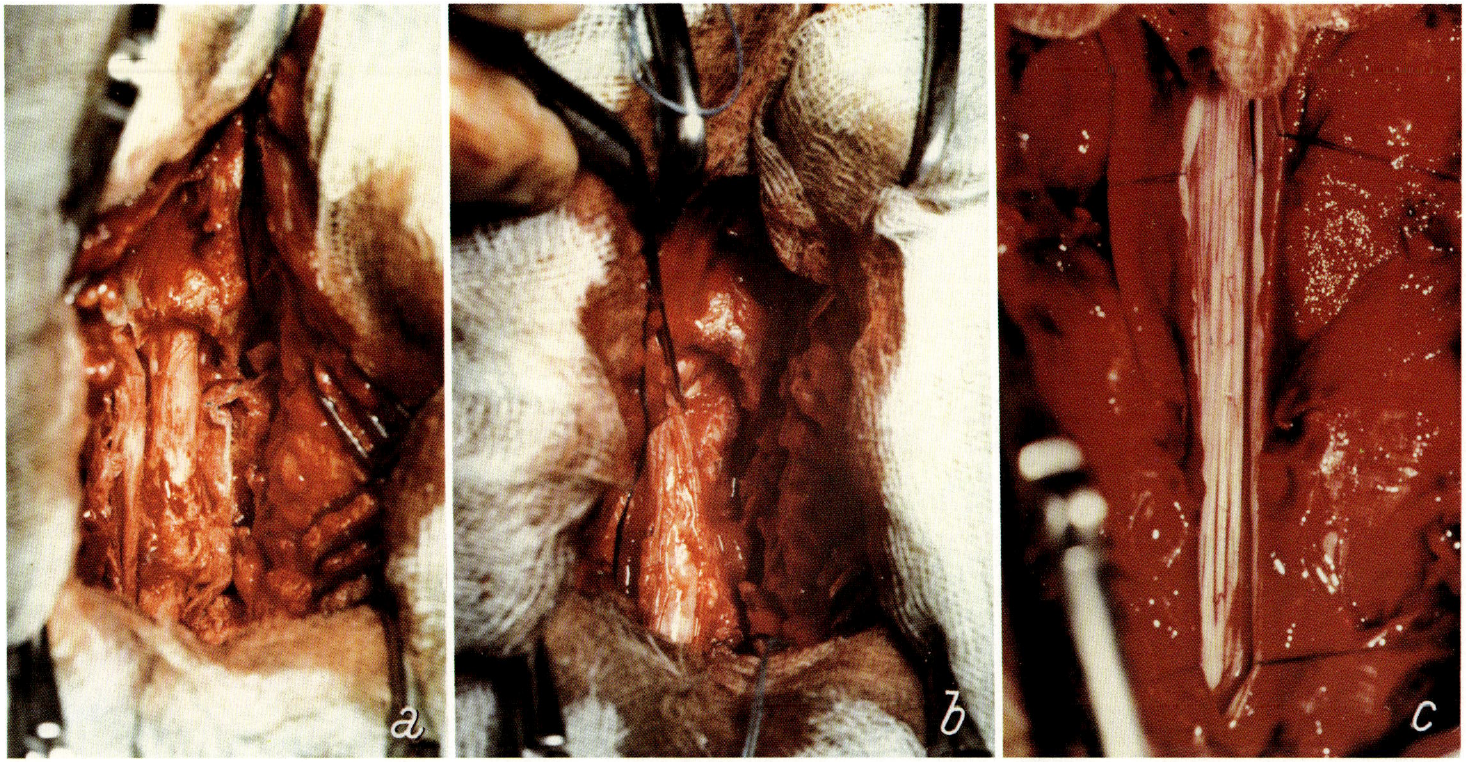

Figures 6.15. a A photograph taken during operation to show the appearance of the dural sac in the lower lumbar spine in the patient whose myelogram is illustrated in Figs. 6.12 a and b. The dura is totally opaque and on digital palpation, in contrast to the normal sensation of feeling a soft balloon, the consistency of the contents can be likened to that of a par-boiled sausage. **b** A photograph taken following opening of the dural sac. Note the markedly thickened glistening arachnoid. It is impossible to identify individual filaments of the cauda equina. **c** A photograph of the cauda equina extending from L 2 to the upper border of L 4 in a woman aged 52 years who presented with a complete block on a myelogram at the level of the lower border of L 2. *Clinically, this patient had severe paraparesis* and at operation, classical features of multi-level lumbar canal stenosis were found along with severe arachnoiditis of the cauda equina. In this photograph, at the top of the picture, it is possible to identify individual filaments of the cauda equina with some blood vessels on the surfaces inside the arachnoid membrane which is normal at this level. In the lower half of the picture, note the thickening of the filaments of the cauda equina and the opacity of the arachnoid. In this remarkable case, when the dura was opened throughout the whole course of the lumbar spine, the cerebrospinal fluid leaked gradually downwards within the exposed arachnoid sheath, until it reached the level of the L 3 vertebral body at its lower border. This patient's paraplegia recovered rapidly following operation for decompression of the canal, the dural sac being left widely opened following operation (see p. 174)

6.6. Results of Surgical Treatment for Arachnoiditis

Twenty cases of severe arachnoiditis of the cauda equina have been treated by this method. Managed post-operatively by early mobilization, the patients have been given Aspirin tablets, four daily, and multi-vitamin tablets, three daily, for three months; the rationale of this therapy being that the fine circulation in the vessels supplying the cauda equina should be thereby enhanced. Two of these patients had been paraparetic before surgery. Many had complained of intractable severe bilateral leg pain, and a number were addicted to narcotics as a result of prolonged usage for pain control.

Both paraparetic patients recovered full motor power in their lower extremities. At least four patients returned to work. Among those apparently addicted to narcotics, only two continued to require non-narcotic analgesics for pain control.

6.7. Recognition and Treatment of Associated Pathological Conditions

In the course of decompression operations in the lumbar spinal canal, particularly in patients with degenerative scoliosis, care should be exercised to ensure that other lesions are recognized and treated, for example:

disc prolapses;
nerve root canal stenosis.

Vertebral instability may occur following removal of a large volume of intervertebral disc tissue, or in rare cases of acute vertebral end-plate necrosis with massive disc sequestration leading to kypho-scoliosis. Only in exceptional circumstances such as these should localized spinal fusion be performed (Fig. 6.3d).

7

Surgery of the Cervical Spine

7.1. Introduction

The surgical management of lesions of the cervical spine is now dominated by the operation of *anterior interbody fusion.* This procedure was introduced for use in the neck in 1955 by Robinson and Smith. Their technique was modified when Cloward introduced special instruments for dowel grafting in 1958.

In the course of performing anterior cervical interbody fusion operations a wide range of pathological lesions can be dealt with safely and effectively. For example, some of the space-occupying lesions which project into the anterior wall of the cervical canal can be removed before the grafts are inserted, lesions such as central disc prolapses, sequestrated disc fragments, or osteophytic bars of bone. The incidence of severe neurological deficits, including quadriplegia, was formerly so high following the use of "laminectomies" for posterior approaches to these lesions that surgery in general–in the cervical spine–had a very poor reputation.

The operation of *cervical laminectomy* still retains an important place for use as follows:

1. For decompression of the spinal canal in cases of multi-level stenosis.
2. For the relief of persistent stenosis of the canal after anterior interbody fusion operations, rarely.
3. For drainage of epidural abscesses.
4. For the treatment of spinal cord tumours.

However, its use to gain access to lesions which lie anterior to the spinal cord has been abandoned.

Posterior cervical spinal fusion between the arch of C1 and the lamina and spinous process of C2–for the treatment of un-united fractures of the odontoid process–remains the treatment of choice for this problem. Apart from this indication, and that of internal fixation following open reduction of some fracture-dislocations in the neck, this operation has been superseded by that of anterior cervical interbody fusion.

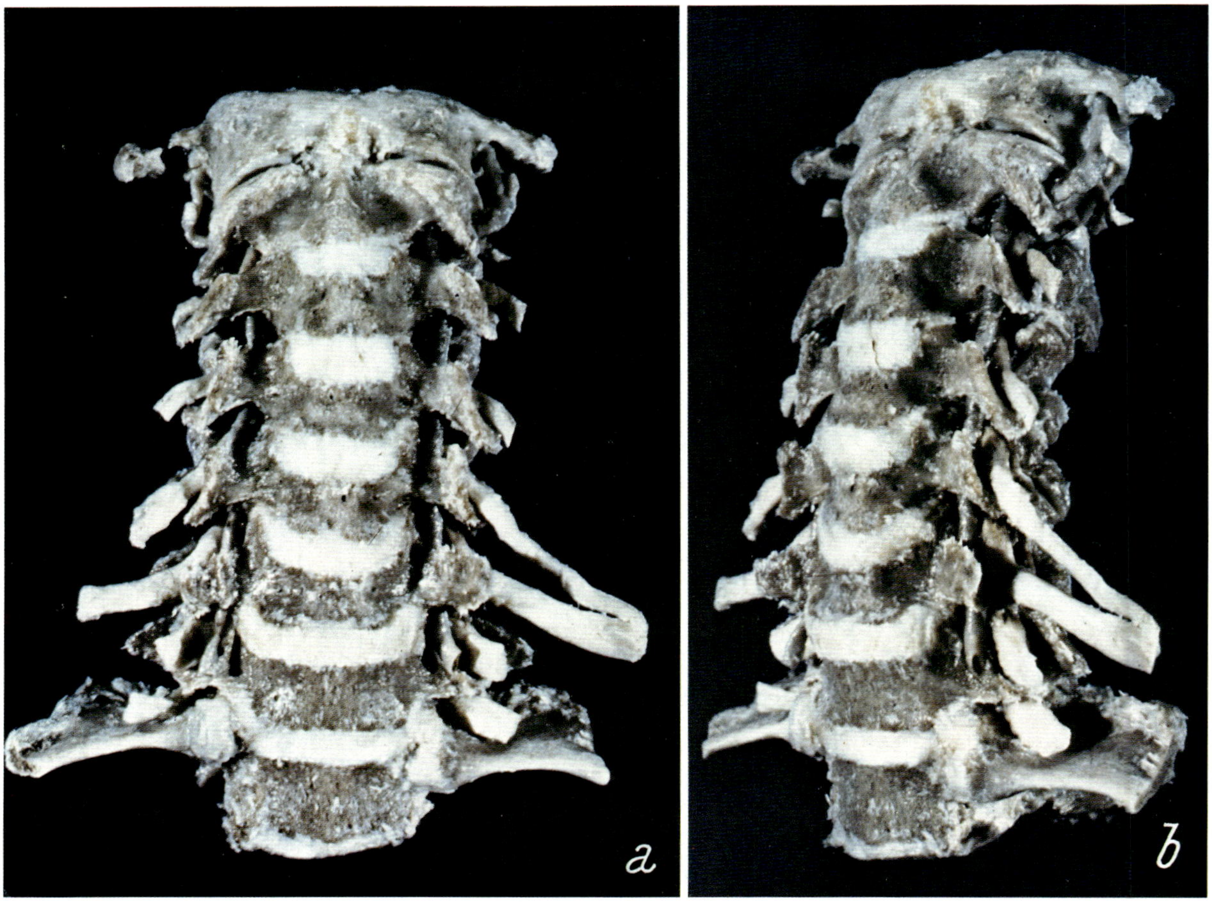

Figures 7.1. **a** A photograph of a dissection of the cervical spine and the cervico-thoracic junction viewed from in front. All the soft tissues have been removed with the exception of the intervertebral discs and the vertebral arteries on both sides. The emerging nerve roots are also shown. Note the proximity of the vertebral arteries to the lateral margins of the intervertebral discs in the region of the unco-vertebral joints. Note also the dimensions of the intervertebral discs particularly in the transverse plane. They increase gradually in size from above downwards (dissected by Dr. M. C. Crock). **b** A photograph of the same specimen viewed obliquely from the left side showing the relationships of the vertebral artery and the emerging cervical nerve roots

7.2. Indications for Surgery

a) Cervical Spondylosis

In the preface to their book "Cervical Spondylosis and Other Disorders of the Cervical Spine", Brain and Wilkinson (1967) wrote: "Cervical spondylosis was hardly recognised twenty years ago". Now, fifteen years later, the most widely accepted indications for surgical treatment in the cervical spine would be for problems complicating that condition. Occurring as a disorder localized to one intervertebral segment or in a more generalized form, it gives rise to a variety of syndromes which can be related largely to the variable pathology resulting from the disc-space narrowing and osteophyte formation which characterize the condition.

Surgical treatment may be indicated in the management of cervical spondylosis as follows:

a) For the relief of persistent or recurrent neck pain, neck stiffness and occipital headache, in the absence of abnormal neurological signs.
b) For the relief of neck pain and brachial neuralgia, with or without abnormal neurological signs.
c) For the relief of symptoms or signs resulting from cervical myelopathy, complicating stenosis of the cervical spinal canal due to the projection of spondylitic osteophytes into the anterior wall of the canal.
d) For the relief of dysphagia. This is a rare complication which may follow the development of a massive osteophyte projecting forwards and compressing the oesophagus. Simple excision of the osteophyte may suffice to relieve the dysphagia.
e) For the relief of stenosis of the vertebral artery or arteries due to mural pressure by osteophytic outgrowths from the regions of the unco-vertebral joints. The results of surgery for this problem are unpredictable and often unrewarding.

b) Cervical Disc Lesions

Cervical disc prolapses are uncommon. Sequestration of relatively large volumes of disc material into the cervical spinal canal may follow manipulation of the spine, performed in the course of conservative treatment for the relief of neck and arm pain. Surgical treatment may be indicated for the management of these lesions and again, there would be general agreement among surgeons on the specific indications for operation. These are in common with those outlined in Chapter 3, p. 103, for the management of lumbar and thoracic disc prolapses.

c) Spinal Injuries

Following spinal injuries, without associated neurological damage, spinal fusion may be required occasionally, as follows:

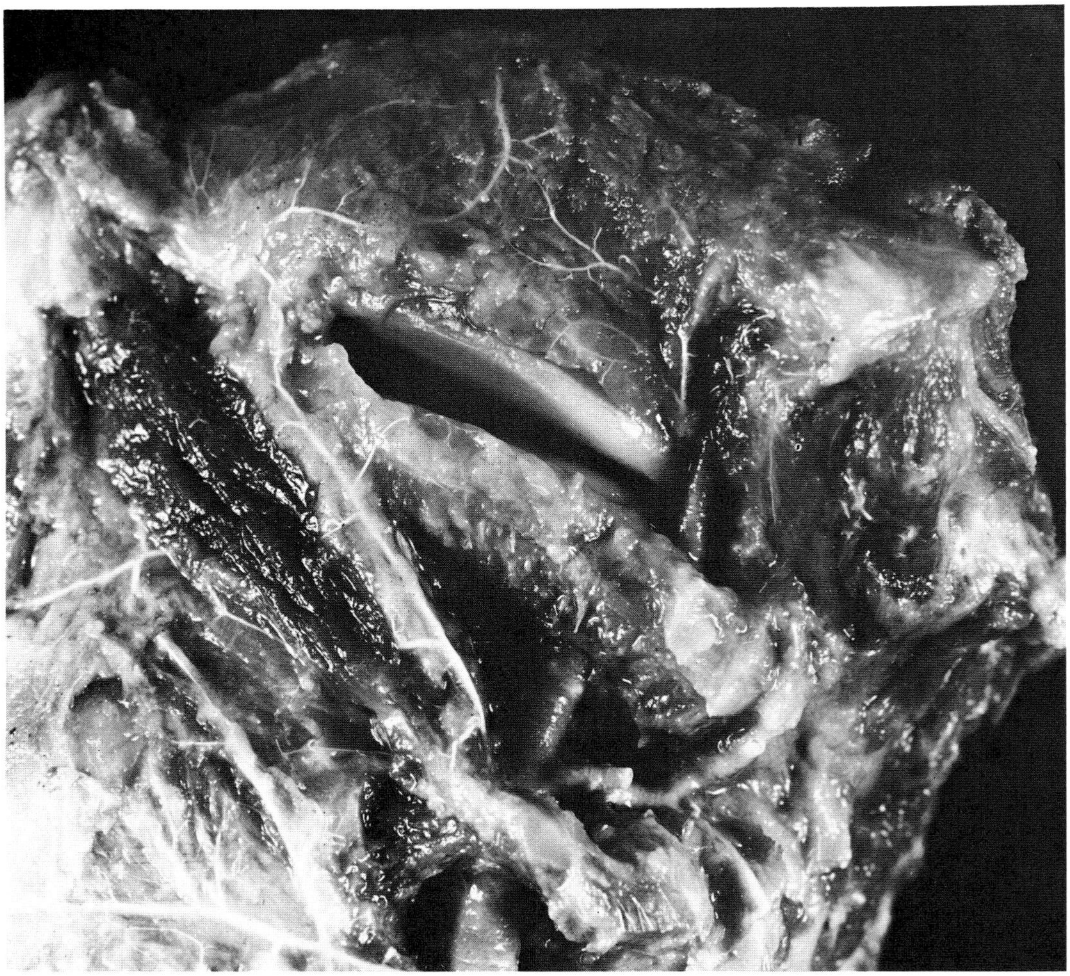

Figure 7.5. A detailed view of the facet joint between C1 and C2 on the left side of the specimen illustrated in Fig. 7.22. Note the relationships of the vertebral artery to this joint, from which the bulk of the capsule has been excised. In the operation of trans-oral fusion of C1 and C2, grafts are inserted into this joint space after removal of the articular cartilage and sub-chondral bone plates. The lateral capsule of the joint should be carefully preserved to avoid damaging the vertebral artery on the lateral aspect of the joint

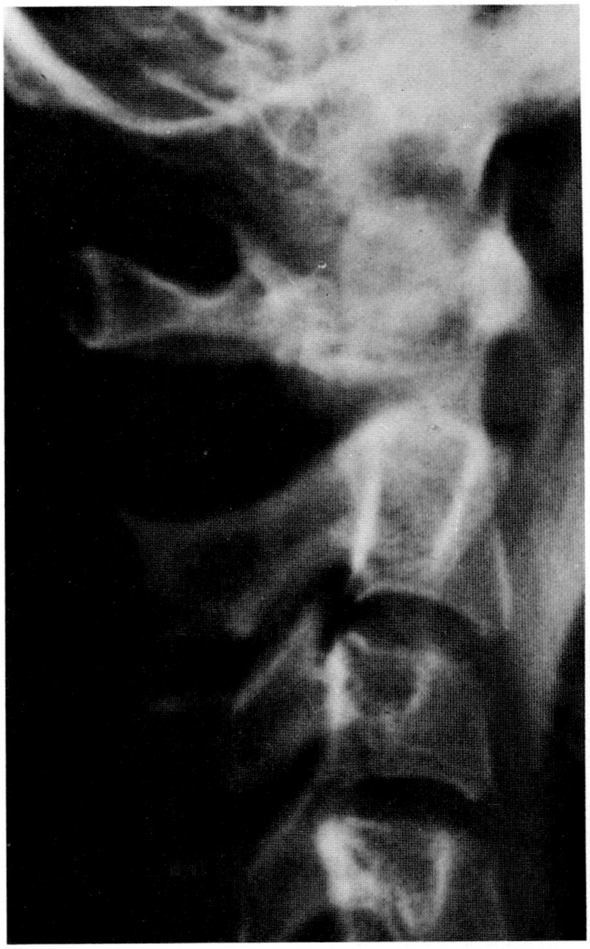

Figure 7.6. A lateral radiograph of the upper cervical spine of the patient aged 22 years, showing an *un-united fracture of the odontoid* following a neck injury sustained in a motor vehicle accident

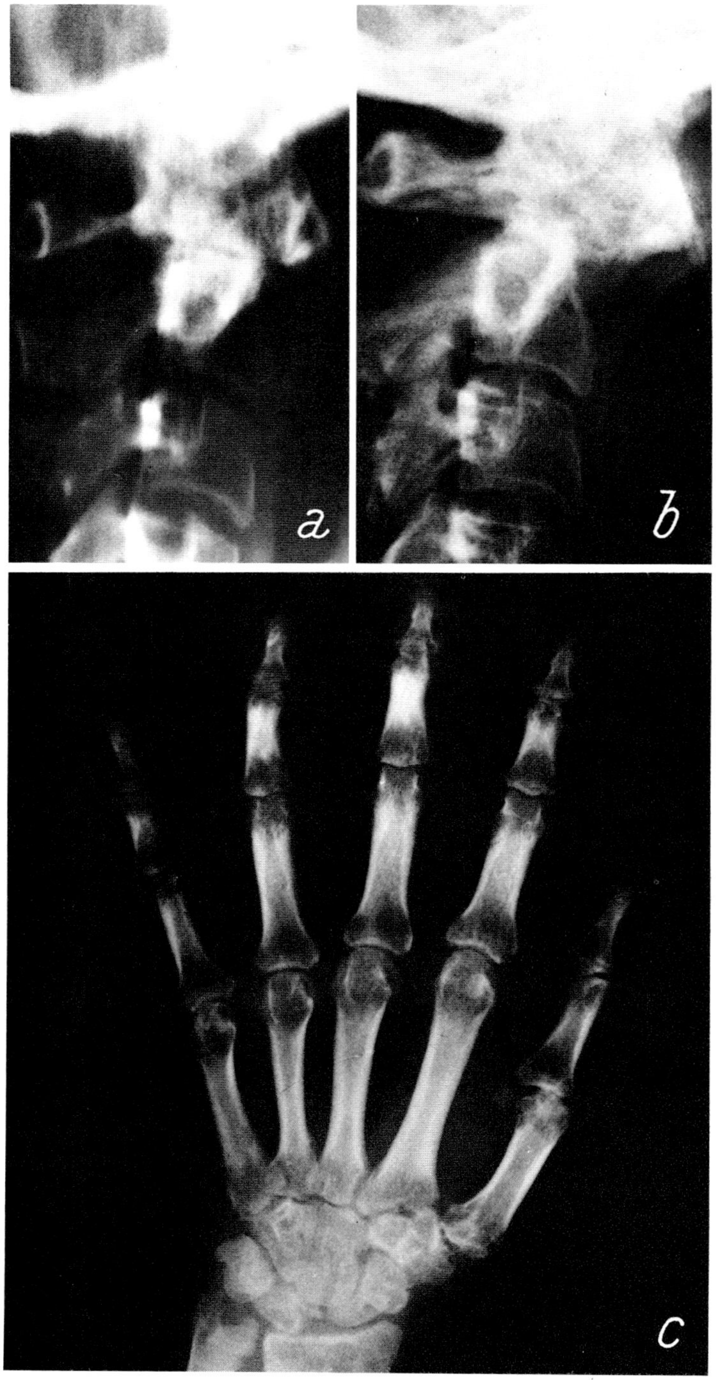

Figures 7.7. **a** A lateral radiograph of the upper cervical spine in a woman aged 30 years, showing erosive changes in the region of the odontoid peg due to rheumatoid disease. **b** A radiograph of the same area of the spine in flexion, showing *instability between C1 and C2 due to rheumatoid joint disease* at that level. **c** A radiograph of the bones of the wrist and hand of the same patient showing the changes of juxta-articular osteoporosis in all the digital joints due to *rheumatoid arthritis*

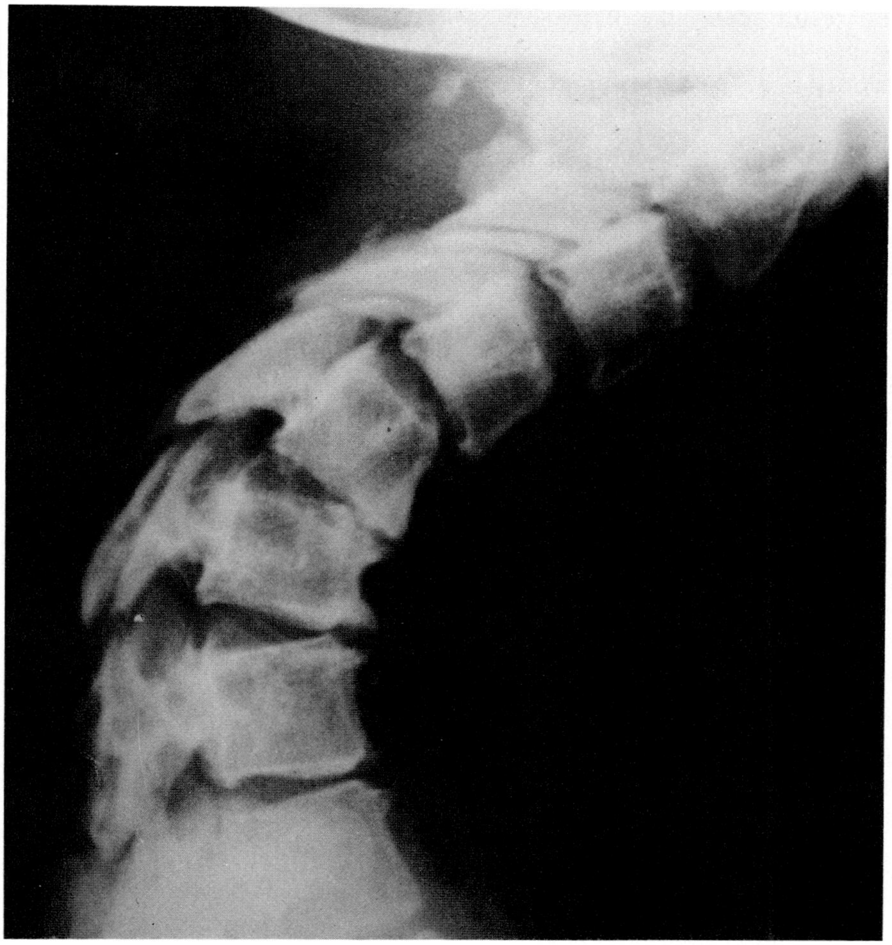

Figure 7.8. A lateral radiograph of the cervical spine of a patient showing *gross kyphotic deformity* with localized degenerative changes between the vertebral bodies of C5/6 and C6/7–*following an extensive laminectomy* for the treatment of syringomyelia

7.3. Controversial Indications for Surgery After Spinal Injury Without Spinal Cord Damage

The incidence of neck injuries following motor vehicle accidents has increased dramatically in the past twenty years. In particular, the number of rear-end collisions, which occur when a moving vehicle strikes the rear-end of a stationary one, has increased enormously in most cities with large numbers of motor vehicles.

The much vaunted "whiplash injury of the neck" is usually sustained by the occupants of stationary cars in accidents of this type. *There is no consensus of opinion among surgeons* about indications for the use of surgical treatment in such patients.

Biomechanical studies have shown that enormous forces are transmitted through the head and cervical spine following this mechanism of injury.

Acting on the results of many of these investigations, car manufacturers have modified seat designs, incorporating head supports and restraining straps for the trunk. Such measures have been quite effective in reducing the morbidity arising from head and neck injuries in many of these accidents.

Despite the improvements in car design and the growing awareness of the hazards of neck injuries that may follow rear-end collisions, many patients still sustain injuries which cause protracted disability. Opinions among doctors vary widely, not only on the question of the causes of the persisting symptoms in these patients, but also on the methods of treatment which should be used to treat them.

The range of symptoms described may include the following:

- Severe neck pain, neck stiffness.
- Occipito-frontal headaches, often with orbital pain.
- Earache and intolerance for loud noise.
- Mental depression.
- Defective memory after the accident.
- Giddiness.
- Varying patterns of arm pain with paraesthesia.
- Feelings of heaviness or weakness of the arms.
- Exacerbation of pain following physical activity or after physical exercise in the course of physiotherapy treatment.

Clinical examination is usually unremarkable. Apart from minor degrees of restriction of neck motion, there may be no objective abnormal physical signs, with particular reference to neurological examination. The only striking findings may be that they appear to be in severe pain, looking pale and downcast.

Having cared for many hundreds of victims of whiplash injuries of the neck in the past twenty years, a number of facts have impressed me:

1. The adverse effects of injuries are likely to be greater and disability more protracted following high speed impacts when the "victims" have been seated in vehicles *without head rests* on their seats.
2. These patients often seek treatment from many different doctors, each of whom may order new X-rays of the spine.
3. Many patients attend specialists only to be discouraged from further attendance if they fail to improve over the course of a few months.
4. The patients are often confused by conflicting advice about the diagnosis of their problems and by diametrically opposed views about treatment as they move from one doctor to another in their search for relief.
5. Despite the fact that abnormal neurological findings are rarely found on clinical examination–many of these patients will be subjected to cervical myelography, which is almost invariably normal. That information is often used, then, to re-enforce the advice that there is no surgical treatment indicated in their case.
6. These patients do not "get better with the passage of time" or after settlement of their court action.
7. Insurance payments to which they are legally entitled may be summarily reduced or stopped on the advice of a doctor acting for the insurance company on the basis of:

   a) Negative physical findings, except for the fact that the patient looks ill and pain-ridden.

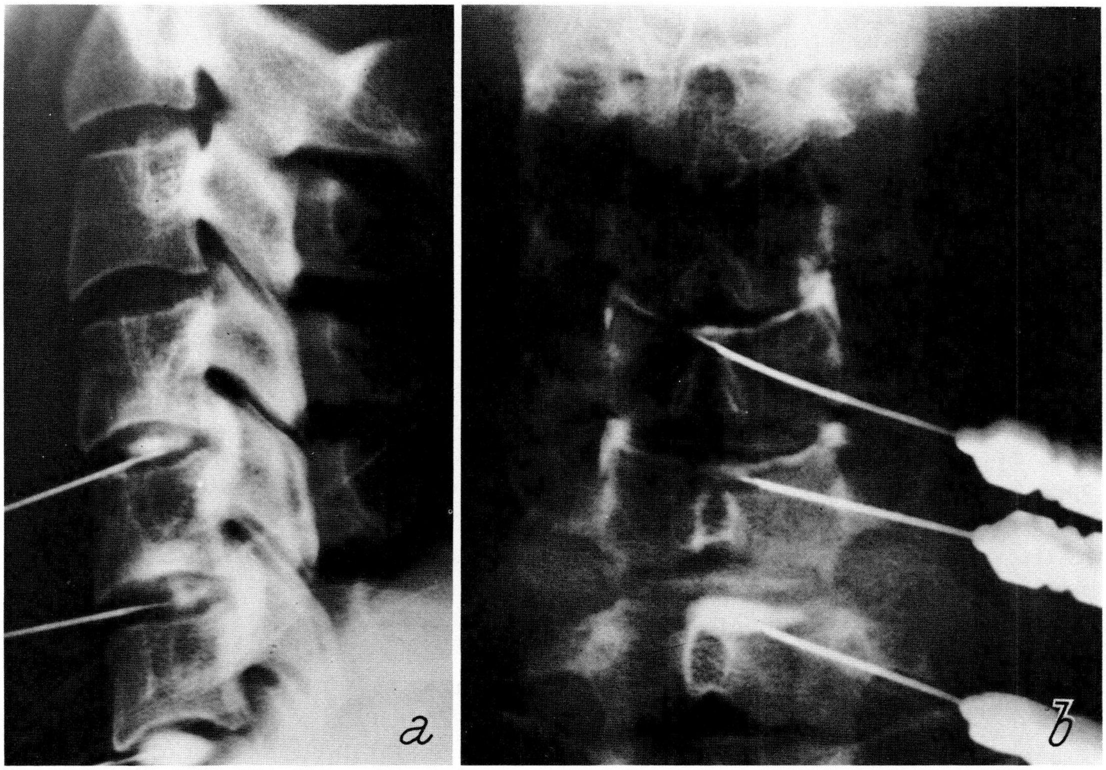

Figures 7.9. a A lateral radiograph of the cervical spine in a girl aged 20 years showing discograms between the vertebral bodies of C4/5, C5/6 and C6/7. Extra-thecal leakage of dye has occurred in both of the upper discs while the C6/7 discogram is of normal appearance. **b** An antero-posterior radiograph of the spine of the same patient, showing a normal discogram at C6/7, with marked disruptive changes at C4/5 and C5/6 discs, in both of which dye leaks transversely across the vertebral interspace towards the unco-vertebral joint regions. This patient was suffering from *post-traumatic internal disc disruption* following a whiplash-mechanism of neck injury. Symptoms of intractable neck pain and occipital headache were relieved by anterior interbody fusions between C4/5 and C5/6. Reviewed 16 years later, she remained symptom free without radiological evidence of disc degeneration above or below the sites of the fusions

  b) Normal spinal radiographs.
  c) Normal myelogram.
8. The only useful diagnostic test, indicated after failure of carefully supervised conservative treatment–in a patient with a history of significant mechanism of injury–is Cervical Discography, to identify the level, or levels, of cervical disc disruption.
9. Many of the patients can be cured after cervical disc excision and interbody fusion.

Neglect of the use of cervical discography has been disastrous for those unfortunate patients suffering from *post-traumatic internal disc disruption* after injuries to the cervical spine (Figs. 7.9a, b).

Unquestionably, soft tissue injuries of the neck may occur in cases following "whiplash injury". Disability from muscle tears, haematomas and ligament "strains" cannot be the cause of protracted disability of the order of magnitude described by many patients. When conservative measures of treatment have been tried for four to six months after injuries of this type, and have proven ineffective, then it is time to think of the possibility of a non-prolapsing disc injury–post-traumatic internal disc disruption–as the underlying cause of the continuing symptoms. Time then to order cervical discograms.

7.4. Cervical Discography

The test is performed on the conscious patient with light sedation. The needles used for this investigation are smaller in calibre than those used in the lumbar spine (Fig. 7.10). They are usually inserted through the right side of the neck, anteriorly, by pushing the mid-line structures of the neck across to the left side with the operator's index finger. Control X-rays are taken in antero-posterior and lateral planes to ensure accurate placement of the tip of each "discogram needle" in the centre of the nuclear zones of the discs before dye is injected (see Chapter 2, pp. 44–56).

Spread of dye beyond the zone of the nucleus pulposus may occur, into the unco-vertebral joint areas on both sides, while leakage backwards into the spinal canal (extra-thecal) may indicate a posterior disc disruption. Spread of dye results from incompetence of annular fibres and is not an indication of disc prolapse as such.

The pain response provoked by injection of dye into the disc is not related to the volume injected or to the resultant increase in intra-discal pressure; rather, it is due

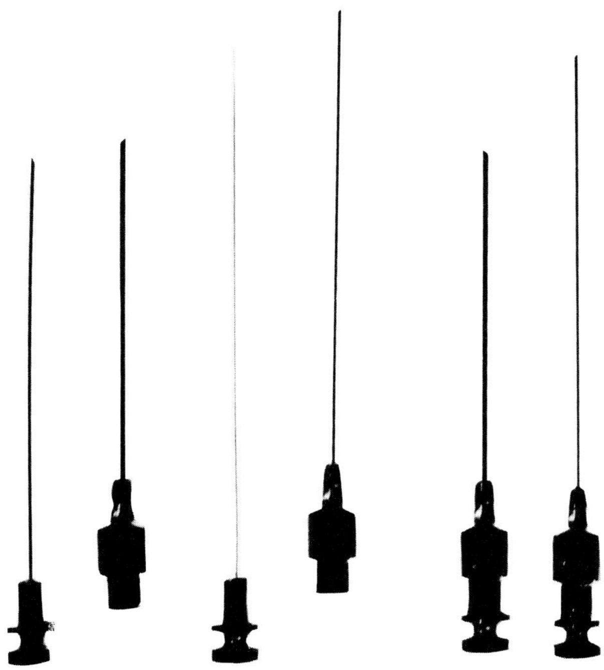

Figure 7.10. A photograph showing a gauge 25 "discogram needle" on the right of the picture with a gauge 22 "guide needle" alongside. On the left of the picture the stilettes are shown alongside their respective needles

to irritation by the dye of the sensitized pain fibres within the disrupted disc itself. Hence, the pattern of pain distribution is not strictly segmental and it does not follow the dermatomes in the upper limbs–as has been suggested by many writers. Use of cervical discography should be reserved for the investigation and demonstration of non-prolapsing disc disorders. By contrast, neither myelography nor C.T. scanning will help to identify the level of a disc with internal disruption. These find their proper application in the investigation of cases with disc pathology producing space-occupying lesions in the vertebral canals.

On December 14, 15, 16 in 1965, Holt performed *30 lumbar discograms* in volunteers at the Menard Penitentiary in Illinois, U.S.A. In a number of "patients" good pictures could be obtained in only two of the lower three lumbar discs.

How is it that the medical profession accepted this *experiment* as evidence that discography was not useful?

The identification of isolated examples of disc disruption, confirmed by discography in patients whose plain radiographs were normal, correlated with the clinical syndromes and relieved by disc excision and cervical interbody fusion should help to cast doubt on the results of that three day sortie into discography performed in patients without symptoms–(for what return?)–in a penitentiary.

7.5. Technique of Anterior Cervical Interbody Fusions

a) Instruments

Dowel cutting instruments permit these operations to be performed accurately at each attempt. Their use in most cases is preferred to the use of chisels or osteotomes for this reason and for the added safety afforded during operation by the safety devices built into the design of Cloward and Crock cutters. Photographs of essential instruments are found in Figs. 7.11–7.16, with descriptive legends outlining details of their assembly and use.

b) Positioning

Patients are placed supine on the operating table. A small wedge-shaped pillow should be placed under the shoulders, with a rolled towel supporting the hollow of the neck, the occiput resting in a rubber ring. The patient's eyes should be protected and the anaesthetic tubes securely fixed to the face (Fig. 7.17).

c) Incisions

Right-sided hemi-collar incisions can be used for approaches to any of the cervical discs, from that between C2 and C3 vertebrae to the lowest in the cervical spine. The use of longitudinal incisions is not recommended as they may result in unsightly scars.

The platysma muscle is exposed by separating subcutaneous fat from its superficial surface before the muscle is cut in the line of the skin incision. Its edges are then under-cut, using blunt dissection to raise flaps for several centimetres

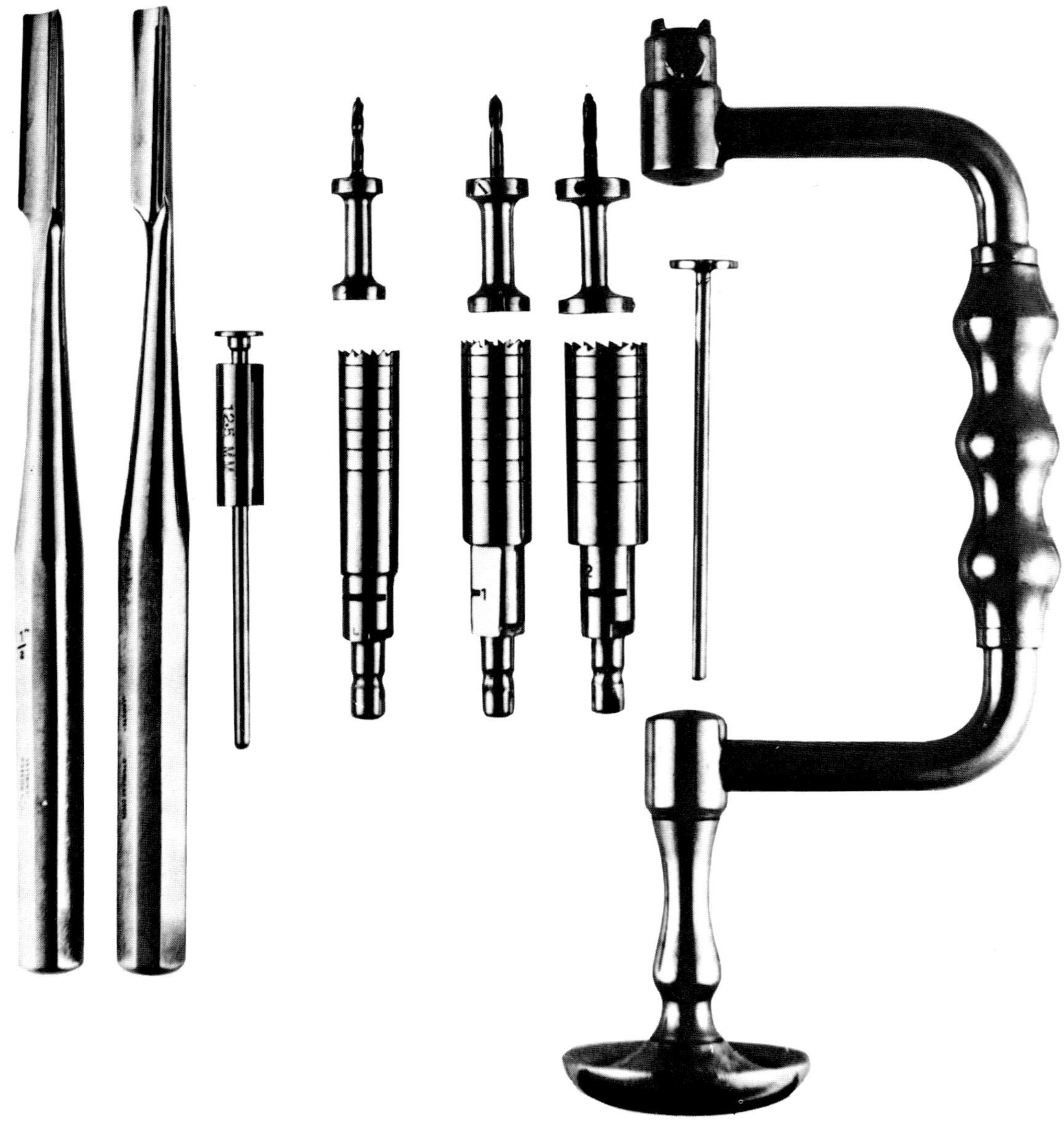

Figure 7.11. A photograph showing the Crock instruments used for dowel cutting in the operation of anterior cervical interbody fusion. On the right of the picture is a Hudson brace. Cutters of three sizes are shown. The starter centre pieces have been removed from each of these. On the right of the cutters is a pusher, which fits inside the cutters and can be used to eject the starter centre pieces or graft bone. On the left of the cutters a pusher is shown with a tubular segment of metal measuring 12.5 mm in depth. When this "dummy" is slotted into the cutter it acts as a guard, preventing the cutter from penetrating deeper than 12.5 mm into the cervical vertebral bodies. Dummies are provided in three sizes, 10 mm, 12.5 mm and 15 mm, for use according to the vertebral dimensions in individual cases. On the left of the photograph, two tooled gouges are shown, which will fit into the cuts made into adjacent vertebral bodies. Their use is illustrated in Figs. 7.20, 7.24a. *Note that the cutters have circular rings marking their outer surfaces, at intervals of 5 mm*. Instruments manufactured exclusively by Thomson & Shelton Instrumentation Company, 6119 Danbury Lane, Dallas, TX 75214, U.S.A.

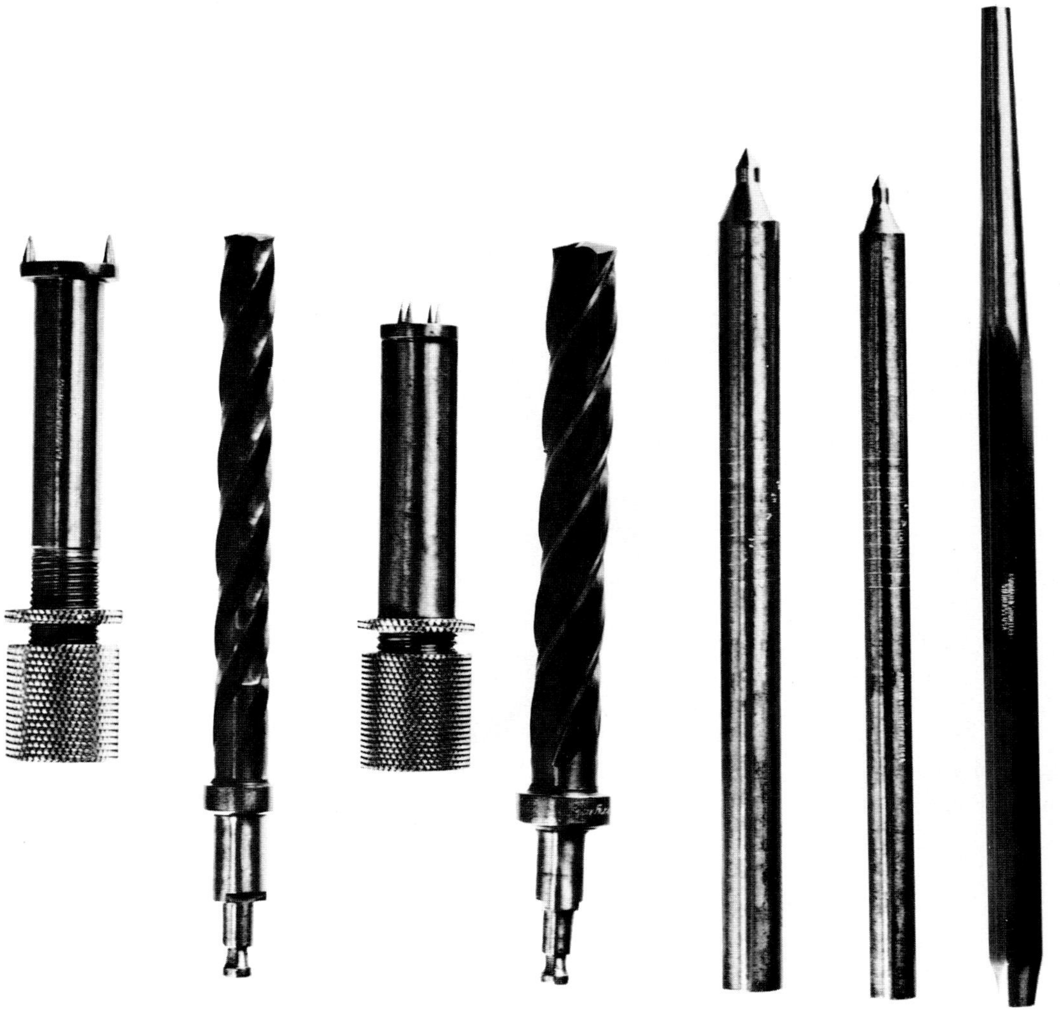

Figure 7.12. A photograph of Cloward's equipment for cervical spine fusion operations, with spiked tubes allowing adjustment to determine the depth of cuts made into the vertebral bodies on either side of the disc space during interbody fusion. Note the twist drills which are used to remove the bone and disc tissue. *With this system* inevitably some *disc tissue is ground into the adjacent vertebral bodies* and *this may lead to non-union of grafts on occasions*

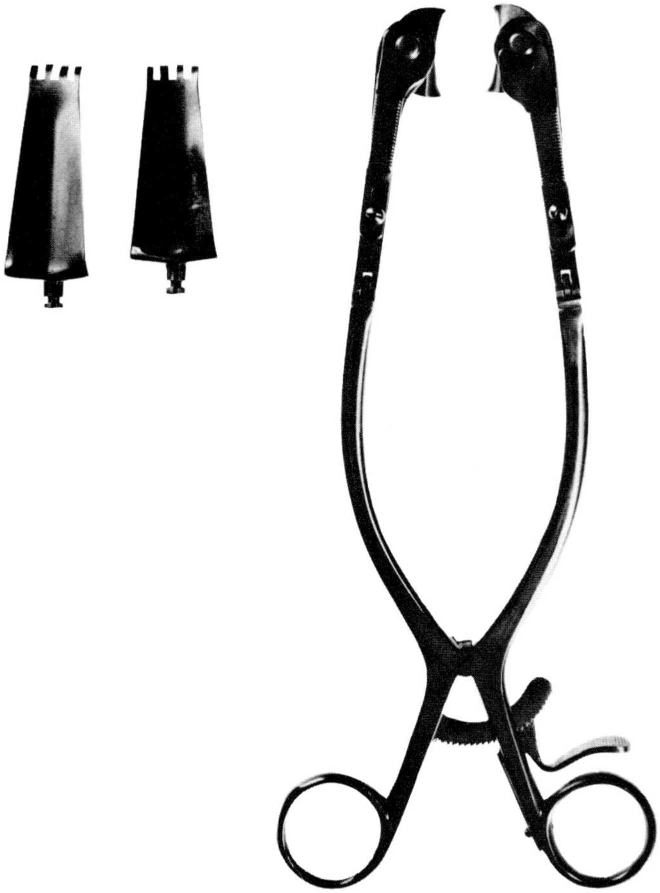

Figure 7.13. A photograph of the self-retaining retractor designed by Cloward for use in anterior cervical fusions

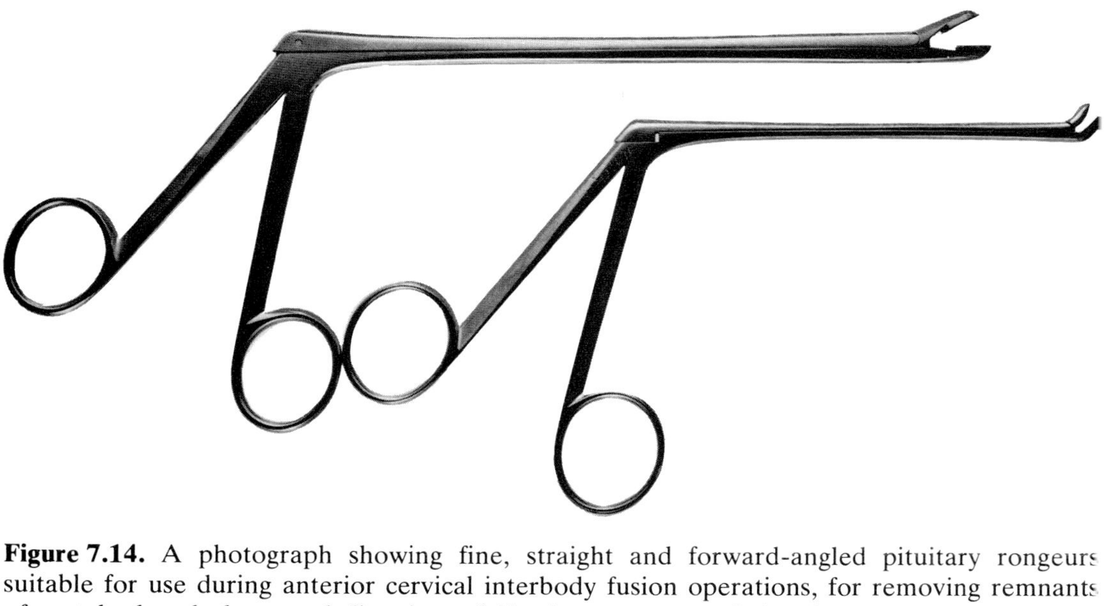

Figure 7.14. A photograph showing fine, straight and forward-angled pituitary rongeurs suitable for use during anterior cervical interbody fusion operations, for removing remnants of vertebral end-plates and disc tissue following curettage of the disc space

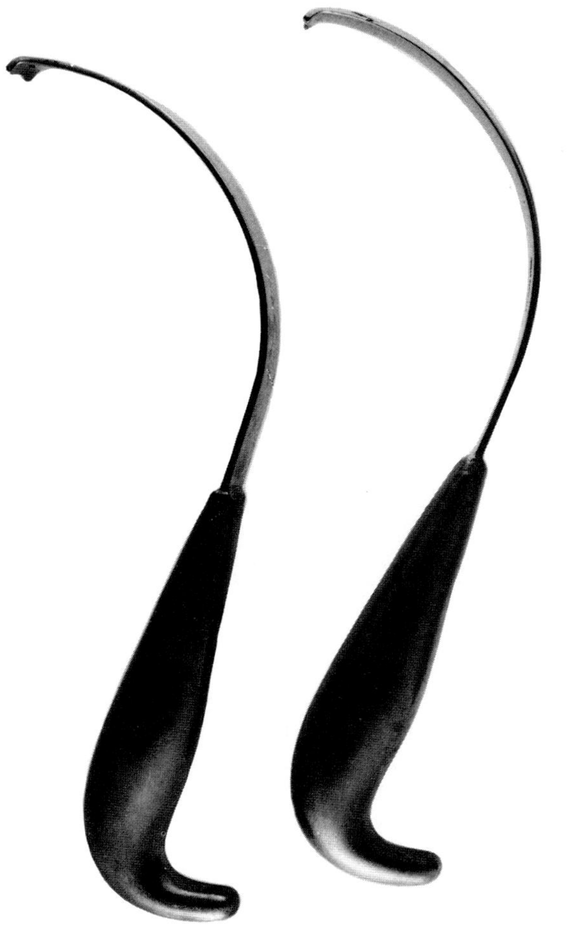

Figure 7.15. A photograph of two cervical retractors with smooth excavated ends designed to be held transversely across the anterior surfaces of the cervical intervertebral discs

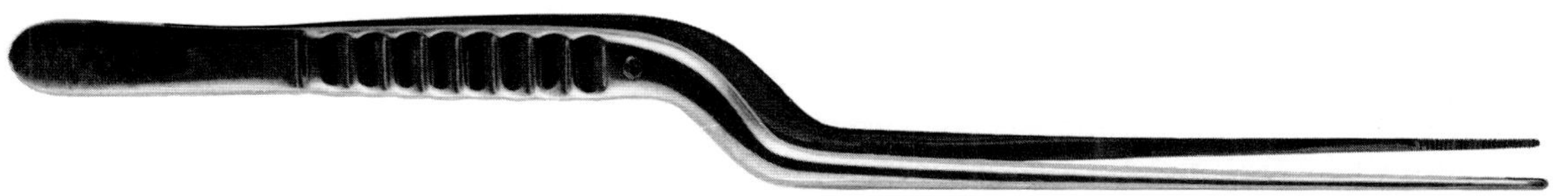

Figure 7.16. A photograph of a Bayonet forceps with a fine tip, essential for use in cervical spine operations

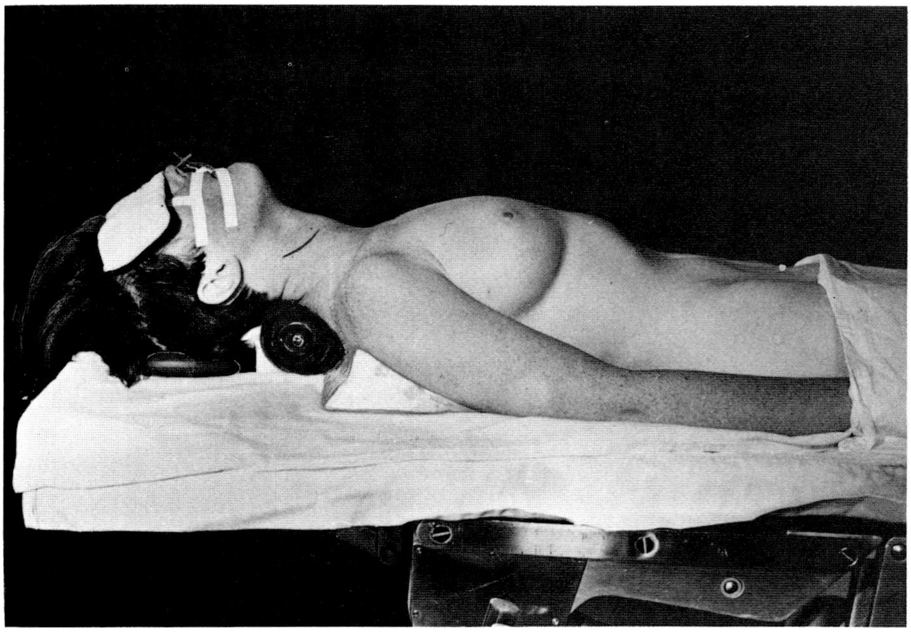

Figure 7.17. A photograph of a patient postured on the operating table for anterior cervical interbody fusion. Note the triangular-shaped pillow underneath the shoulders, the rolled towel (in black) under the neck, and the rubber ring on which the occiput rests. The endotracheal tube and the reinforced rubber airway adjacent to it are strapped to the patient's face. Note the pad covering the eyes, to prevent pressure on the orbits during surgery. Assistants have been known to press on the eyes during anterior cervical interbody fusion operations. *Irreparable ocular damage has been reported from this cause.* Note also the outline of the hemi-collar incision extending from the anterior border of the sterno-mastoid muscle to just behind the mid-line. Through this incision two or three cervical discs can be exposed. For exposure of the disc between C2 and C3 vertebral bodies, the incision needs to be placed in the sub-mandibular region, care being taken to avoid damaging the mandibular branch of the facial nerve. Note that both arms are by the patient's side, to allow traction on the hands for lowering the shoulders while control X-rays are being taken during the operation

upwards and downwards. The encircling layer of deep cervical fascia is then incised along the anterior border of the sterno-mastoid muscle, allowing access to the space between the carotid sheath laterally and the mid-line structures of the neck medially. The fascia along the lateral edge of the superior belly of the omohyoid muscle is cut with Metzenbaum scissors until the lateral edge of the oesophagus can be seen. Inserting his index finger into the space now created, the surgeon can palpate the front of the vertebral column. By moving his finger deliberately and carefully along the antero-lateral margin of the vertebrae, a plane of cleavage can be opened easily in the loose fascia between the carotid sheath and the mid-line structures of the neck over a distance sufficient to allow exposure of one, two or three of the cervical intervertebral discs.

Most cervical fusions are performed at the levels of C4/5, C5/6 or C6/7. Having cleared the space as indicated, retractors may then be inserted, orientated transversely and applied to the anterior aspect of one of the intervertebral discs. Up to this point the only major anatomical structures encountered will have been the ones already mentioned. Only occasionally will it be found necessary to ligate and divide an anterior cervical vein or some un-named venous tributary of the internal jugular vein. The superior thyroid vessels may be seen, but it is rarely necessary to ligate and divide them.

The pre-vertebral fascia, that thin, filmy, opalescent membrane which sheaths the paravertebral muscles and the cervical column itself, is split longitudinally in the mid-line and the retractors re-positioned to give a clear view of the intervertebral discs and anterior aspects of the vertebral bodies. The medial edges of the right and left-sided longus colli muscles can be seen clearly and, using fine bayonet forceps (Fig. 7.16), the vessels related to the muscles at their attachments along the antero-lateral aspects of the vertebral bodies are coagulated with diathermy. These muscular attachments are then separated from the vertebrae and discs, so that the cervical retractors may be replaced once again, to provide definitive clear exposure of the disc or discs to be removed. The risk of obstructing the carotid vessels during operation is reduced by this method.

d) The Thyroid Gland

Before planning cervical discography and anterior cervical spine surgery in any patient, the surgeon should examine the patient's thyroid gland. On three occasions in twenty years of practice, I have had patients in whom thyroidectomy has been required before satisfactory access to the anterior aspect of the cervical vertebral column was possible.

e) Control X-Rays to Identify Individual Intervertebral Discs

The use of a specially bent disposable needle is recommended before lateral X-rays are taken. The needle serves a dual purpose, allowing also the precise measurement of the antero-posterior width of the disc space (Fig. 7.18). Never remove the needle before the control X-ray has been exhibited in the operating room.

f) Preparation of the Dowel Cavity

The relevant anatomy of the spine and the steps in this critical phase of the operation are illustrated in detail in Figs. 7.18–7.24. Once cutting instruments have been applied to the vertebral bodies *the potential hazards of injuring the vertebral arteries or the neural structures in the spinal canal must be borne in mind* (Figs. 7.1a, b).

Having made the preliminary cut across the disc space, the starter centre piece is removed from the cutter. The surgeon then selects the "safety dummy" of pre-determined size, by re-checking the antero-posterior measurements of the disc space. He then personally assembles the cutter ready for use by inserting the "dummy", which is held in place by the "pusher device". Both the assistant surgeon and theatre sister should check the preparation of the cutter with the "dummy" and cross-check the disc space measurements before the surgeon re-inserts the cutter–after stage one–to commence the final preparation of the dowel cavity.

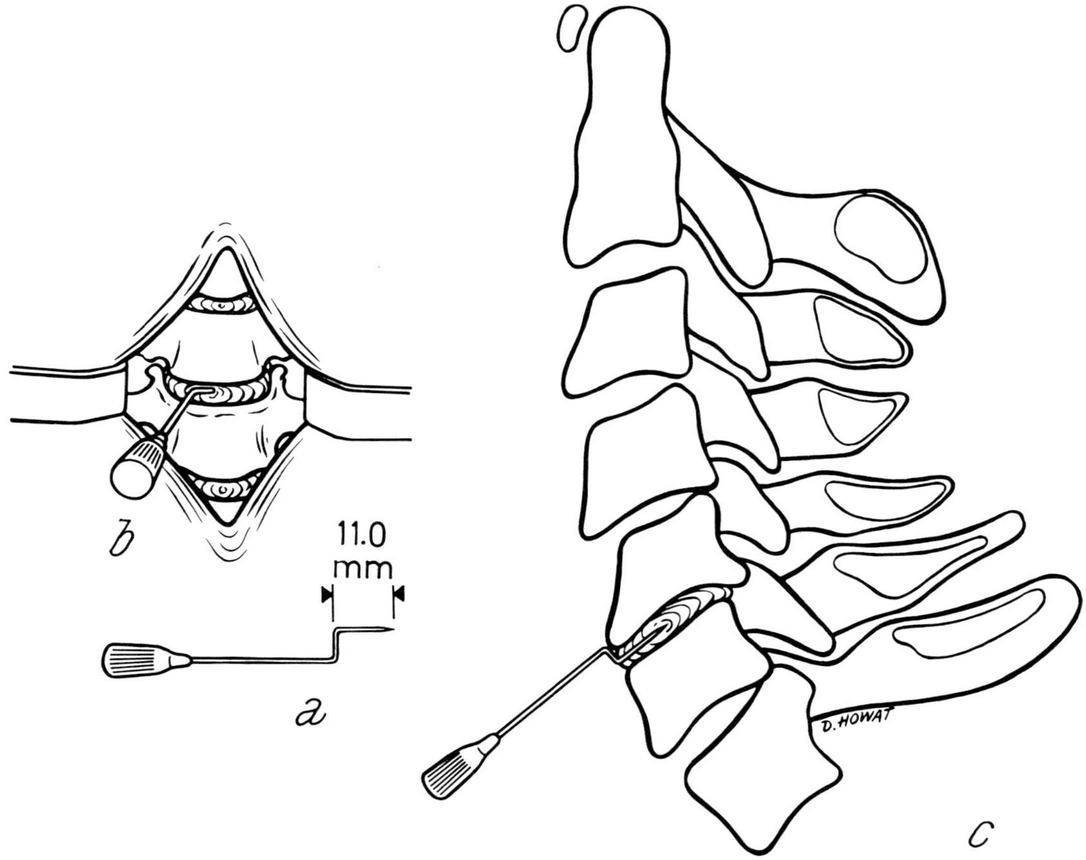

Figures 7.18. **a** A drawing to illustrate the use of a bent needle recommended by the author for use during control X-rays in the neck. A disposable 19 gauge needle is prepared by bending it in the jaws of an artery forceps. A right-angle bend is made near the tip and the measurement between the tip and the first right-angle bend taken. Usually 11.0–12.5 mm is satisfactory, depending on the size of the patient. **b** A drawing to depict the front of a cervical intervertebral disc with the needle in place for control X-ray during operation. **c** A drawing of the cervical spine shown from the side depicting the use of the bent needle for control X-ray. The right angle bend *prevents penetration of the needle into the cervical canal,* a potential risk if a straight needle is inserted. *It has the added advantage of allowing precise measurement of the intervertebral disc space on the control X-ray* when it is brought back into the theatre

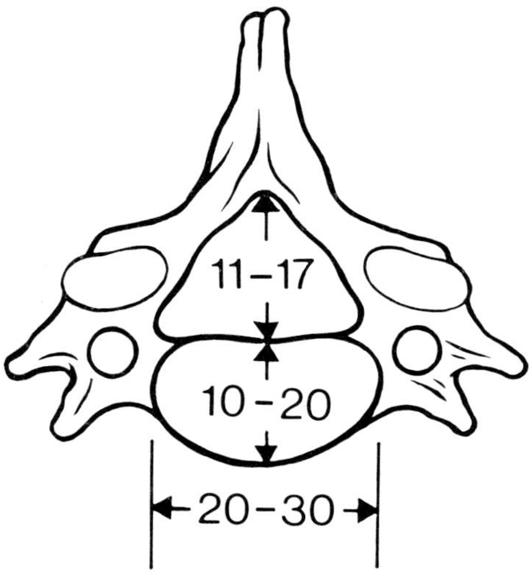

Figure 7.19. A drawing of a typical cervical vertebra *with the ranges of measurements in millimetres* of the transverse and antero-posterior diameters of the vertebral body and the antero-posterior diameter of the cervical canal

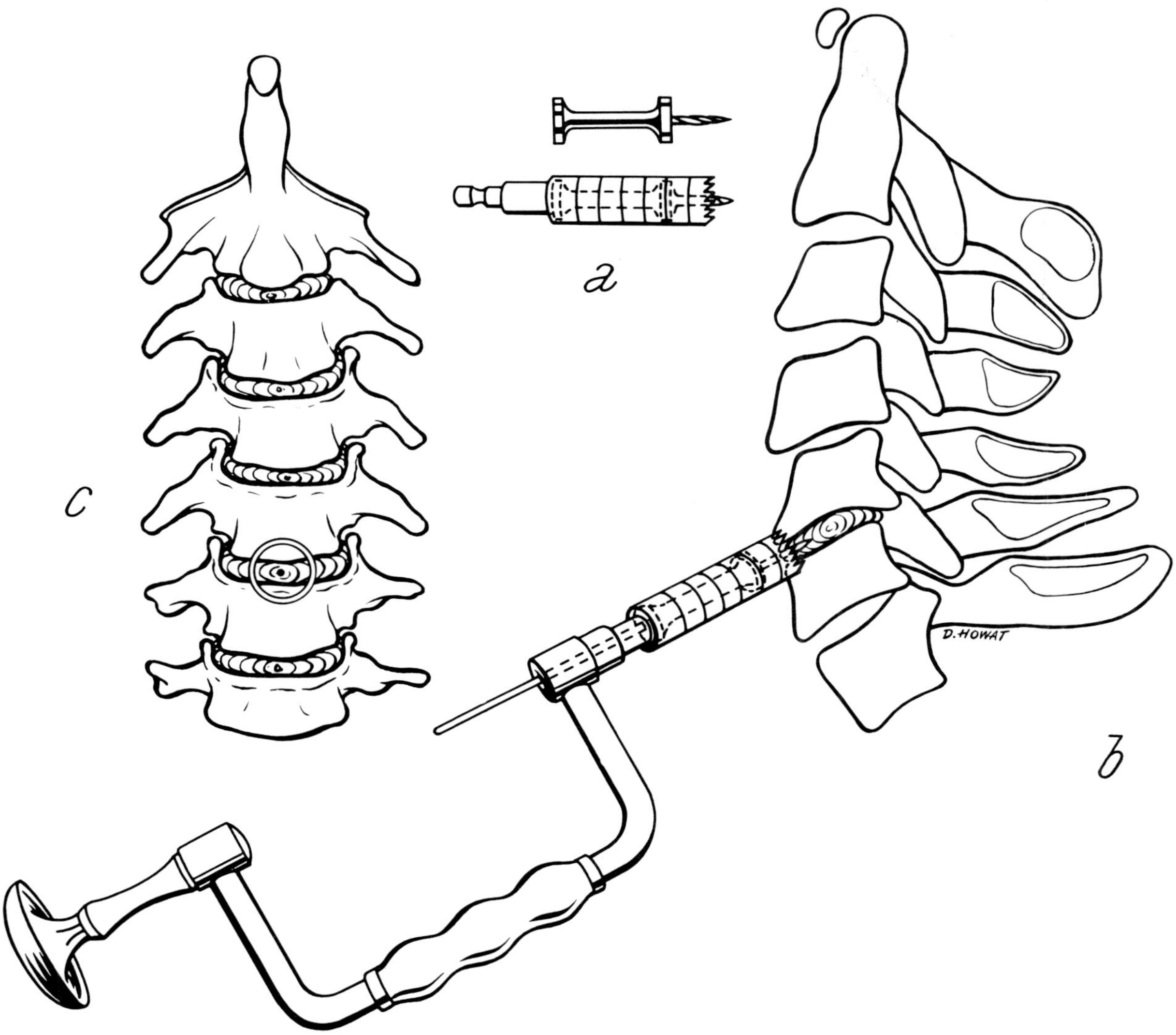

Figures 7.20. **a** A drawing showing a starter centre piece at the top. Below it, the starter centre piece is shown in outline, assembled in the zero-size cutter. Note the circumferential markings on the cutter, each separated from the other by 5 mm. **b** A drawing of the cervical spine, viewed from the side, showing the cutter assembled on a Hudson brace with the starter centre piece in position and the pusher within the tube. The drawing depicts the method of commencing the preparation of a dowel cavity between the vertebrae of C5 and C6. **c** A drawing of the cervical spine viewed from in front, showing the outline of the cut in the mid-line between the vertebral bodies of C5 and C6, at the first stage of preparation of the dowel cavity

Errors made at this stage may lead to catastrophic accidents during the operation.

Having re-fitted the cutter into the preliminary circular slot cut during stage one (Fig. 7.20), it should be oscillated clockwise and counter-clockwise, avoiding wobbling motion as the Hudson brace is being rotated. No force is to be exerted on the proximal end of the brace, other than that required to steady it with one hand, while the surgeon's other hand holds the off-set central bar through which the oscillating motion is transmitted to the cutter.

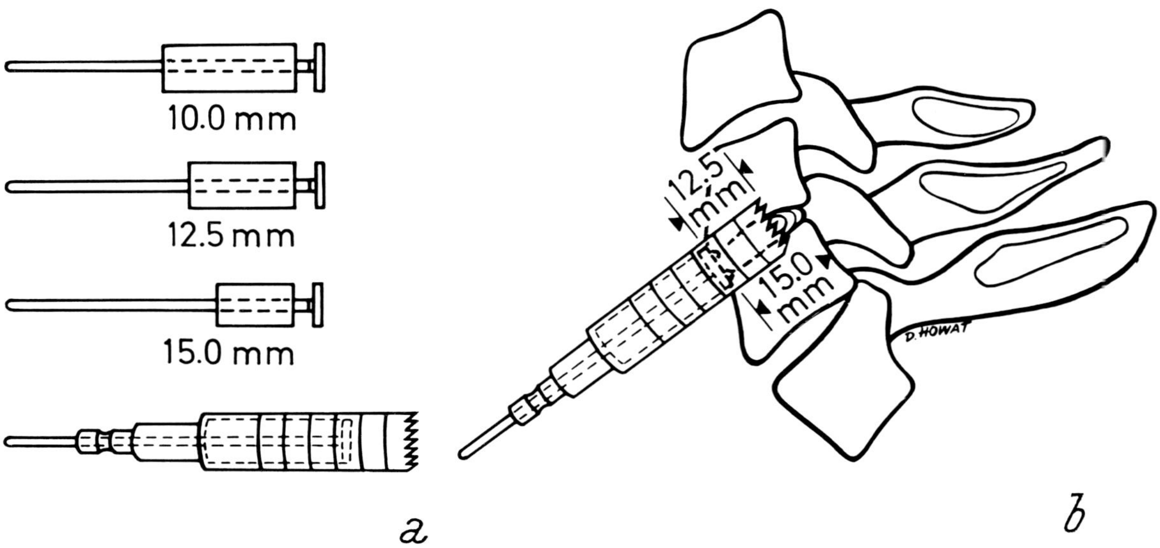

Figures 7.21. **a** A drawing to show the range of metal dummies available for insertion into the zero-size cutter, allowing the preparation of dowel cavities of pre-determined depth, depending on the depth of the disc space in individual patients. *The depth of the space is checked at operation by control X-ray with the use of the bent needle as indicated in Fig. 7.18.* At the bottom of the drawing, note the dummy assembled inside the cutter. **b** A drawing to depict the cutter in use, *demonstrating the mechanism of safety protection provided by the 12.5 mm dummy* which has been inserted after removal of the starter centre piece. *Note also that the surgeon is able to count the rings on the outer side of the cutter, providing a double safety factor.* (See pp. 199–202 for a detailed description of the technique for cutting the dowel cavity)

As the cutter advances slowly into the vertebral bodies and intervening disc tissue, *the operator becomes aware of a grating sensation* at its cutting end, from which an audible grating sound is emitted. The "dummy" inside the cutting cylinder will abut against the anterior surface of the disc and adjacent vertebral margins when the cutter has reached the depth that is determined by the length of the "dummy" (Fig. 7.21). Further penetration of the cutter into the vertebral bodies is thereby prevented. At this stage, the grating sensation ceases and the cutter spins smoothly and silently. For added safety, while the cutter is being oscillated, the surgeon may check the measurement of its advancement by counting the rings on its outer surface.

In the third stage of the preparation of the cervical dowel cavity, special tooled gouges are used to displace the fragments of vertebral bodies and intervertebral disc

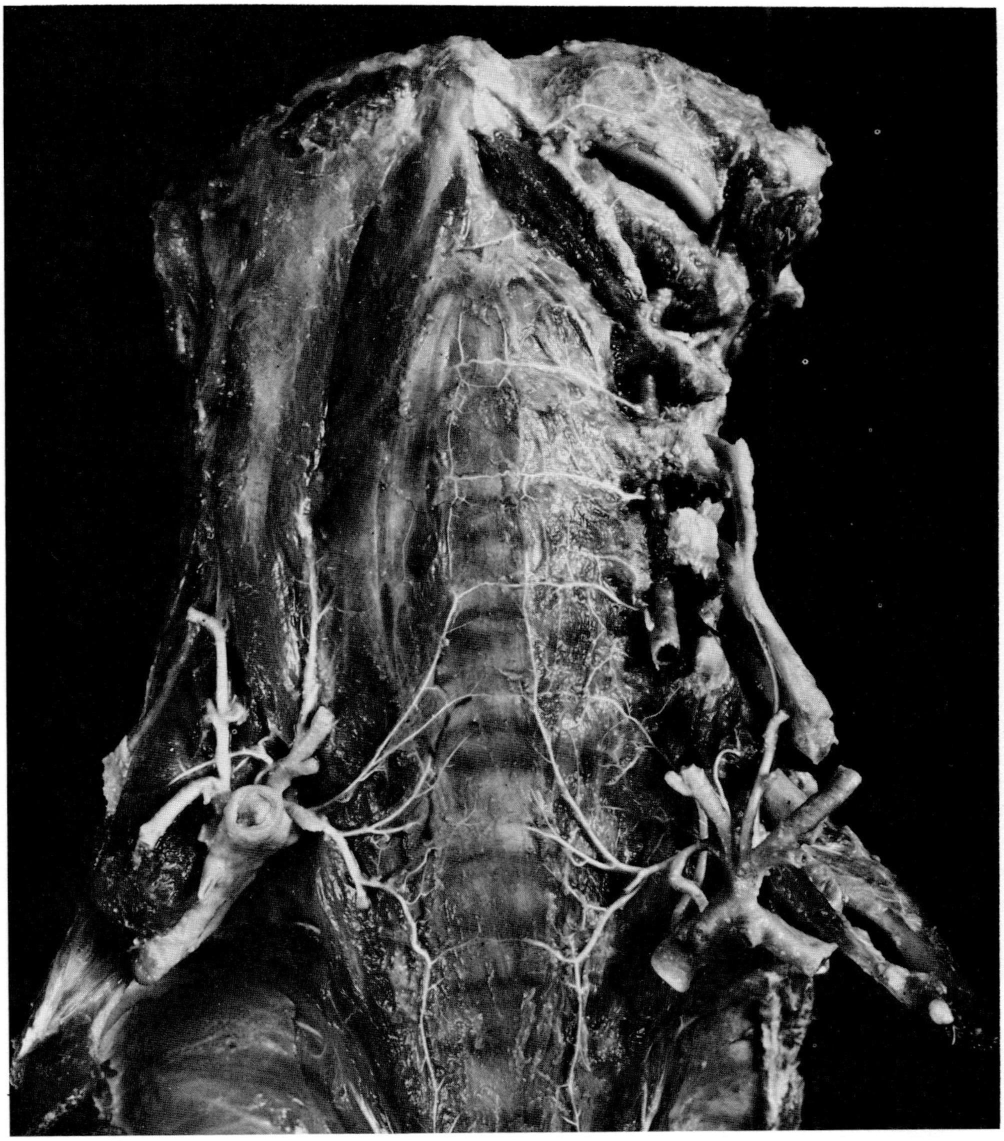

Figure 7.22. A photograph of a dissection of the anterior aspect of the cervical and upper thoracic spine of a female child aged $3^1/_2$ years, showing the origins and courses of arteries supplying the antero-lateral aspects of the vertebral bodies. The longus colli muscles have been removed from the left side of the specimen. The pre-vertebral fascia has also been removed but the anterior margin of the longus colli at its attachment to the antero-lateral aspects of the vertebral bodies on the right side is intact. Note the vertical chain of arterial anastomoses running along the margin of this muscular attachment, forming a parallel vascular channel with corresponding vessels on the left side of the vertebral column. (Dissected by Dr. H. Yoshizawa, reproduced from: Crock, H.V., Yoshizawa, H.: The Blood Supply of the Vertebral Column and Spinal Cord in Man. Wien-New York: Springer. 1977)

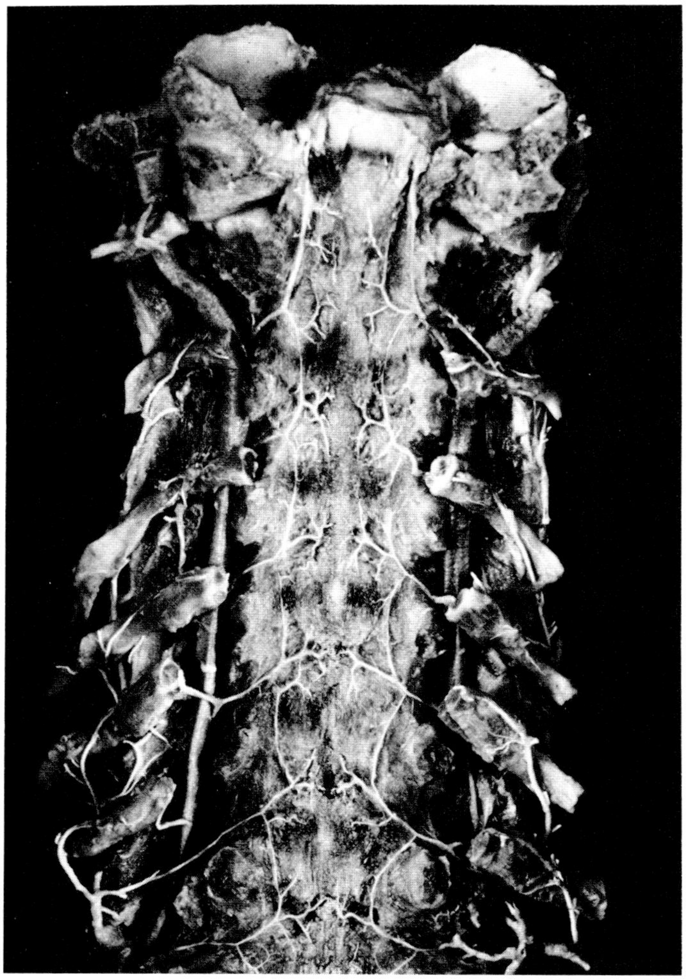

Figure 7.23. A photograph of a dissection of the posterior aspect of the cervical and upper thoracic spine of a male aged 34 years. The posterior aspects of the vertebral bodies have been exposed and portions of the posterior longitudinal ligament have been removed from a number of vertebral bodies in the lower part of the specimen. In the upper part of the specimen on both sides, the origins of the anterior spinal canal branches of the vertebral arteries can be seen. In the neck, these vessels form the familiar arcuate arterial pattern on the anterior surface of the spinal canal which is found along its length. The vessels contribute to the intra-osseous arterial supply of the vertebral bodies, anastomosing with branches from the vascular chains demonstrated in Fig. 7.22 on the anterior aspect of the vertebral column. In the operation of anterior cervical interbody fusion the blood supply of the vertebral body remains largely intact, ensuring rapid vascularization of grafts

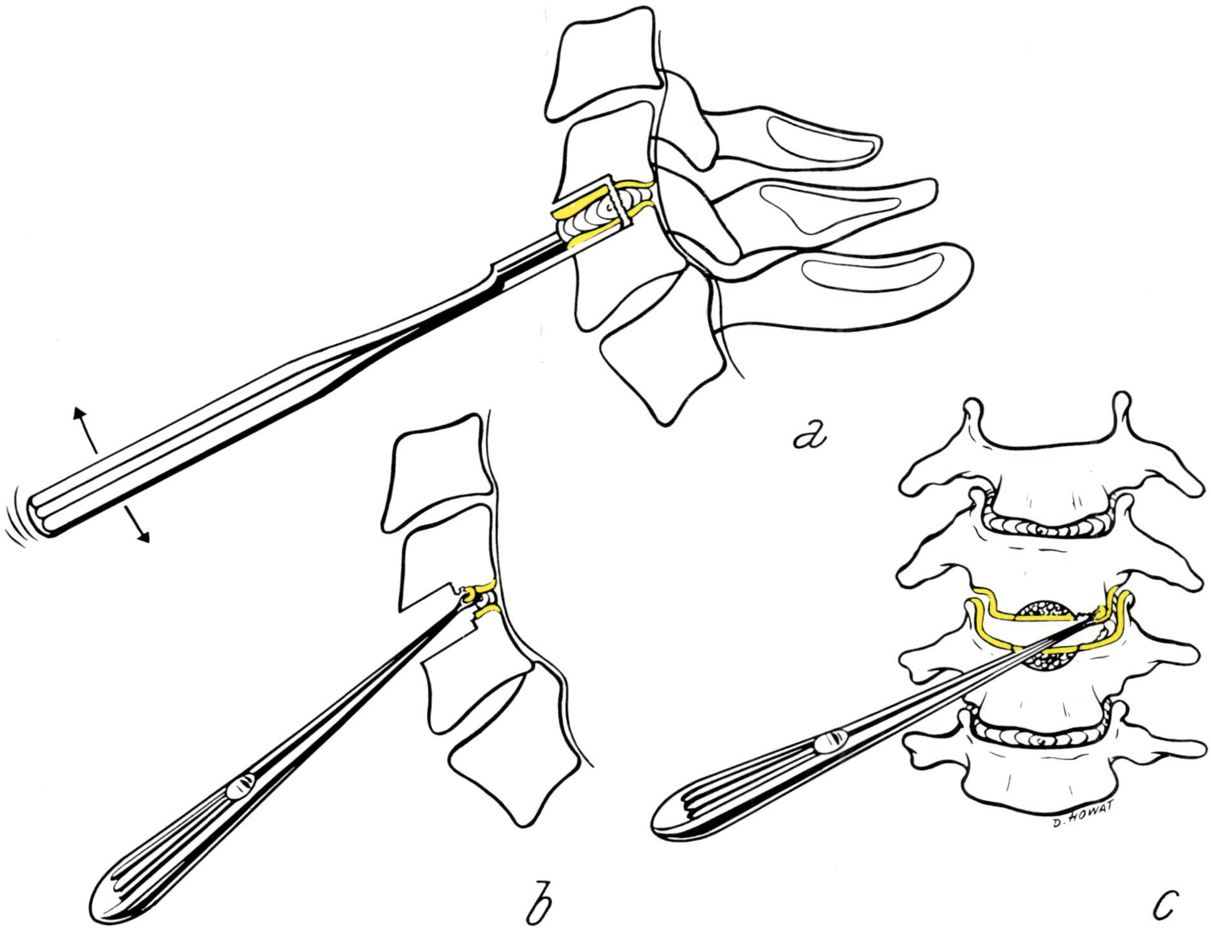

Figures 7.24. **a** A drawing to show the method of use of the tooled gouge for removal of the plug of the vertebral bodies and disc following the use of the cutter as depicted in Fig. 7.21b. **b** A drawing to illustrate the use of a fine curette (2 mm cup) for removal of the vertebral end-plate remnants shown in yellow–after the plug of disc tissue sandwiched between vertebral end-plate margins has been displaced with the gouge and removed with a straight pituitary rongeur. **c** A drawing depicting the use of the fine curette (2 mm cup) showing the prepared dowel cavity from in front with the curette removing remnants of vertebral end-plate cartilage and disc tissue in the region of the left-sided unco-vertebral joint. It is possible to remove virtually all disc tissue and vertebral end-plate remnants in this manner

from the spine (Figs. 7.24a–c). If the disc has been of normal dimensions, after using the gouge in the manner illustrated, first on one side of the disc, then on the other, it is usually possible to remove the plug of bone and intervening disc tissue in one piece.

In cases of advanced spondylosis, where the opposing vertebral end plates are sclerotic, being separated by thin unyielding remnants of disc tissue, it may be necessary to curette the remnants of the disc tissue from between the arcuate segments of vertebral bodies before these bony fragments can be displaced with the gouges.

When the base of the dowel cavity has been exposed, brisk haemorrhage may occur from arteries and veins in the vertebral bodies. This is controlled easily by applying small quantities of bone wax to the cut surface of the vertebral bodies, only at the site of bleeding.

The fourth and final stage of preparation of the intervertebral space now commences, leading up to the actual impaction of the bone graft. Vertebral end-plate cartilage remnants are removed with a fine curette (1 or 2 mm cup)–disc remnants attached–as illustrated in Figs. 7.24b, c. Care is taken to avoid damaging the vertebral arteries (Figs. 7.1a, b).

Longitudinal traction applied to the skull by the anaesthetist will result in opening up of the intervertebral space, allowing the surgeon to see the posterior longitudinal ligament in the depths of the dowel cavity. Through visible defects in this ligament in cases of sequestration of disc fragments into the cervical spinal canal, it is possible to remove the displaced disc tissue from the canal.

Excision of osteophytic bars of bone from the anterior aspect of the cervical spinal canal may be required in cases of cervical myelopathy. Depending on the transverse width of the disc, two overlapping dowel cavities may be cut, allowing a wider exposure for this delicate–and potentially dangerous–task. The use of high speed drills is recommended by some surgeons. My personal preference is for the use of strong fine angled curettes to fragment these bars, allowing their removal piece-meal with the help of fine pituitary rongeurs. One should aim to make the initial entry into the cervical canal from the side of the intervertebral disc space.

g) *Graft Preparation*

While waiting for the control X-ray film to be developed, autogenous grafts should be cut from the anterior third of the iliac crest. If only a single graft is required, this may be cut through a small vertical skin incision placed 2 or 3 cms behind the anterior superior iliac spine, splitting the fibres of tensor fascia lata in the line of the

---

Figures 7.25. a A drawing of the cervical spine, viewed from the side, showing a prepared dowel cavity between two vertebral bodies with a *depth gauge inserted to measure the depth of the cavity before the graft is inserted.* **b** A drawing of the pelvic crest to show the site of removal of a plug of bone which is cut from the outer table and through the inner table. The measurement of this graft between the two cortical faces varies, depending on the size of the patient's pelvis. Grafts should be trimmed so that the anterior and posterior margins are parallel. The depth of the anterior iliac crest between the inner and outer cortical tables varies between 5 and 15 mm. In patients in whom the pelvis is thin (3–5 mm between outer and inner cortices), it may be necessary to cut grafts vertically downwards from the top of the crest, by the method used in lumbar interbody fusions. **c** A drawing to show the initial stages of impaction of the graft, *the measurement of which has been checked carefully with the measurement of the prepared dowel cavity. At this stage the anaesthetist is asked to elongate the neck by applying traction under the angles of the mandible.* **d** Final seating of the graft is sometimes necessary if the anterior margin is not flush with the anterior vertebral margins after the use of the initial impactor which has a central nipple on it, as illustrated in (c) above. The manoeuvre shown is performed with a plain-ended impactor and *it is important to note that the impactor is placed half-way across the graft and half-way across the adjacent vertebral body so that when a blow is struck with the hammer it is impossible to drive the graft too deeply into the dowel cavity,* the impactor coming to rest on the anterior vertebral margin, thus it is prevented from plunging too deeply into the prepared dowel cavity. *Accurate seating of the graft is essential if the complications of graft rotation or post-operative prolapse are to be avoided*

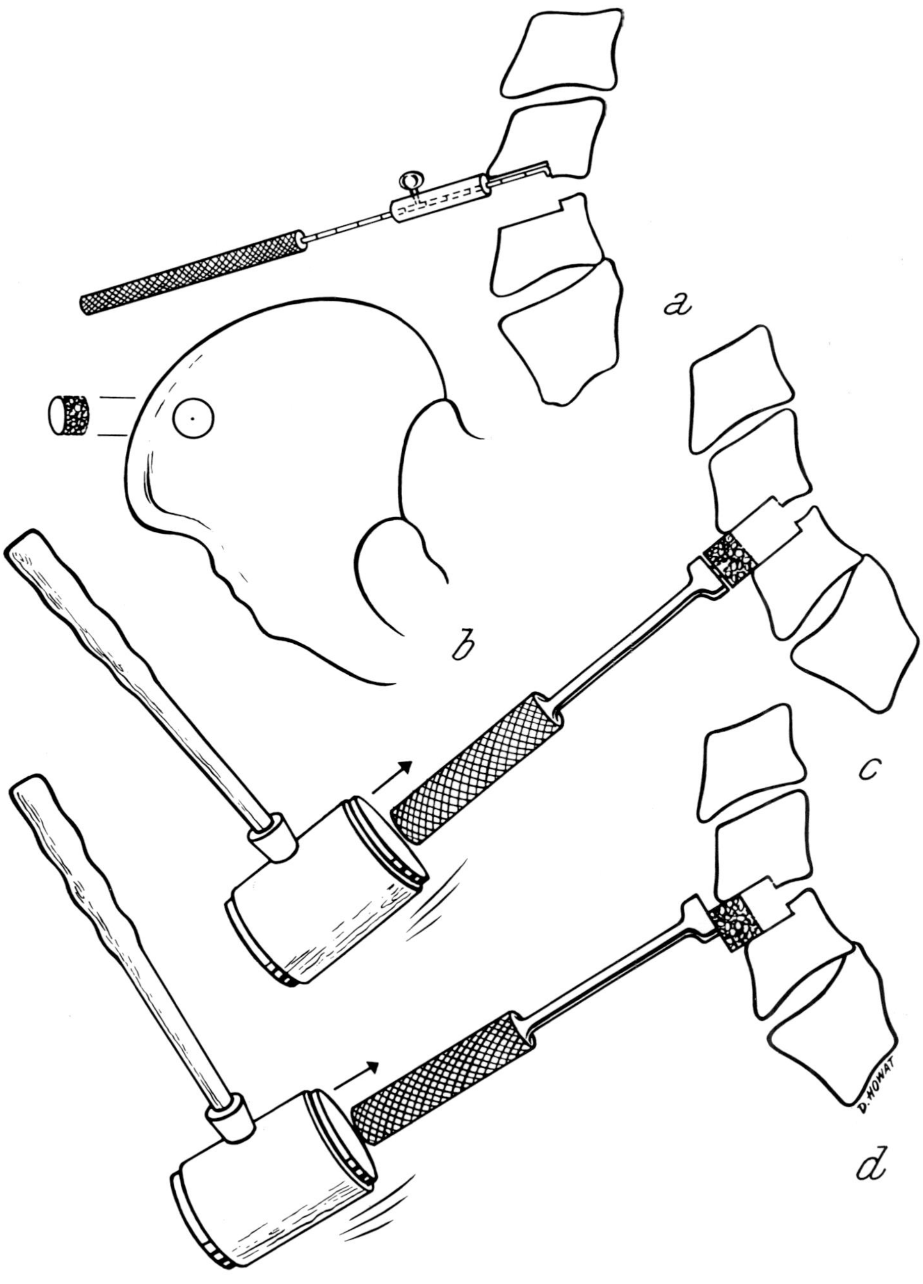

Figures 7.25

skin cut. *The cutting cylinder must be one size larger than that used to prepare the dowel cavity in the neck.*

When more than one graft is required, the skin incision should run parallel to the iliac crest about 1 cm below it. The fascia lata is cut 1 cm below its upper attachment to the iliac crest and the muscles of the outer table of the ilium stripped down sufficiently to allow easy access for removal of the desired number of grafts. During wound closure, a suction drain tube should be inserted. The sutures should be placed deeply into the muscle mass from within-out, allowing the bulky muscle to be pulled up towards its former site of attachment on the outer wall of the iliac crest. If the sutures approximate only the fascial coverings near the margins of the incision, a noticeable ugly defect results in the muscle bulk below the iliac crest.

For rare indications, long stout grafts may be required to bridge multiple vertebral levels, where, for example, a cervical kyphotic deformity is being corrected (Fig. 7.8), or after excision of vertebral bodies for tumour or infection. Fibular grafts have been advocated for use in such circumstances. In my view, it is preferable to use long grafts cut from the ilium, to include both cortical surfaces, with cancellous bone between. These grafts will vascularize more rapidly than full fibular grafts, the latter being useful only in exceptional circumstances.

h) Graft Impaction

The final critical manoeuvres required to seat the graft in the dowel cavity are illustrated in Figs. 7.25 a–d. Before insertion of the graft, the surgeon must always measure the depth of the dowel cavity and the depth of the graft. *Great force is never required during impaction.* Soft tissue should be carefully retracted from the margins of the cavity and the neck should be gently elongated by traction applied to the skull before the graft is inserted.

i) Wound Closure

After the grafts have been inserted, a careful inspection should be made of the anterior aspect of the vertebrae; any bleeding points should be coagulated, especially along the medial margins of the longus colli muscles.

The neck wound may be closed then, without drainage, except after multi-level fusions or in rare circumstances after associated thyroid surgery.

j) Post-Operative Management

Patients complain of little pain after this operation–in contrast to those who have had cervical laminectomies.

Nursed with the head raised on two or three pillows, they should have collars fitted after returning to bed from the operating room (Figs. 7.26, 7.27). Patients are more comfortable when they wear an appropriate neck support after cervical fusion.

Dysphagia is common in the first few days after surgery; restriction of the intake of solid foods is advisable, but special measures in management are rarely required. During an anterior cervical interbody fusion at the C2/3 level, in one case, a small pharyngeal laceration occurred. This was sutured. Nothing was given to the patient by mouth for three days, intravenous fluid replacement being administered during that time, with prophylactic chemotherapy and no ill-effects resulted.

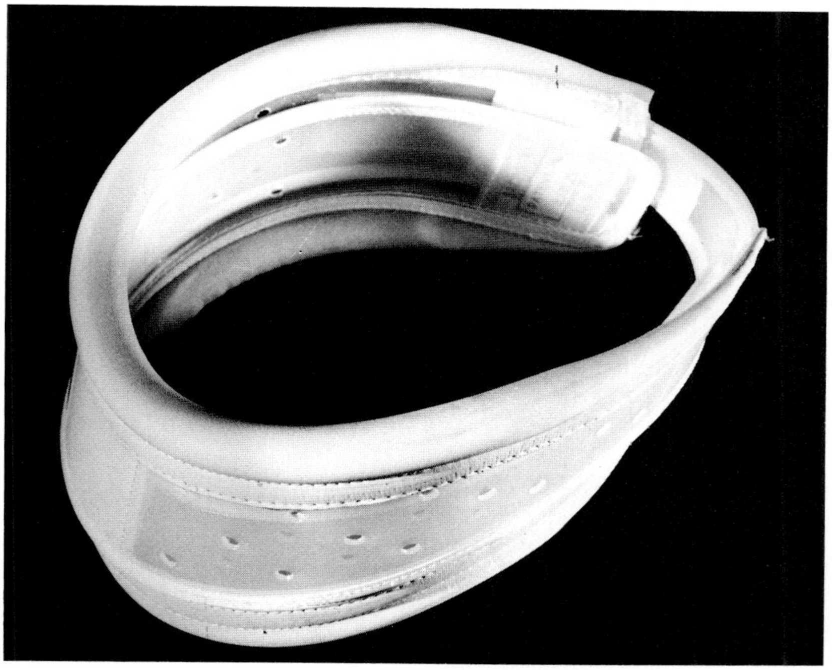

Figure 7.26. A photograph of a light plastic collar of adjustable height suitable for use in the post-operative period after single level anterior cervical fusion operations. This type of collar is also suitable for use in the conservative management of patients with neck pain after neck injuries, or for the treatment of recurring symptoms of neck pain and occipital headache due to cervical spondylosis

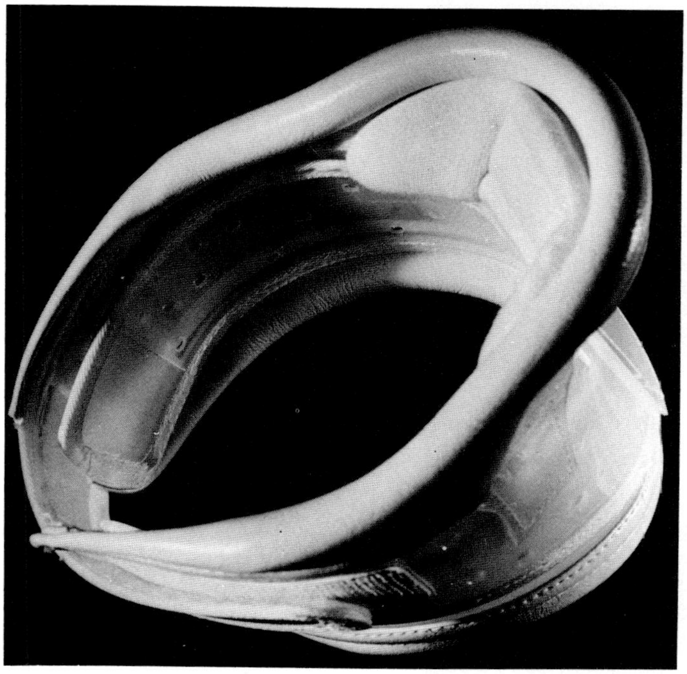

Figure 7.27. A photograph of an adjustable plastic cervical collar with supporting chin piece suitable for use after multi-level cervical fusions

Within twenty-four hours of operation, patients should be encouraged to get out of bed and to walk short distances. Their stay in hospital averages 12 days.

Travel by car should be avoided for six weeks and then allowed only in vehicles with head rests fitted or built into the seats. Until the graft or grafts have incorporated with the vertebrae, a collar should be worn at all times when travelling.

7.6. Radiological Changes After Interbody Fusion

The appearances of grafts at different levels in the neck and at varying periods after operation are shown in Figs. 7.28–7.31.

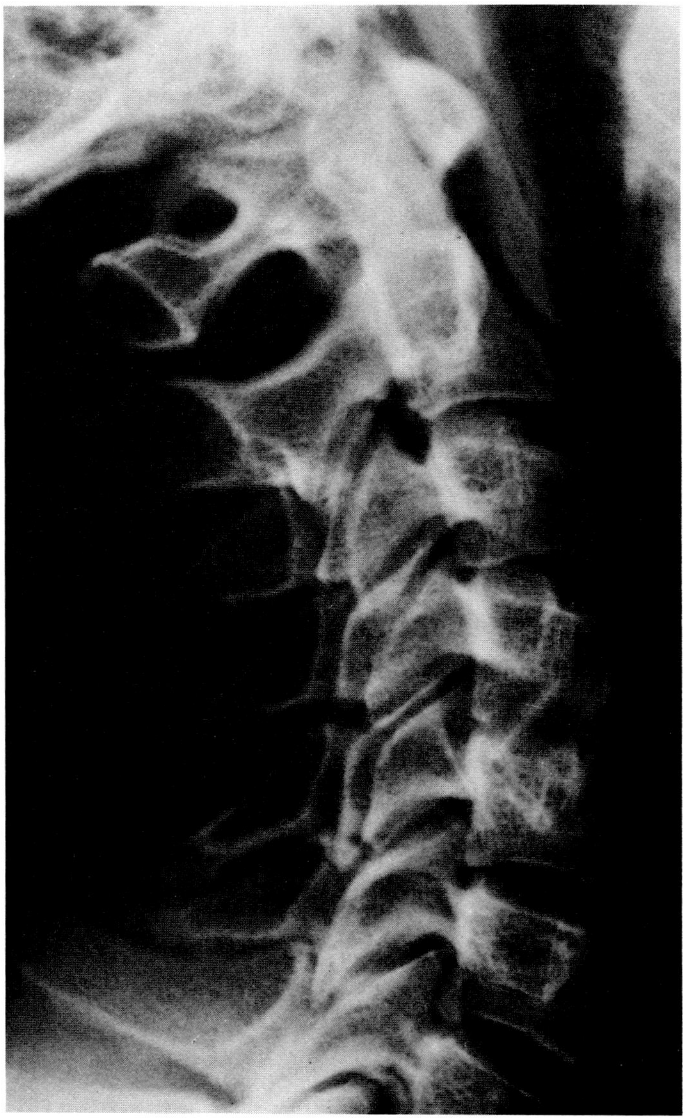

Figure 7.28

Union with this method can be expected in about 96% of cases. Mal-union with kyphosis may occur, if the shape of the grafts at the time of operation was unsatisfactory because of the size and contour of the pelvis at the donor site. In such cases, X-rays should be taken at intervals of one, two and four weeks post-operatively. If the grafts rotate during that time, with resultant kyphotic deformity of the neck, the patient should be re-admitted to hospital and nursed with the head in traction and the neck in extension for several weeks. A collar of the

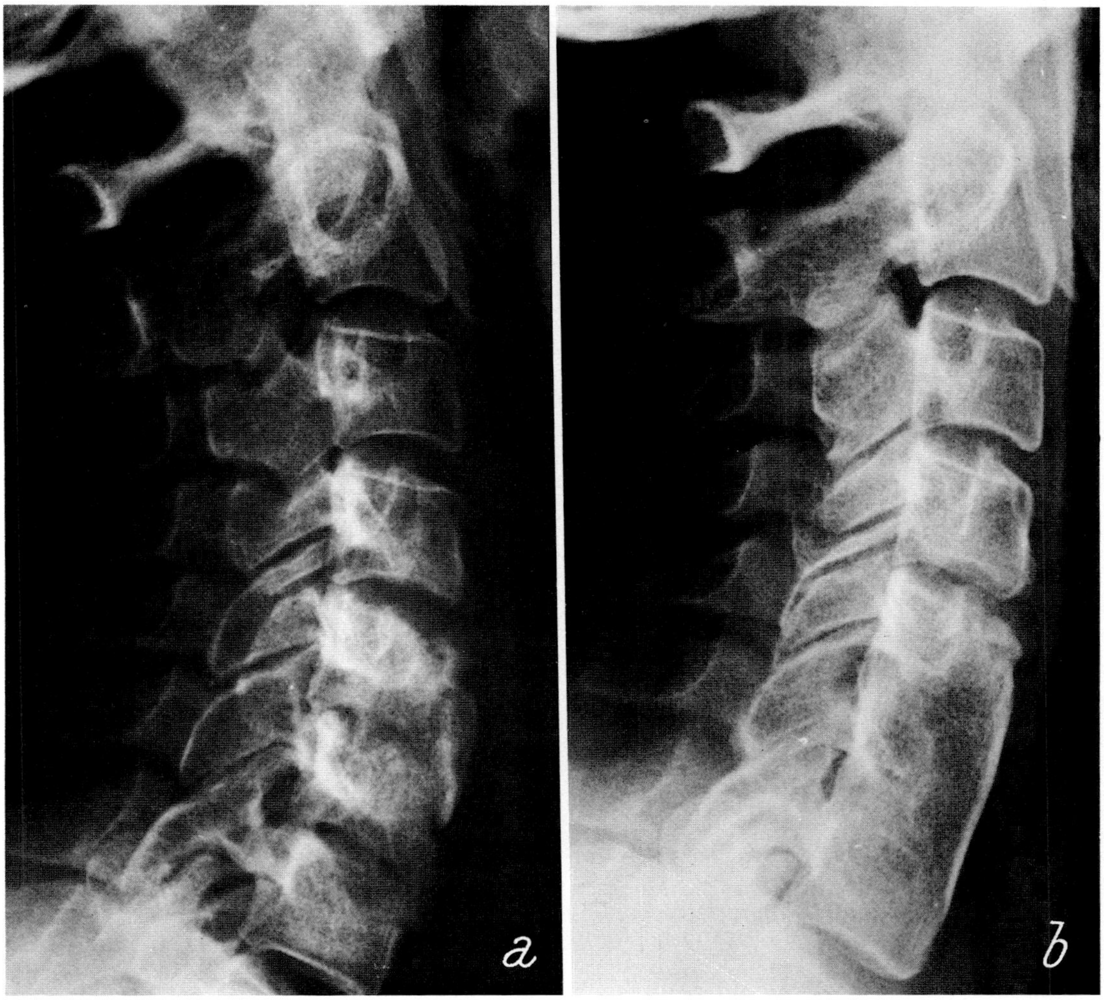

Figures 7.29. **a** A lateral radiograph of the cervical spine of a man aged 34 showing the appearance at three months following anterior interbody fusions at C5/6 and C6/7. Early incorporation of the grafts in satisfactory position is evident. The indication for the operation in this case was to control intractable neck pain and headache with some referred shoulder pain *following post-traumatic internal disc disruption demonstrated by discography.* **b** A radiograph of the same spine taken five years later showing complete remodelling of the fused segments between the vertebral bodies at C5/6 and C6/7

Figure 7.28. A lateral radiograph of the cervical spine of a man aged 24 years taken five months after an anterior *cervical fusion* performed at the C4/5 level for *post-traumatic internal disc disruption.* The fusion is solid and union has occurred without spinal deformity

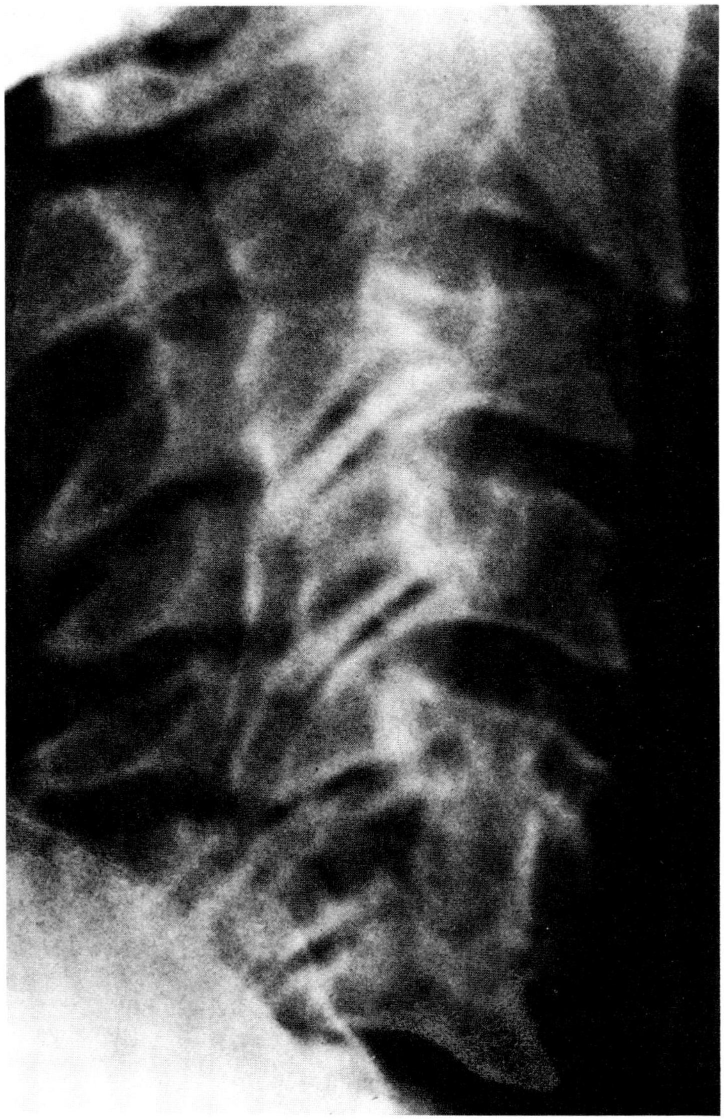

Figure 7.30. A lateral radiograph of the spine of the patient whose pre-operative films are illustrated in Figs. 7.4 a and b. *This patient had clinical evidence of cervical myelopathy* with a spastic gait and weak upper extremities. Note the positioning of the interbody graft which is already incorporating. *Note also that the large osteophyte has been excised completely from the front of the cervical vertebral column*

Zimmer or SOMI type should be fitted thereafter, with the neck held in the corrected position, checked by lateral X-rays taken with the collar applied.

In general, collars should be worn for two or three months, until early union of the grafts can be expected. Instruction in the use of gentle mobilizing neck exercises should be given at that time. Should restriction of neck movements persist beyond six months after fusion, the neck may be manipulated with gentle longitudinal traction and rotatory motions to right and left, under a short-acting general anaesthetic.

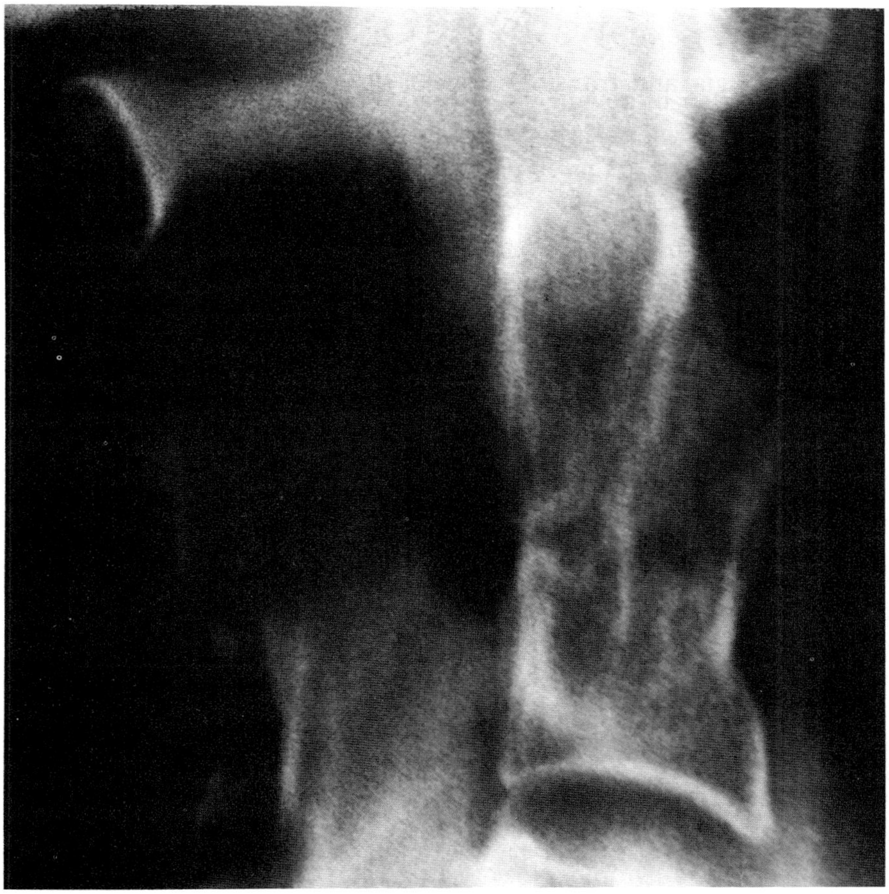

Figure 7.31. A lateral tomogram of the upper cervical spine in a man aged 24 years showing an *anterior interbody fusion at the C2/3 level* six months after operation. The indication for treatment was for *persisting subluxation of C2 on C3 following a neck injury* sustained in a motor vehicle accident when his car overturned

7.7. Complications

The list of *potential complications* following anterior cervical interbody fusion operations includes:

1. Quadriplegia.
2. Unilateral blindness produced by the pressure of an assistant's hand resting on the globe.
3. Vascular catastrophes involving the vertebral or carotid arteries.
4. Severe venous haemorrhage following damage to the jugular vein.
5. Oesophageal laceration.
6. Horner's syndrome.

Reviewing my own experience with the use of this operation during twenty years, I have had to deal with a range of minor problems and with only a few serious complications.

7.9. Posterior Cervical Spinal Fusion

The indications for these procedures have been set out above. Details of surgical technique will not be discussed as they involve simple manoeuvres which are in common use. However, radiographs showing the appearance of conditions requiring these procedures, with post-operative X-rays are found in Figs. 7.6, 7.33, and 7.34, together with photographs of suitable braces and a Minerva jacket which may be used post-operatively (Figs. 7.35–7.37).

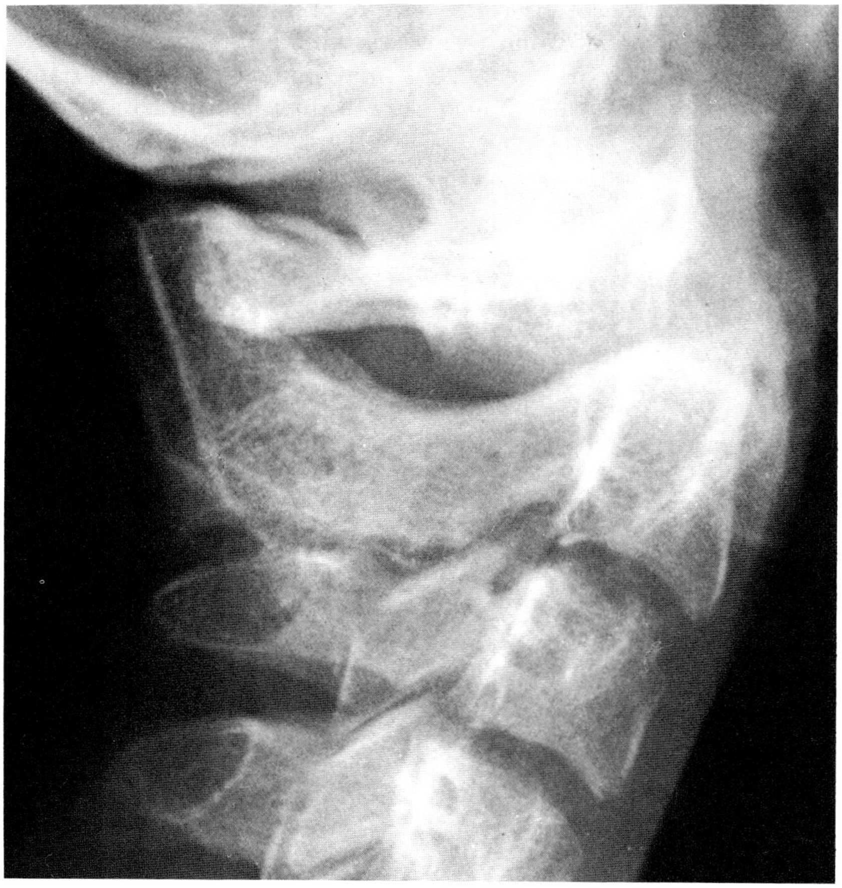

Figure 7.33. A lateral radiograph of the upper cervical spine of a man aged 22 years who sustained a severe head injury following a motor vehicle accident in which the odontoid peg was fractured. C1/2 fusion is solid, though the reduction of the odontoid fracture is incomplete. The patient had no neurological signs or symptoms following union of the graft. At operation the grafts were held in place with heavy braided nylon which does not appear on the X-ray film

---

Figure 7.34. A lateral radiograph of the upper cervical spine showing an extensive occipito-cervical fusion performed for the treatment of an un-united fracture of the odontoid. The film was taken three months after operation

Figure 7.35. A photograph of an adjustable cervical collar of the Zimmer type, providing more effective immobilization following multi-level cervical fusions or in the later stages of management of C1/2 fusions after removal of halo-jackets or Minerva jackets

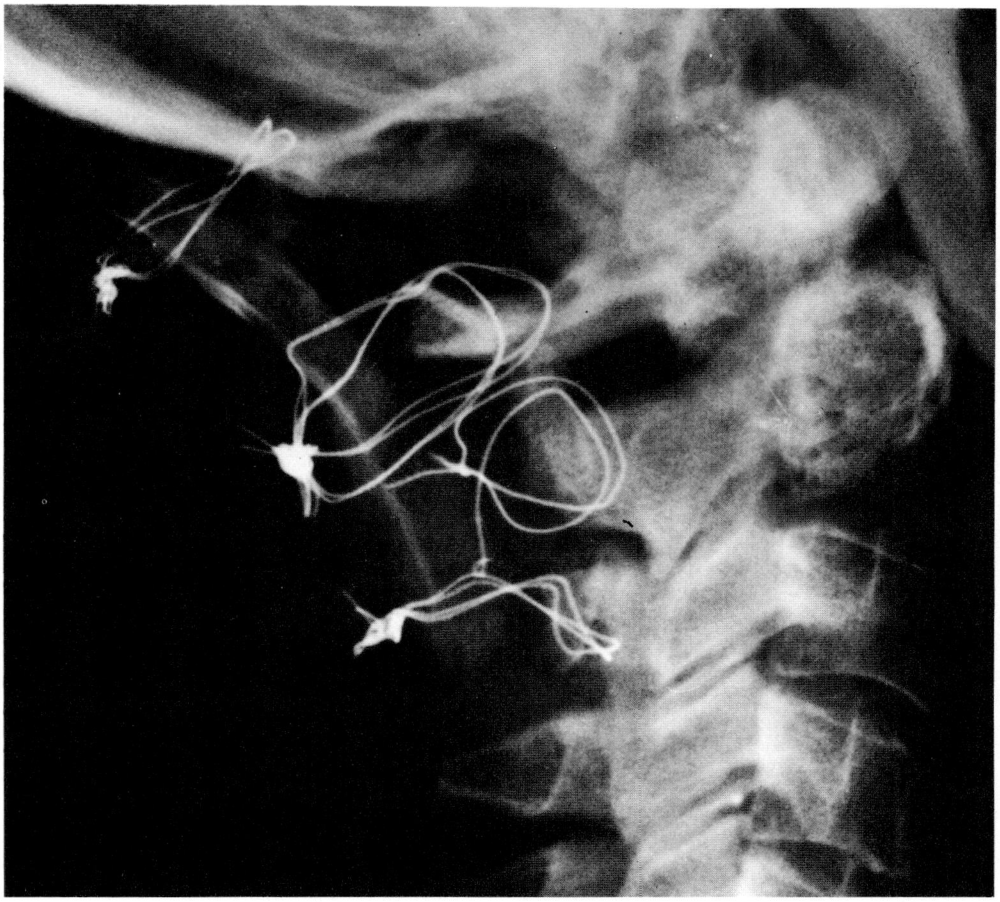

Figure 7.34

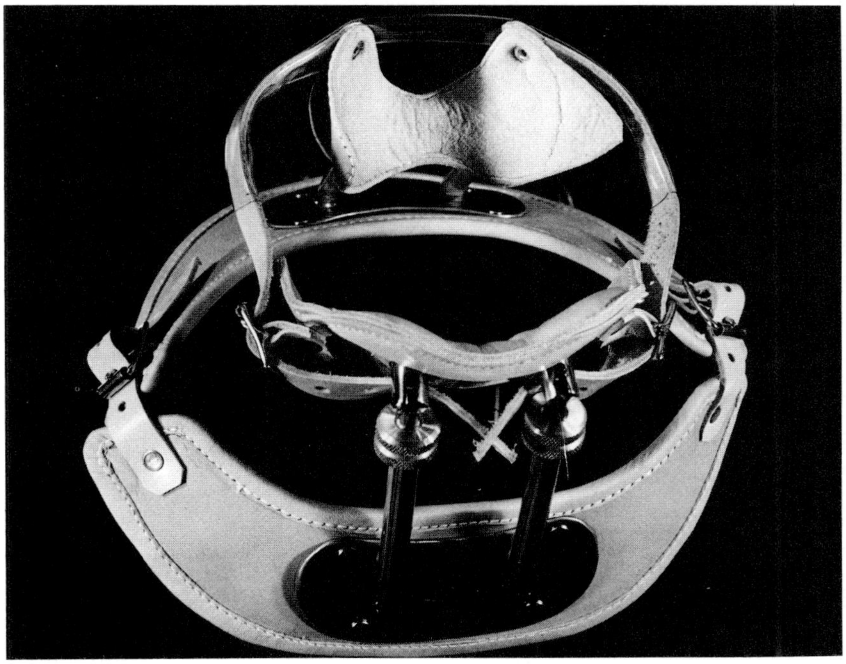

Figure 7.35

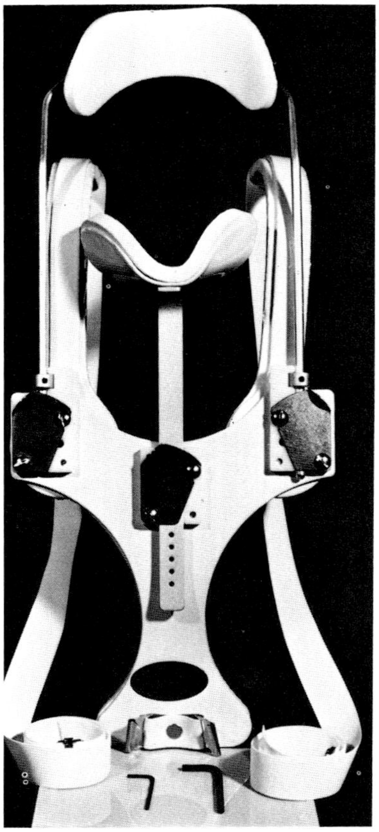

Figure 7.36

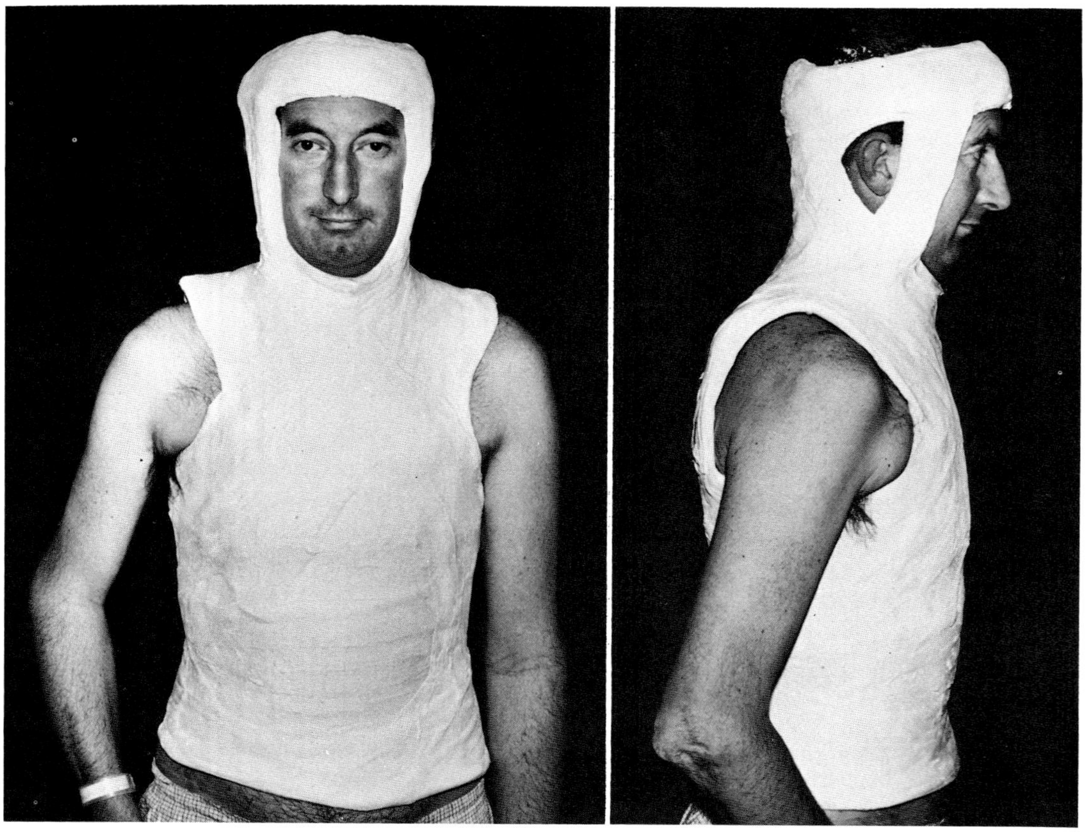

Figure 7.37

7.10. Cervical Laminectomy

a) Positioning (Fig. 7.38)

The prone position, using a neurosurgical headrest, provides satisfactory conditions for operation.

b) Exposure

The techniques used in this approach to the laminae are identical to those described for exposure of the lumbar spine, except that the scale and mobility of the bones is different, the cervical spine being small and very mobile. Smaller instruments are therefore required for use in this area (Fig. 7.39).

Having identified the lamina or laminae to be removed, the spinous processes should be excised. Then, using a Leksell-type rongeur, with thin cutting blades, the inferior surface of the superior lamina at the interspace can be removed piece-meal, while the thin ligamentum flavum is still intact. Having enlarged the inter-laminar space, the ligamentum flavum can be reflected and excised, after passing a small moistened patty beneath it, propelled gently laterally on the tip of the curved end of a Watson-Cheyne dissector. This done, on both sides of the canal, preparation is then made to perform a foraminotomy. The soft tissues and veins are separated carefully from the remnants of the roof of the spinal canal, one side at a time. The pedicles can be identified using the curved tip of the Watson-Cheyne probe. Venous bleeding should not obstruct the surgeon's view, unless the manoeuvres just described have been carried out carelessly or too quickly.

Using a forward-angled 45° rongeur with a 1 or 2 mm cup, it is then possible to open the roof of the intervertebral foramen, protecting the dura and nerve root sleeve with a patty on the end of a fine sucker. When this has been done, the regional veins will distend remarkably–if a stenosis in the region has been relieved. Some brisk venous haemorrhage may then occur. This is best controlled by the application of small fragments of gelfoam (or its equivalent) packed lightly in place with an overlying moist patty. The use of coagulating currents, through low voltage diathermy machines, is still widespread. However, I have not found it necessary to resort to this method of haemorrhage control, which I believe to be potentially dangerous if used at multiple levels in the cervical spine. There is a significant risk of damaging the fine

---

Figure 7.36. A photograph of a *SOMI brace* which provides an adjustable occipital support and an adjustable mental support fitted to a sternal plate which is suspended over the shoulder and fixed firmly to the trunk with adjustable straps. On cine-radiography this is one of the most effective devices for immobilizing the cervical spine. However, there are problems with its management as it tends to ride up when the patient lies in bed

Figure 7.37. A photograph showing a patient viewed from in front and from the side, fitted with a Minerva jacket for immobilization of the upper cervical spine following occipito-cervical fusion. Although variations of halo-jackets are available, *this useful method of spinal immobilization is illustrated for the benefit of surgeons who do not have access to more expensive commercially available braces such as the halo with thoracic jacket and pillar supports.* Before the Minerva jacket is fitted, the patient should be placed on a tilting bed so that he is used to standing in a vertical position, and then the jacket can be put on when he is able to stand without dizziness for periods in excess of 30 minutes

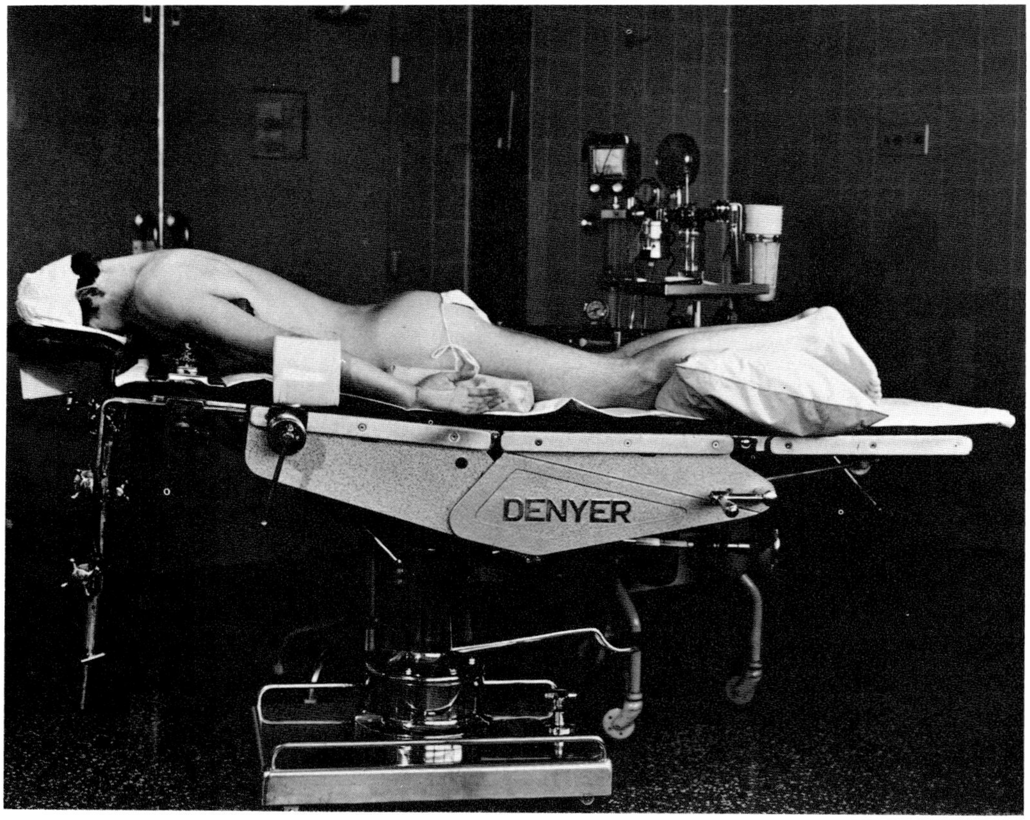

Figure 7.38. A photograph to show the arrangements for posturing the patient on an operating table for posterior approaches to the cervical spine. When the patient is in the prone position for operations on the cervical spine, particular precautions must be taken to ensure that the anaesthetic tubes and airways are securely fastened, with all their linkage points strapped to prevent accidental separation during the surgery. When the patient is in this position, the skin of the neck is often lax. Strapping should be applied across the hairline transversely and fixed to the head support. Further strapping is then attached across the vertex of the skull running from the transverse strapping to the front of the headrest. In addition, long strips of strapping should be applied just lateral to the spinous process of C7 on both sides, running down the back to the buttocks. This will ensure that the skin of the neck is tightly stretched and it makes the incision and its subsequent closure much easier. Note also the inclination of the table. If the head is raised any further, then *the potential risk of air embolism must be borne in mind*

segmental arteries which join the anterior median longitudinal arterial channel of the cervical spinal cord if diathermy is used to excess in the region of the intervertebral foramina within the cervical canal (Crock and Yoshizawa, 1977).

On completion of the "laminectomy" and foraminotomies, the partes inter-articulares of the laminae being preserved, along with the bulk of the facet joints, the wound should be closed with suction drainage. Before this is done, all haemorrhage should be controlled, using haemostatic agents in the cervical canal as described, and diathermy in the muscle layer.

Facets should be preserved, except in cases of trauma, when facetectomy may be required to allow reduction of a fracture-dislocation. Localized inter-laminar posterior cervical fusion should be performed then, using inter-spinous wire fixation.

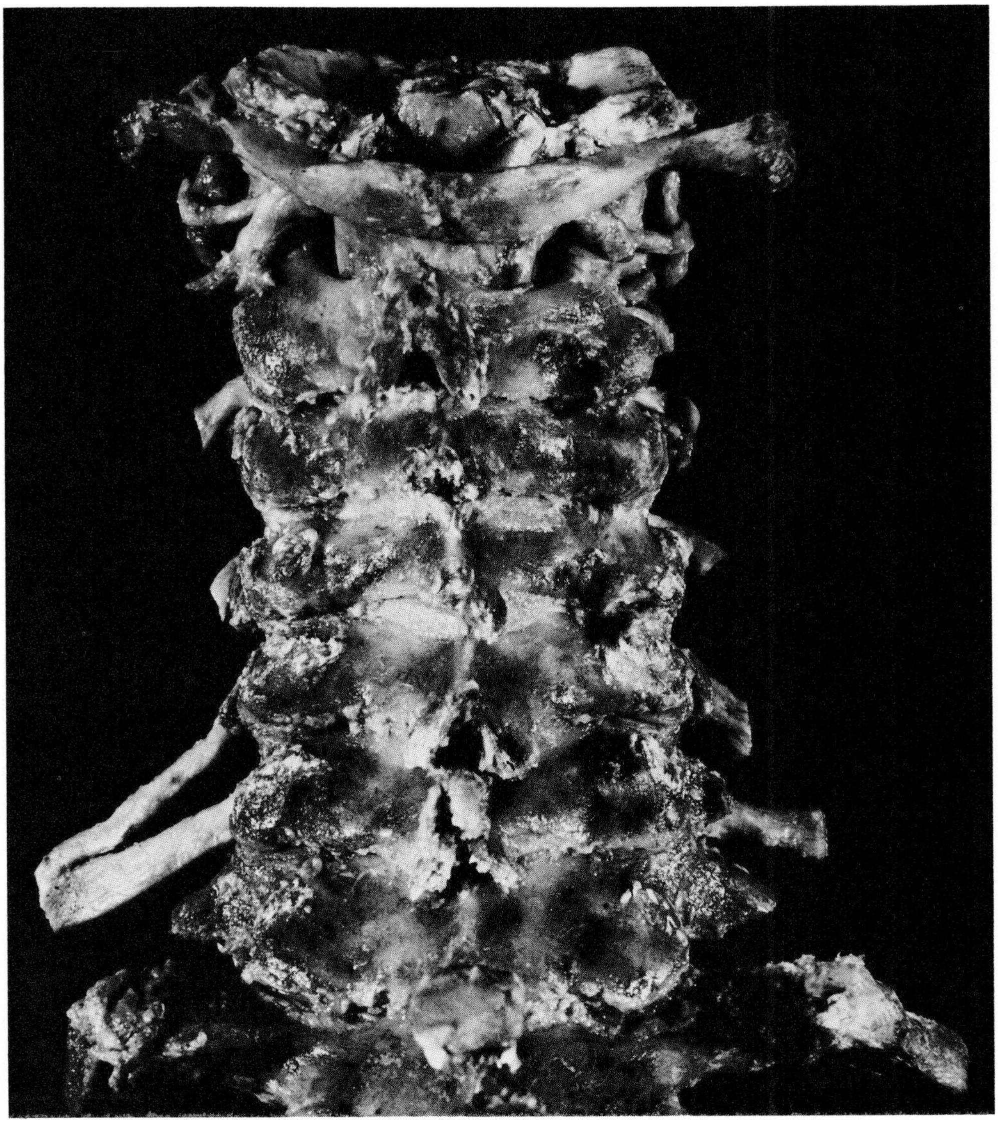

Figure 7.39. A photograph of a dissection of the cervical spine viewed from behind. All the soft tissues have been removed except the ligamenta flava, the dural sac and the emerging nerve roots. At the level of C1 and C2, note the relationships of the emerging nerve roots to the vertebral arteries on both sides. The facet joints from C2 distally can be seen orientated in the coronal plane. In the cervical spine the inter-laminar spaces are very narrow at all levels, and only a few millimetres of ligamentum flavum can be seen in the normal state. (Dissected by Dr. M. C. Crock)

c) Post-Operative Care

Patients complain of severe pain after posterior cervical spinal operations. Adequate analgesia should therefore be ordered.

The use of soft collars for short periods can be recommended after decompressions of the cervical canal.

8

Spinal Infections

8.1. *Acute Vertebral Osteomyelitis*

a) Introduction

In clinical practice, acute inflammatory lesions of the spine are relatively uncommon. For this reason alone, diagnosis of vertebral osteomyelitis is often delayed, so that patients may not receive specific treatment for the disease until they present with major complications.

The virtues of specialist hospitals are often hailed but cogent arguments favour the retention of specialist units in large general hospitals, where orthopaedic surgeons and neurosurgeons can be consulted readily about the surgical problems relevant to bone disease, not the least important of which are infective lesions of the spine.

Most referred cases of vertebral osteomyelitis will come from physicians. Vertebral infections follow repeated episodes of bacteraemia or septicaemia which may occur in many debilitating medical diseases such as: pneumonia, chronic bronchitis and diabetes mellitus (Figs. 8.1a, b). One of the most elusive causes of pyrexia of unknown origin is sub-acute bacterial endocarditis. Acute vertebral osteomyelitis may complicate the course of this disease before the underlying pathology of the cardiac valvular disease is recognized and even before positive blood cultures have been obtained.

Some cases will be referred from general surgical wards, having been admitted with abdominal pain and fever (Fig. 8.2).

A third significant source of referred cases in general hospitals is from the urology department. Following urethral or bladder surgery, some patients will present with spinal pain due to vertebral osteomyelitis following gram-negative septicemia.

Some general hospitals in particular localities in large cities often admit many drug addicts and alcoholics, in whom complaints of severe spinal pain should raise the suspicion of underlying vertebral infection. A wide range of organisms, including fungi, may be identified either in blood cultures or from needle biopsy specimens in the drug-addicted patient.

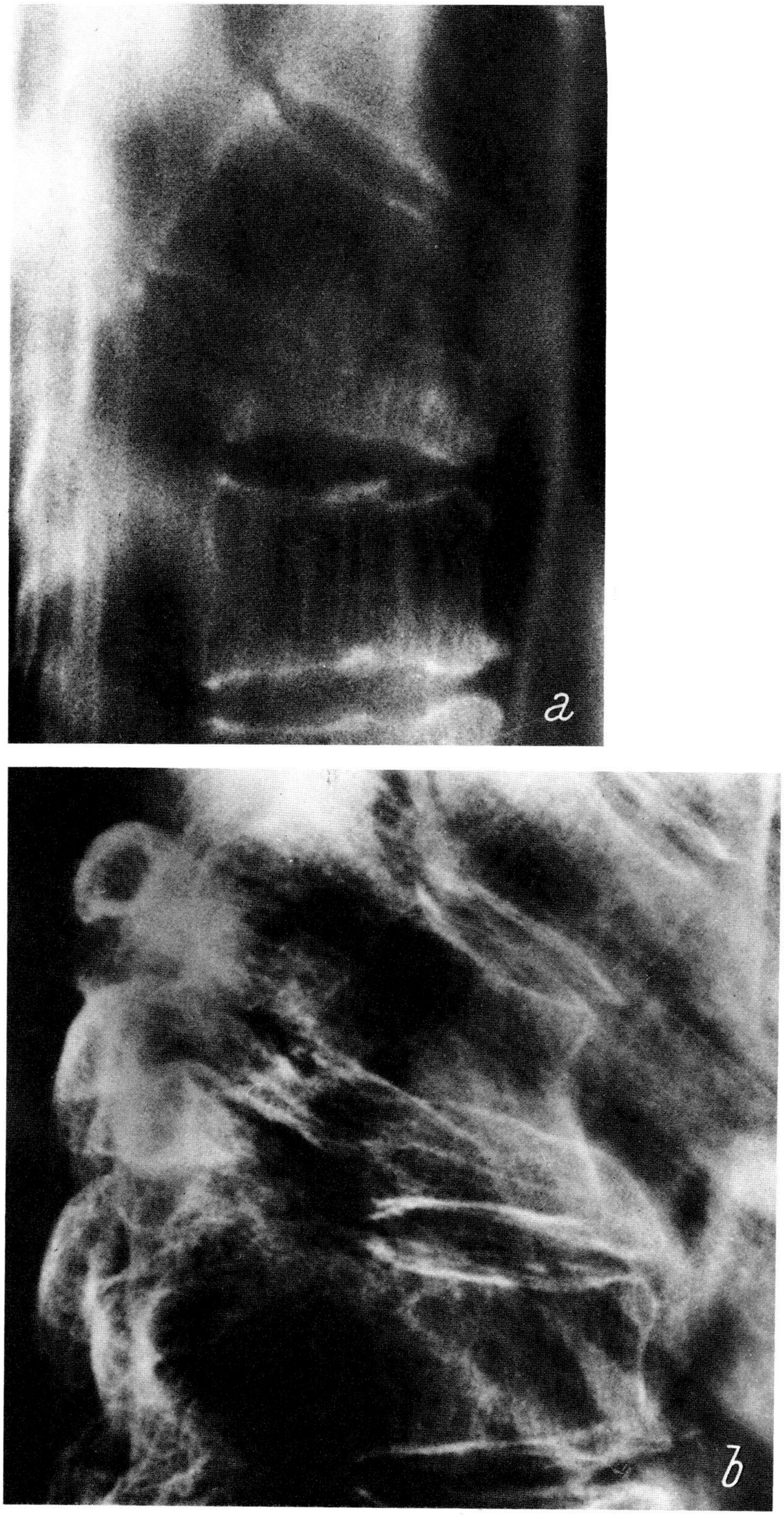

Figures 8.1

Organisms lodge in the complex vascular bed, in the region of the vertebral end-plates, in children and adults (Crock and Yoshizawa, 1977). The pathological changes induced vary enormously depending on the bacteriological characteristics of different organisms.

Although the radiological appearances may be similar, in the case of staphylococcal infections chondrolytic activity destroys cartilage and disc tissue, whereas in tuberculous disease these tissues are not destroyed. The loss of disc height shown on X-rays in cases of spinal tuberculosis is due to osteitis with pathological fracture, the disc tissue simply collapsing into the adjacent carious vertebral bodies (Figs. 8.3a, b).

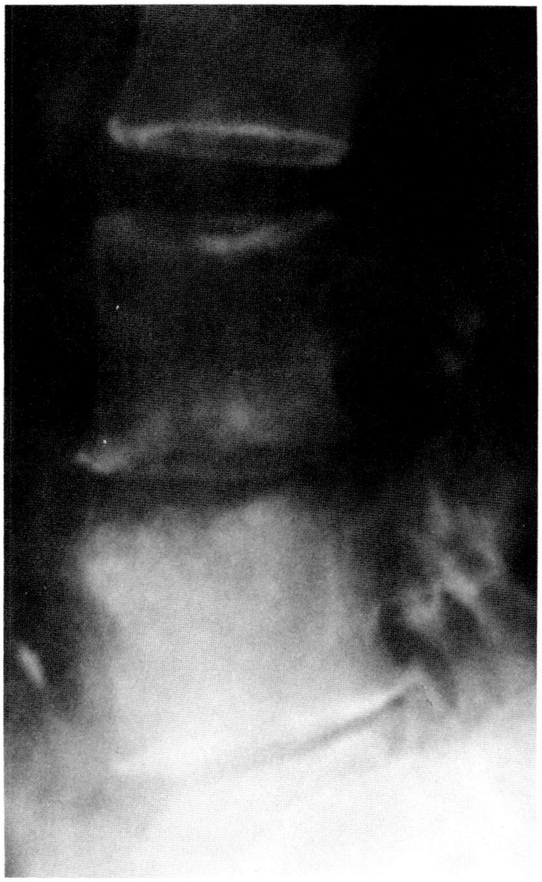

Figure 8.2. A lateral tomogram of the lower lumbar spine of a woman aged 59. Note the changes in the upper half of the body of the 5th lumbar vertebra in the region of the vertebral end-plate, with erosion and narrowing of the intervertebral disc space. The patient presented with acute abdominal pain, overshadowing back pain. The lesion was due to an acute osteomyelitis of the body of L5 complicating bronchitis

Figures 8.1. a A lateral tomogram of the mid-thoracic spine of a woman aged 66 who had been under treatment for chronic bronchitis for three months prior to her presentation with back pain and paraplegia. Gross destruction of the vertebral body of T7 is noted with pathological fracture-dislocation. **b** A lateral X-ray of the same area taken four years after conservative treatment of this lesion with long-term chemotherapy. Considerable remoulding of the vertebrae at the site of the dislocation had occurred and the paraplegia had recovered in part

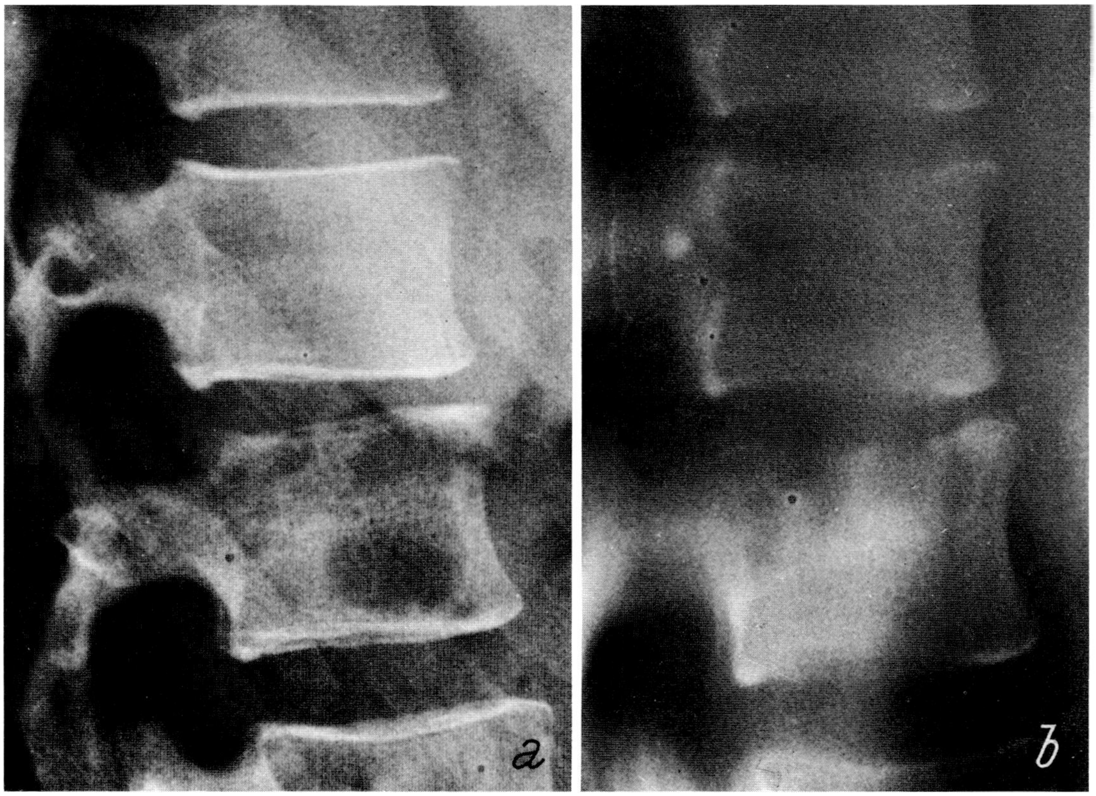

Figures 8.3. **a** A lateral radiograph of the lumbar spine of a 32 year old patient who presented with a history of *low back pain and weight loss.* She had not complained of pain in the region of this lesion. The film is centred on the disc between T12 and L1 at the thoraco-lumbar junction. Note the narrowing of the disc space. **b** A lateral tomogram of the same area of the spine in the same patient. Note the extensive erosive changes in the upper vertebral end-plate of the lower vertebra at the level of the narrowed disc space. *This lesion was tuberculous* and, at operation, intact disc tissue was found within the cavities of the lower vertebral body

b) Clinical Findings

The sudden onset of excruciating spinal pain in a febrile patient, should immediately arouse the suspicion of the diagnosis of vertebral osteomyelitis. Physical signs include:

- marked local tenderness in the spine;
- paraspinal spasm and rigidity, or psoas spasm causing fixed flexion deformity of the hip;
- local spinal deformity;
- rapidly advancing neurological deficits in cases with spinal epidural abscesses (Figs. 8.4a–c).

c) Investigations

Full *blood examination* should be carried out urgently, and repeated samples of blood taken for bacteriological cultures, both aerobic and anaerobic.

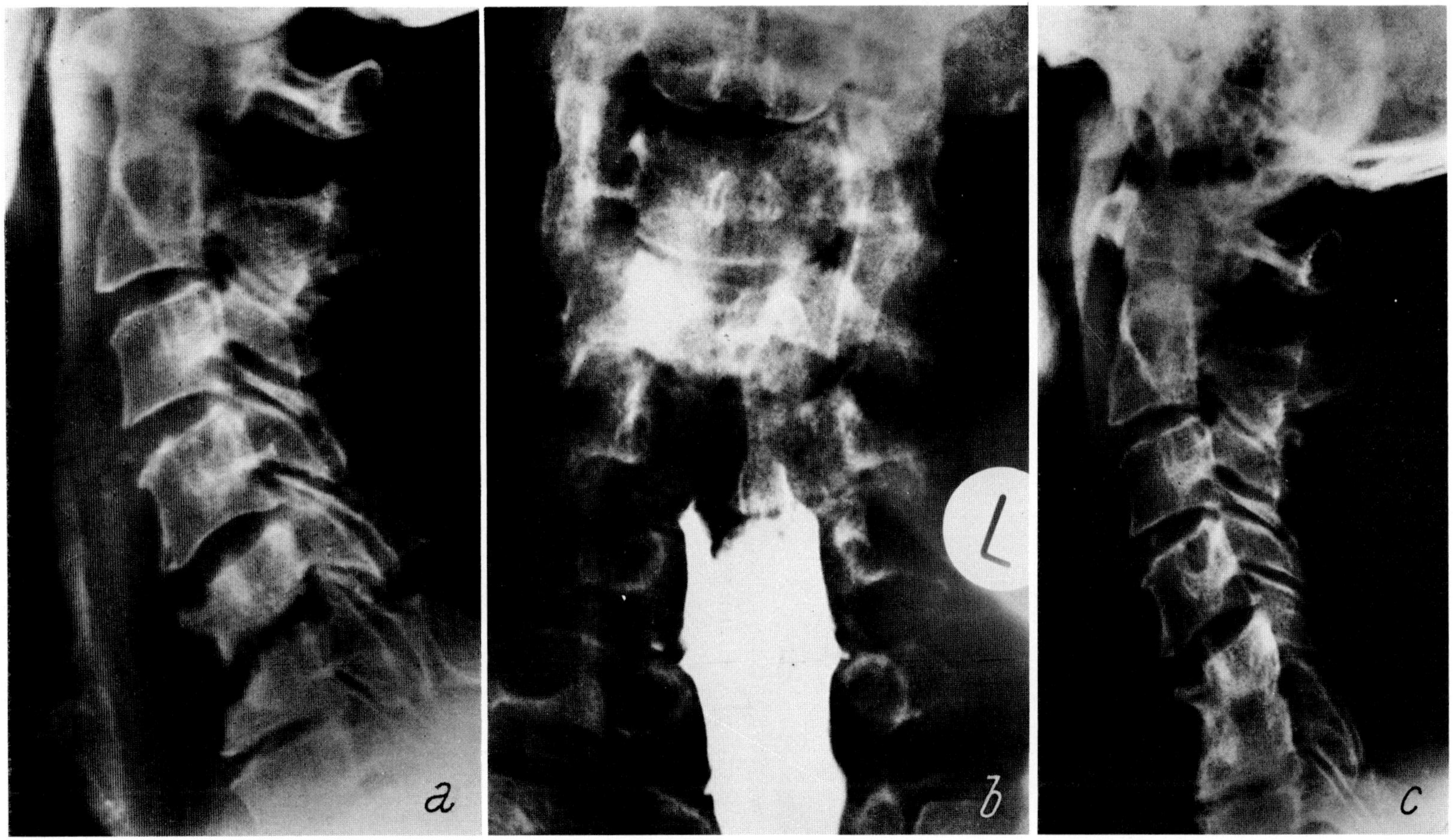

Figures 8.4. **a** A lateral radiograph of the cervical spine of an alcoholic male patient aged 54 years who presented with severe neck pain of sub-acute onset. Note the extensive changes in the vertebral bodies of C5 and C6 with vertebral end-plate erosion in the adjacent vertebral margins of these vertebrae; the disc space is also reduced in height. Note in particular the wide separation of the gas shadow in the pharynx and oesophagus from the anterior aspects of the cervical vertebral bodies, indicating the presence of a pre-vertebral abscess. This patient became quadriplegic within 48 hours of presentation. (By courtesy of Mr. B. J. Dooley and Mr. J. K. Henderson.) **b** An antero-posterior radiograph of the spine of the same patient showing complete obstruction to the flow of a Myodil column upwards at the level of C6 and C7. **c** A lateral radiograph of the spine of the same patient taken 15 months after operation. The spinal canal was decompressed from behind and a large epidural abscess aspirated. Treatment then consisted of splinting the neck in traction with hyperextension; chemotherapy was administered for twelve months. Note the restoration of the normal relationships between the pharynx and oesophagus and the anterior surfaces of the vertebral bodies

Other cultures may be taken from infected skin lesions, sputum, urine or faeces, depending on their predicted relevance on clinical grounds.

The significance of the results of many of these tests is that they may form the basis for decisions in the differential diagnosis between infections, acute and chronic, and neoplastic diseases. In addition, the critical choice of appropriate chemotherapeutic agents will depend on some of them.

d) Radiological Examinations

i) Plain X-Ray

Plain X-rays and tomograms will demonstrate a variety of changes in the bones and soft tissues, pointing to their likely inflammatory basis.

ii) Computerized Axial Tomography

C.T. Scanning has been of inestimable value in demonstrating the relationships between pathological changes in the vertebrae and in the related soft tissue structures. Paravertebral and spinal epidural abscesses may be mapped accurately using this technique.

iii) Myelography

Myelography may be essential to identify the level of obstruction in the spinal canal caused by vertebral collapse or epidural abscess.

e) Needle Biopsy

The use of needles or small trephines inserted into vertebrae under X-ray control represents one of the most significant advances in management of patients with neoplastic or inflammatory lesions (Fig. 8.5). In parts of Asia, where infective lesions of bone are still common, the use of this method to obtain samples both for histological and bacteriological examination has improved the accuracy of diagnosis in many cases of non-tuberculous spinal infections which would have been classified previously as tuberculous (Chari, 1979).

f) Treatment

i) Bed Rest and Chemotherapy

Many patients will respond satisfactorily to conservative treatment. Spontaneous spinal fusion often follows healing of lesions in staphylococcal osteomyelitis.

Problems arising in cases of osteomyelitis due to staphylococcal infections vary with the virulence and sensitivity of the particular organisms. The use of chemotherapy continuously for more than six months may be necessary in patients who have developed multiple bone lesions complicating septicemia (Figs. 8.6a–d).

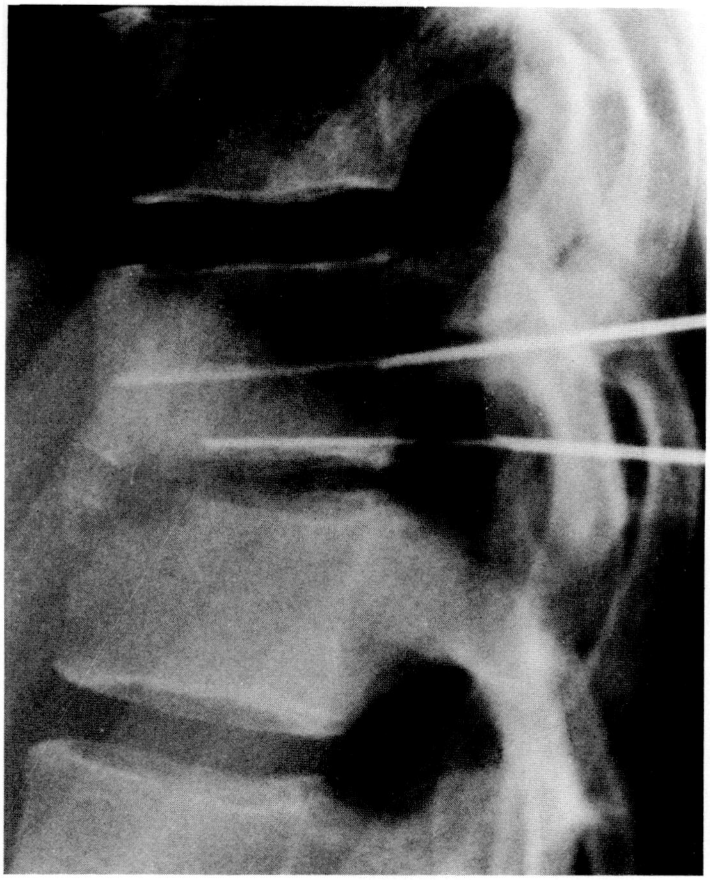

Figure 8.5. A lateral radiograph of the thoracic spine showing a lesion between the vertebrae of T11 and T12 from a woman aged 27 years who had presented with acute thoracic pain and upper abdominal pain some weeks after a gynaecological infection. Note the erosion of the vertebral end-plates in the anterior thirds of the adjacent vertebral margins together with the narrowing of the disc space. Needles used for vertebral biopsy are shown in place. Positive culture of a streptococcal organism was obtained

ii) Drainage of Abscesses

Emergency surgery is required for decompression of the spinal canal in cases developing tetraplegia or paraplegia due to the formation of epidural abscesses.

Occasionally drainage of psoas abscesses may be required, even in cases of non-tuberculous infections (Figs. 8.6c, d).

Surgical treatment of this type is recommended early in the management of vertebral osteomyelitis in drug addicts, because of the high resistance of organisms in these cases to chemotherapy alone (Hartman, 1978).

Even after extensive destruction of vertebral bodies due to staphylococcal infection, spontaneous spinal fusion usually occurs. Supplementary bone graft operations should not be required, providing sharp contrast with the requirements in the surgical management of Pott's disease.

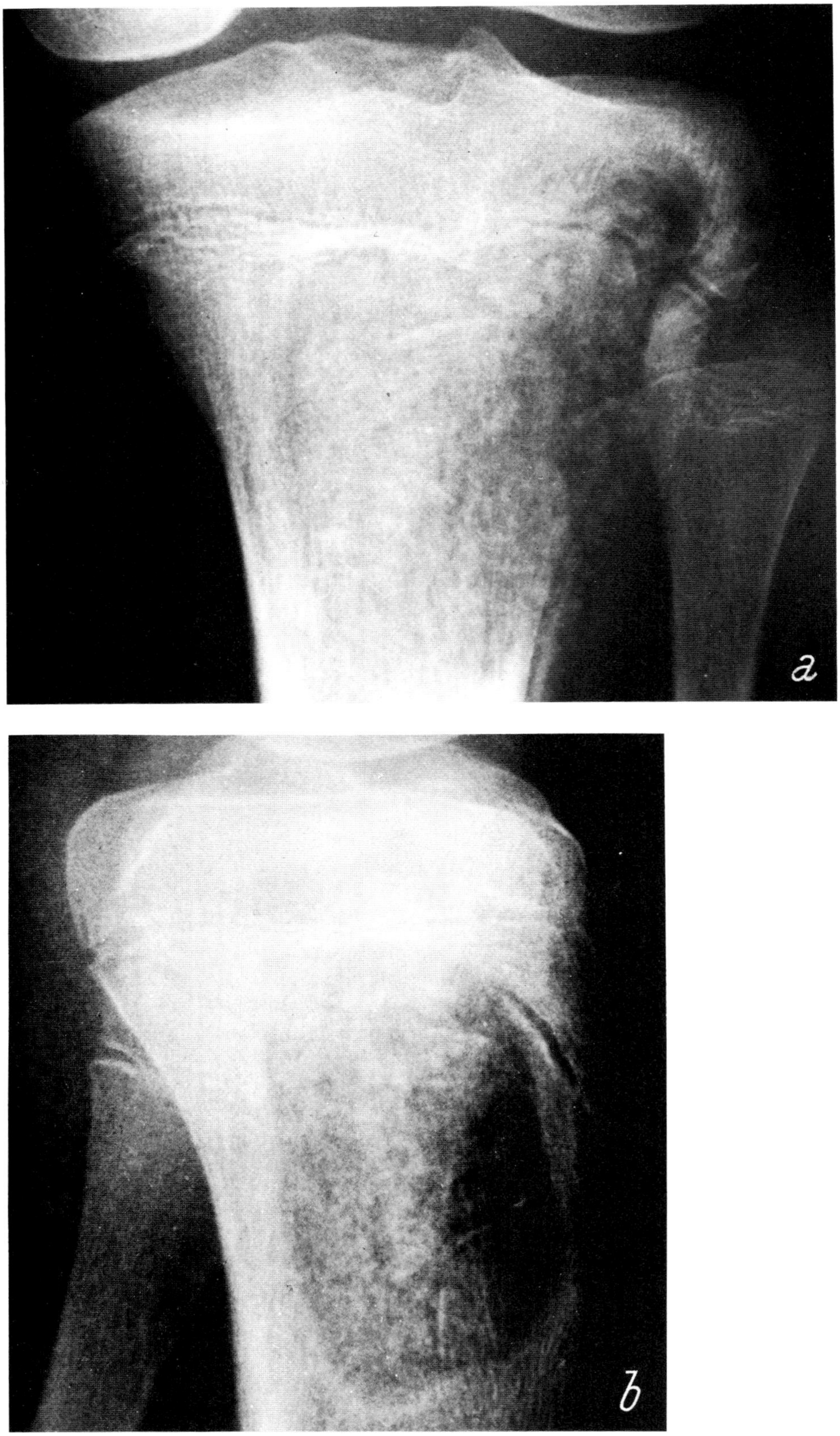

Figures 8.6a and **b.** Antero-posterior and lateral radiographs of the upper end of the tibia of a boy aged 14 years showing a large cavity in the upper metaphysis of the tibia resulting from acute haematogenous osteomyelitis. This enormous cavity had been drained and packed open until granulation covered its walls. Fragments of bone grafts can be seen in both views, these had been inserted when organisms had failed to grow in cultures taken from the cavity

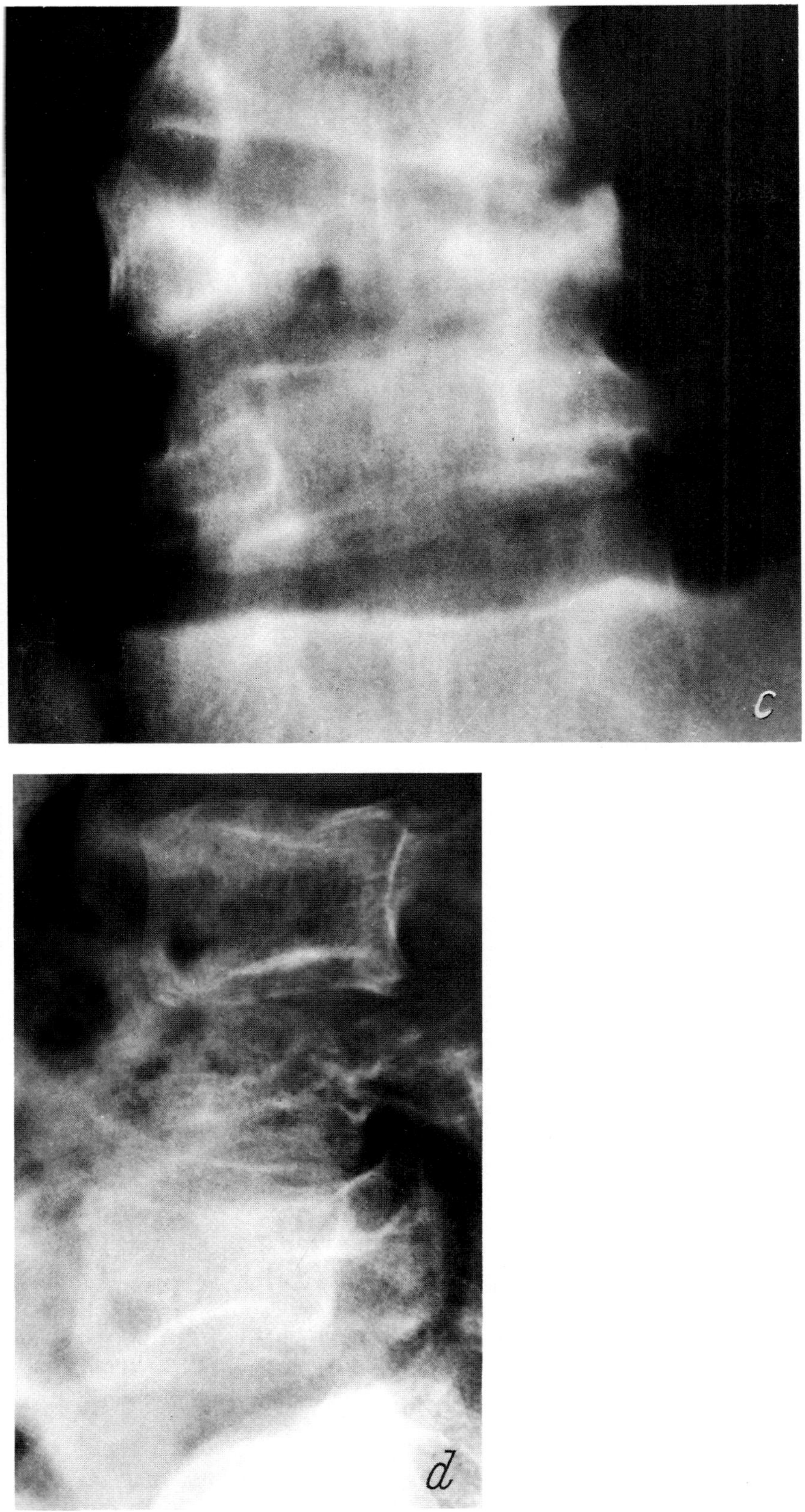

Figures 8.6 c and **d.** Antero-posterior and lateral radiographs of the lower lumbar spine showing the 3rd, 4th and 5th lumbar vertebrae and the 1st sacral vertebra. Extensive destruction of the vertebral body of L4 is noted. This lesion developed in the spine twelve months after the boy had been treated for the acute lesion shown in Figs. 8.6a and b in the upper end of his tibia. This vertebral lesion required extraperitoneal drainage of a large paravertebral abscess. The organism was a Penicillin-sensitive staphylococcus aureus

8.2. Tuberculous Disease of the Spine

The surgical treatment of tuberculosis of the spine has attracted widespread interest in the past twenty years. During that time, the most authoritative accounts of the various surgical procedures which may be required in dealing with the spinal complications of this disease have come from the East, especially from Hong Kong (Hodgson, 1956).

Tuberculosis is now seen only rarely in Western communities, being found occasionally in migrants.

The illustrations in this chapter have been chosen simply to draw attention to some of the outstanding features of this disease as it affects the spine (Figs. 8.7–8.10).

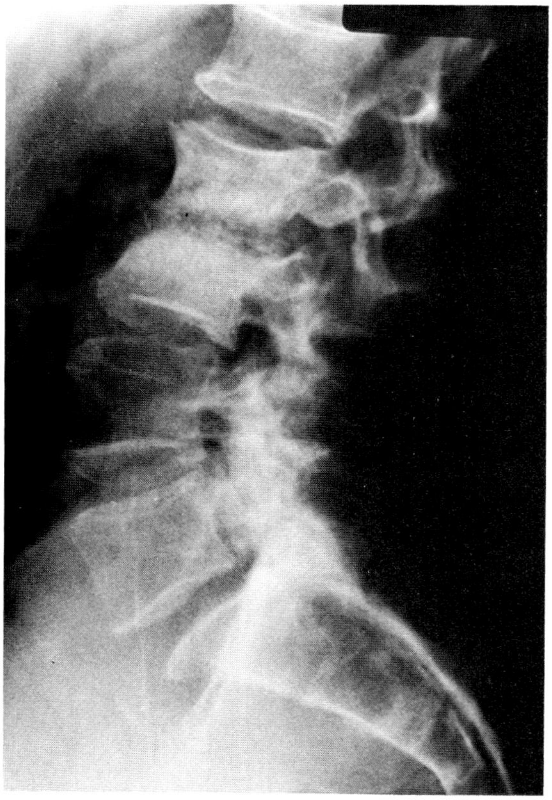

Figure 8.7. A lateral radiograph of the lumbar spine of a man aged 54 who presented with severe low back pain. Note the loss of disc space with erosive changes in the adjacent vertebral bodies at the level of the disc between L2 and L3. The body of L4 is somewhat osteoporotic. In the antero-posterior view the classic deformity of the psoas shadows indicated the presence of bilateral psoas abscesses. This is an example of relatively localized tuberculous disease with minimal spinal deformity at the time of presentation

Figures 8.8. a A lateral radiograph of the thoraco-lumbar junction of the spine of a man aged 24 years who presented with complaints of spinal pain and increasing weakness of the lower extremities. **b** A lateral tomogram of the same area of this patient's spine following debridement and bone grafting of the area for active Pott's disease. No attempt was made to correct the deformity. The patient was managed post-operatively in a plaster bed and anti-tuberculous chemotherapy administered

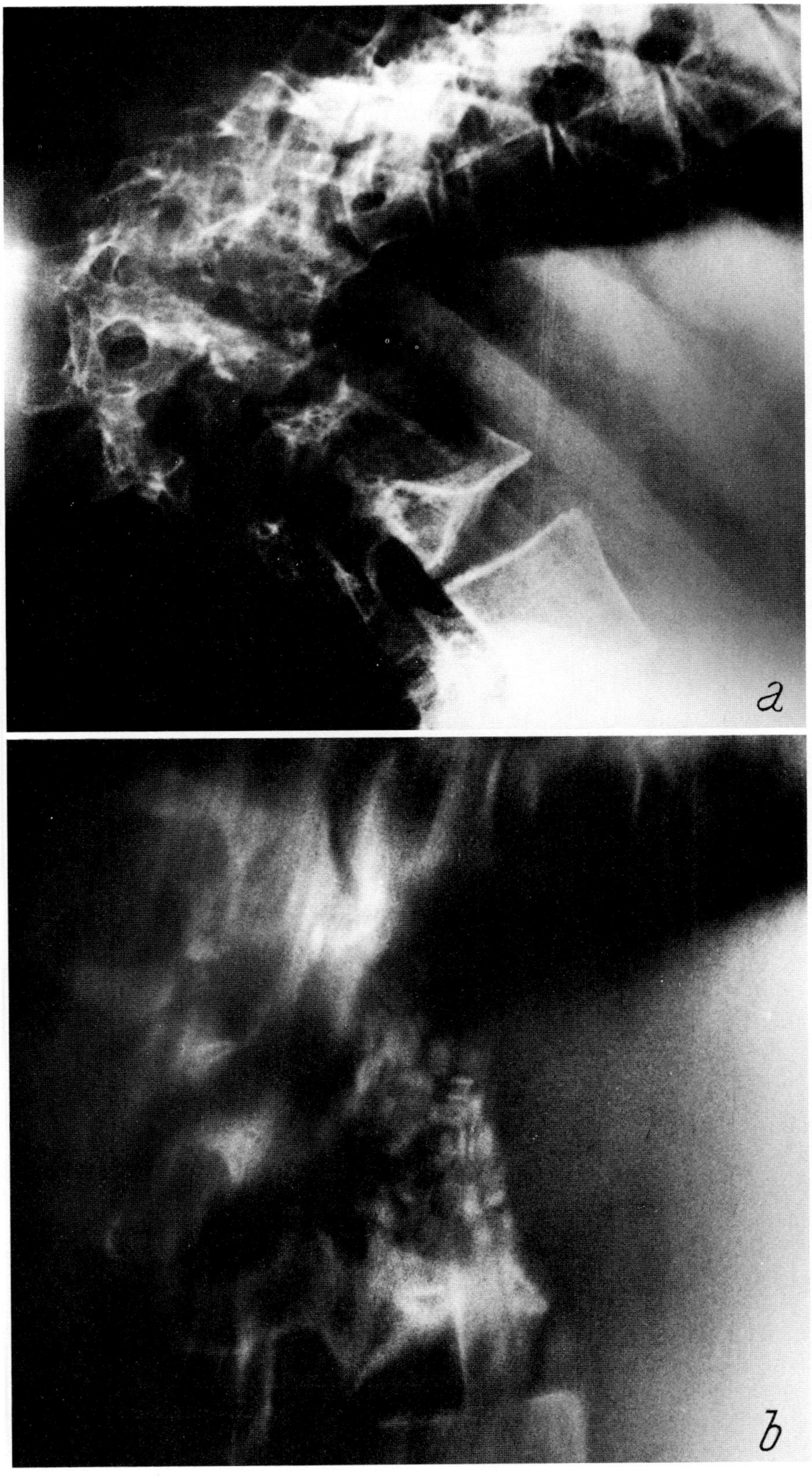

Figures 8.8

Publication of these records may serve a useful purpose for those readers whose experience of this disease has been limited, reminding them of the magnitude of the problems which may occur in spinal tuberculosis.

Surgical treatment has been dominated by the use of interbody fusion operations, performed through anterior approaches at every level of the vertebral column, allowing debridement of carious debris and necrotic bone fragments before the insertion of strut grafts (Figs. 8.11–8.13).

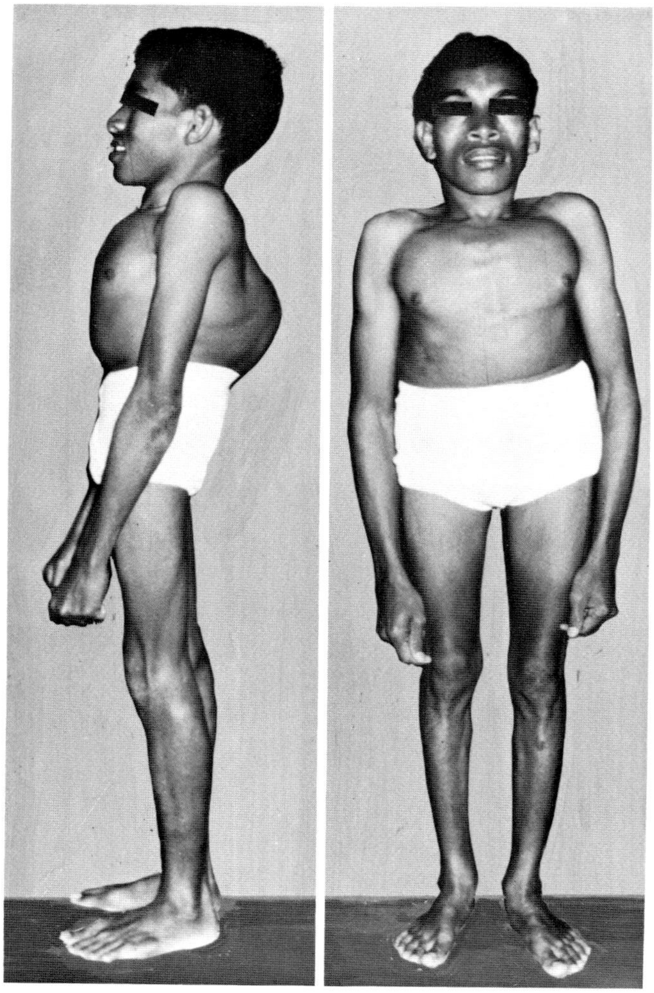

Figures 8.9. Lateral and anterior photographs showing the gross deformity of the spine resulting from Pott's disease at the thoraco-lumbar junction. The X-rays of this patient are shown in Figs. 8.8a and b

Figures 8.10. a A lateral tomogram taken four months after operation showing the incorporation of grafts inserted for the treatment of tuberculous disease in the patient whose pre-operative films are illustrated in Figs. 8.3a and b. Note the fragment of rib graft adjacent to the spinal canal. **b** An antero-posterior tomogram of the same spine showing sound interbody fusion with no lateral deformity of the spine

Figure 8.11. A photograph of a Stryker rotor bed suitable for nursing patients following spinal surgery for infective or neoplastic lesions

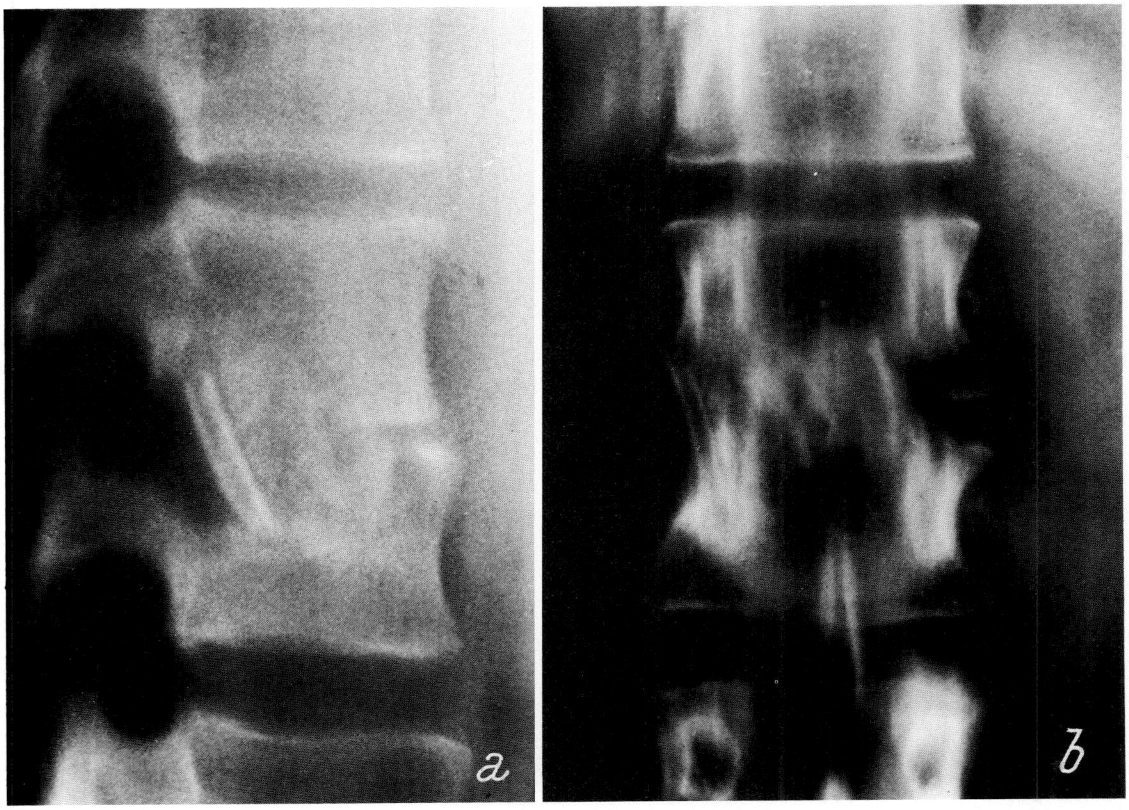

Figure 8.10

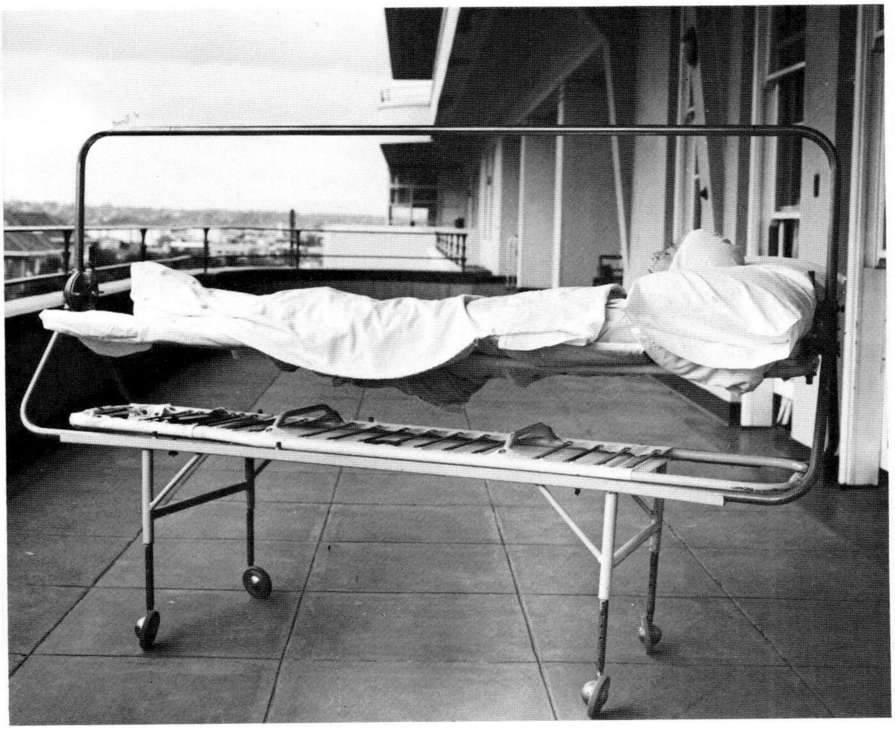

Figure 8.11

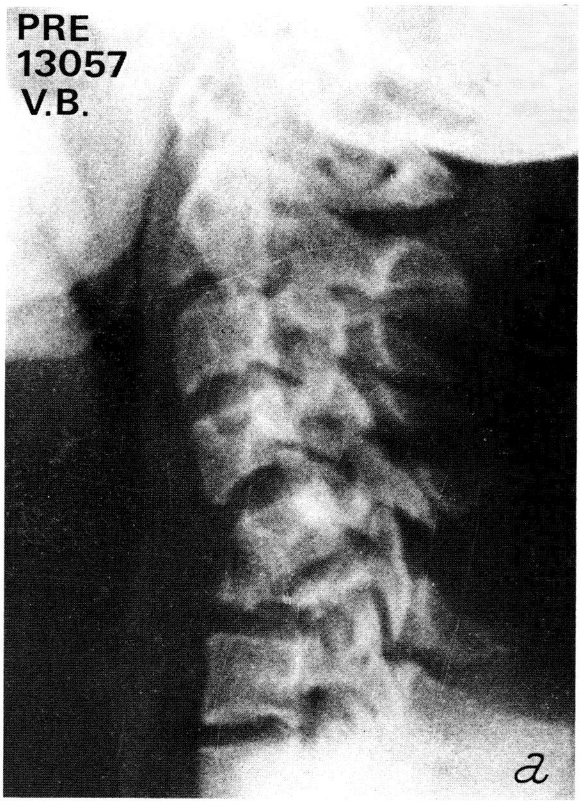

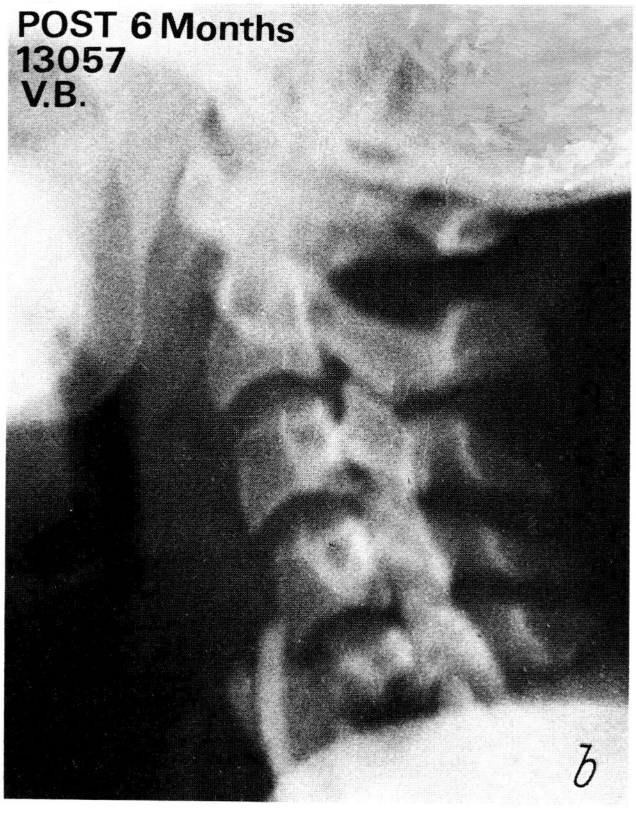

Figures 8.12. a A lateral radiograph of the cervical spine showing gross vertebral destruction at C6 with subluxation of the spine complicating tuberculous infection. **b** A lateral radiograph of the same spine six months after operative treatment for debridement and anterior interbody fusion. Note the correction of the deformity and the presence of a uniting interbody fusion

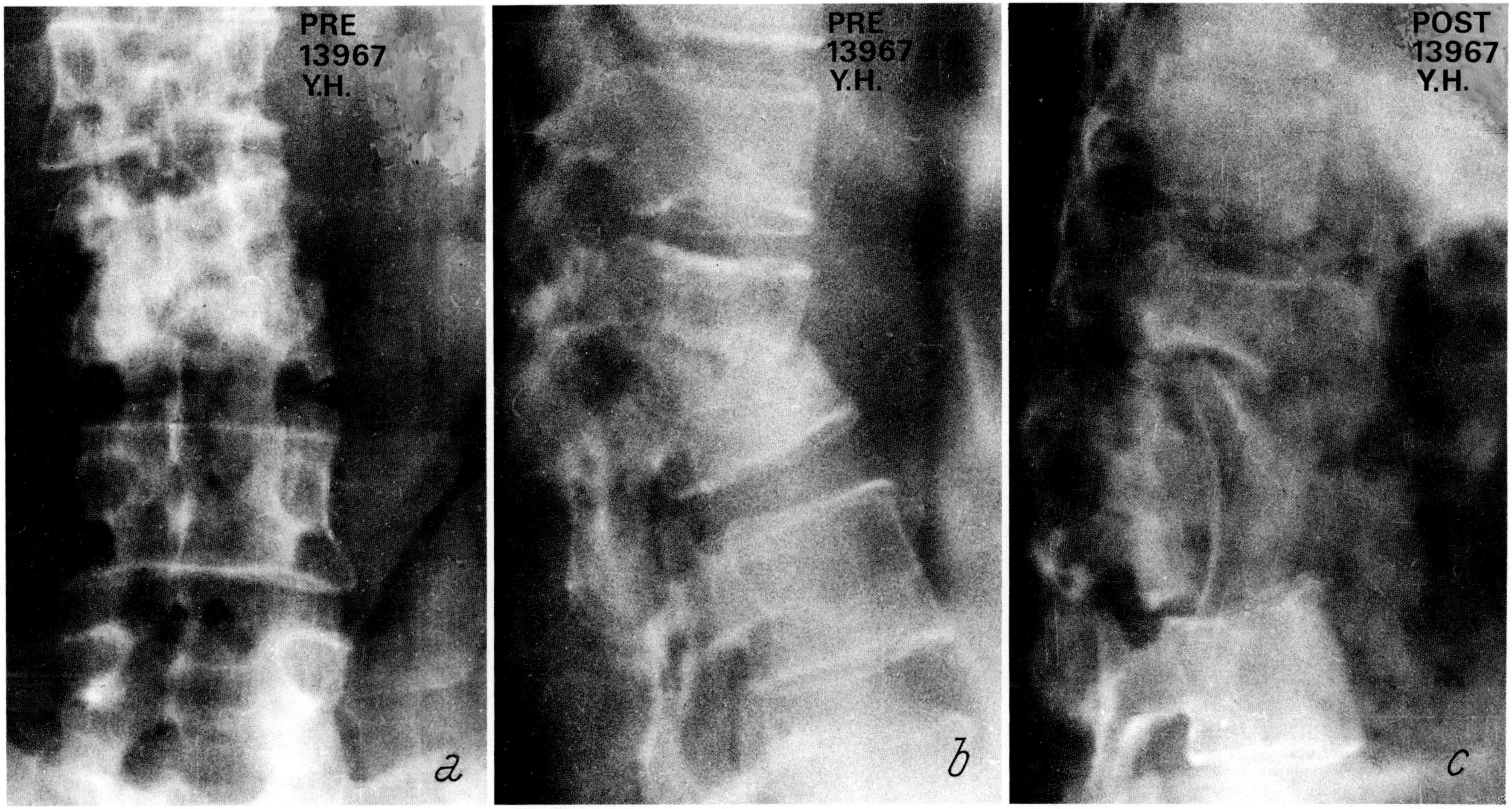

Figures 8.13. **a** An antero-posterior view of the lumbar spine of an adult patient with destructive changes in the vertebral bodies of L 2 and L 3 with a minor scoliosis. The psoas shadow is distorted on the right side of the picture. **b** A lateral radiograph of the same spine showing a kyphotic deformity developing at the site of the tuberculous lesion affecting the adjacent margins of the L 2 and L 3 vertebral bodies. **c** A lateral radiograph of the same spine taken following extensive debridement of the tuberculous lesion with the insertion of a large graft cut from the iliac crest. Post-operative management either in a plaster bed or on a rotor bed is essential for at least three months before the patient can be fitted with a plaster jacket or suitable brace. (The illustrations in Figs. 8.12 a and b and 8.13 a–c are provided by courtesy of Professor P. R. Chari, formerly of the Osmania Medical College, Hyderabad, India)

Correction of kyphotic deformities of the spine due to Pott's disease has been undertaken with considerable success in a limited number of special centres in the world.

A surgeon who has had no special experience in the management of post-infective kyphoses should avoid "trying his hand" on such cases. Should he be obliged to operate on a patient with a gross spinal kyphosis, with active tuberculous disease and clinical evidence of spinal cord dysfunction, he should treat the case by anterior decompression and anterior interbody fusion, making no attempt to correct the deformity. The patient should be nursed in a plaster bed for three months after surgery.

8.3. *Post-Operative Infections*

Some of the surgical aspects of the management of post-operative infections following spinal operations are discussed in Chapters 7 and 9.

Fortunately, serious infections are uncommon. Surgeons, therefore, have a natural tendency to hope that wound infections may subside with the use of chemotherapy alone. They may be reluctant to explore the wound early after the onset of infections.

Clinically, distinction should be drawn between superficial and deep wound infections. In patients with a thick layer of subcutaneous fat between skin and lumbo-dorsal fascia, fat necrosis and infections in the haematoma between the skin and the underlying paraspinal muscle layer will give rise to the appearance shown in Fig. 8.14. The patient's temperature will be only slightly elevated and local pain in the wound will not be severe. Although slow to heal, this type of infection is not serious. It will respond to limited local drainage, following removal of a few sutures, and the use of chemotherapy.

On the other hand, with deep infections, patients become febrile and ill, and they complain of extremely severe pain. Prompt surgical drainage should be carried out under anaesthesia. All sutures should be removed from the skin and deeper structures, so that the vertebral column can be re-explored. Infected blood clots and free pus should be aspirated, and material sent for further detailed bacteriological tests.

The whole wound should be washed out with a solution of hydrogen peroxide. Dry packing should then be inserted. Secondary suture of the wound can be performed when cultures from the granulating wound surfaces have become sterile.

If deep infections, either in the neck or elsewhere in the spine, are treated promptly in this way, the dreaded complications of vertebral osteomyelitis, epidural abscess formation, or even meningitis should not develop (Figs. 8.15a–d).

Patients who present with persistent severe spinal pain (with or without small discharging sinuses) some months after treatment for post-operative wound infections, will require very careful re-assessment. In this group, chronic osteomyelitis and chronic spinal epidural abscesses may be discovered resulting in crippling and prolonged illness (Fig. 8.16).

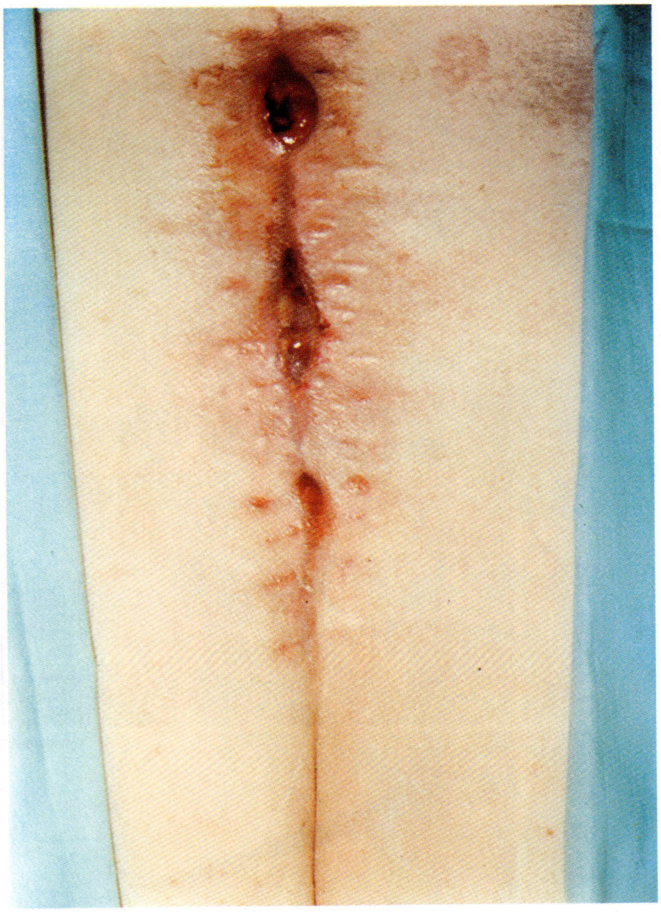

Figure 8.14. A photograph of the incision used for lumbar laminectomy in a young woman in whom the subcutaneous fat layer between skin and lumbo-dorsal fascia measured 9 cms. Serous fluid containing fat droplets leaks from the wound. The incision was re-opened in the mid-line but extensive dissection was not necessary, the problem being confined to the sub-cutaneous layers of tissue superficial to the lumbo-dorsal fascia, as is usual in this type of wound infection

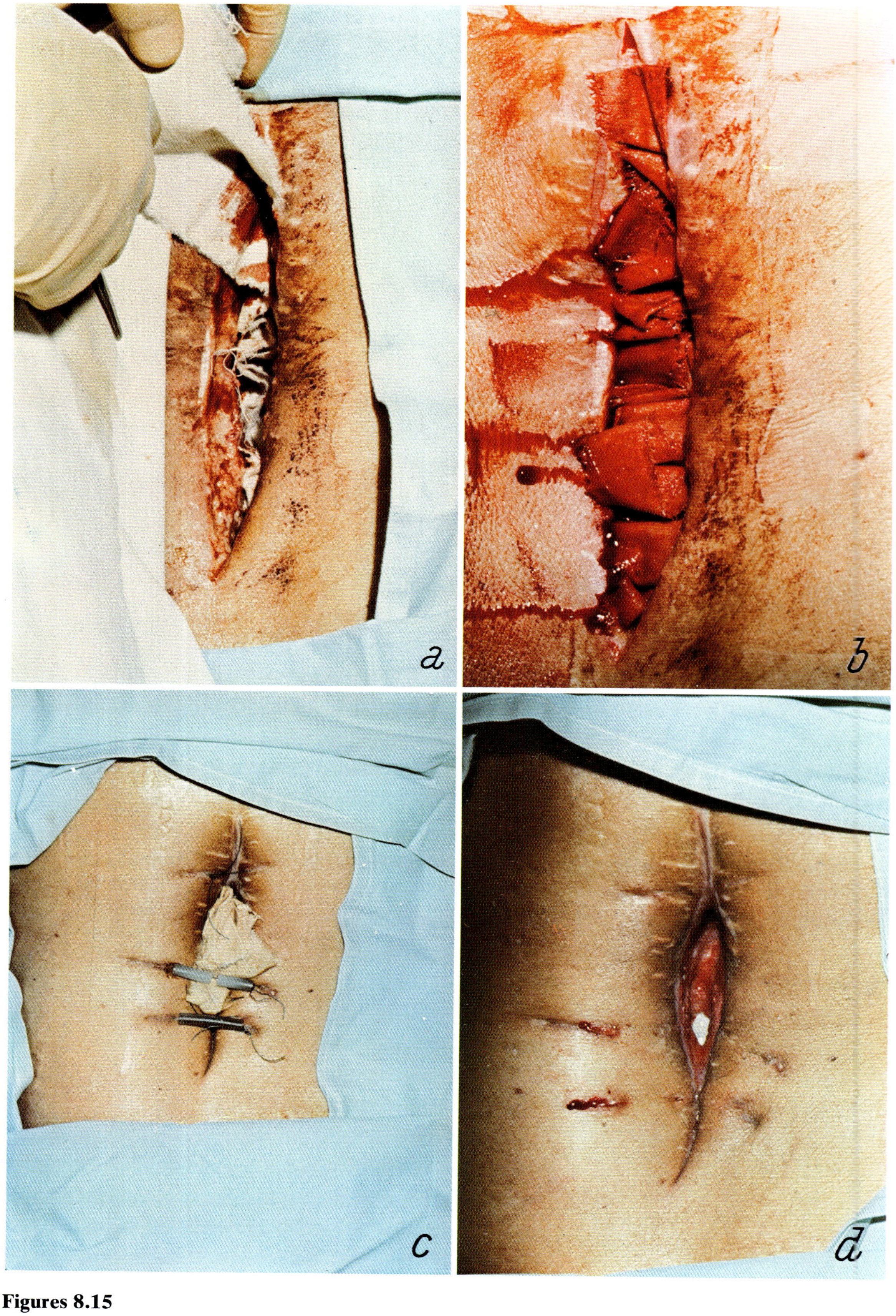

Figures 8.15

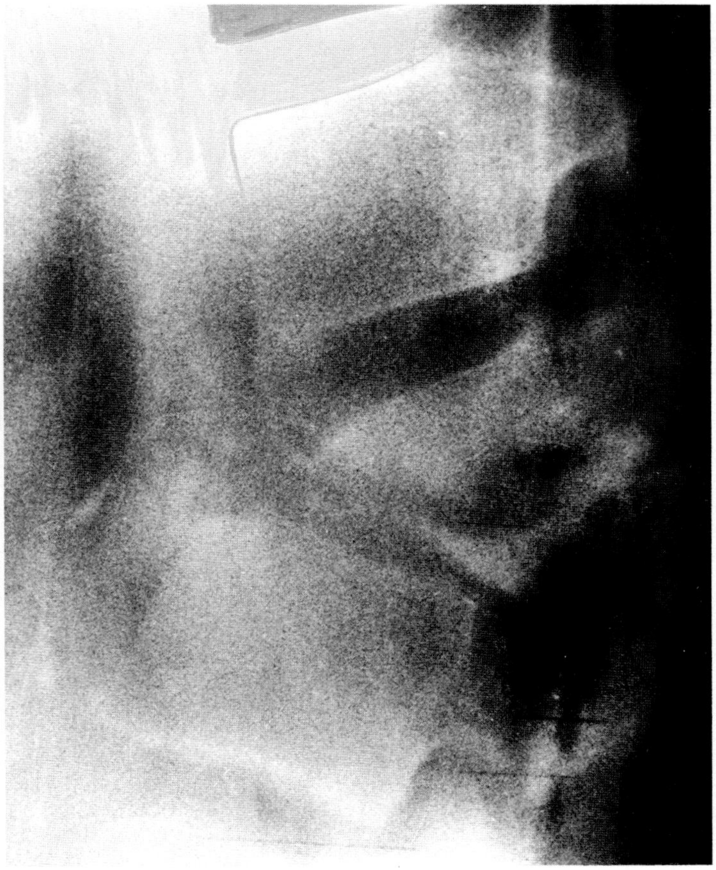

Figure 8.16. A lateral tomogram of the mid-lumbar spine of a woman aged 58 years. Note the gross destruction of two adjacent vertebral bodies and the resultant marked kyphotic deformity. This patient developed an epidural abscess following infection of a laminectomy wound with secondary vertebral osteomyelitis

---

Figures 8.15. Photographs illustrating progressive stages in the management of chronic osteomyelitis of the spine following posterior bone grafting for spondylolisthesis 15 years earlier. This patient had had a discharging sinus in his back with intractable back pain for many years. **a** The problem was treated by radical excision of the graft and packing of the cavity with calico. **b** The appearance of the wound three days after the operation for graft excision. **c** The appearance of the wound at the time of secondary suture when cultures from the granulating surfaces were sterile. **d** The appearance of the wound following removal of the tension sutures after secondary suture. Note the dural tissue in the base of the wound. The wound healed completely and epithelialized four weeks after this photograph was taken. The patient was treated with appropriate chemotherapeutic agents for more than one year

9

The Management of Failed Spinal Operations

9.1. Introduction

Waddell *et al.* (1980), painted a gloomy picture of the outcome for patients who have had multiple back operations. Little wonder that patients with persisting serious spinal problems are often given dire warnings about further operations, not only from non-medical sources but even from some specialist surgeons. There are certainly daunting problems in their management. These patients are often debilitated and demoralized. Family breakdown, financial stress, drug dependency and frank persecution by insurers, examining doctors and employers constitute some of their difficulties–leaving aside the question of the actual physical causes of their persisting disability.

This is one of the most challenging fields of spinal surgery and there is no place in it for a surgeon who is sceptical or suspicious of his patient or whose attitudes are in any way defeatist.

9.2. Investigation

The cornerstone of management is to investigate these problems with great care and with compassion, before recommending further surgery. The surgeon must establish a competent team of consultants to help him, though he should remember the aphorism which guided Harry S. Truman, the U.S. President: "The buck stops here"; a saying applicable to decision making in the context of divided responsibility. The team should include the following people:

general practitioner, psychologist, psychiatrist, social worker, physiatrist, physiotherapist, neurologist, radiologist–providing each has a declared interest in this type of work.

Before outlining a simple system for the analysis of failures after spinal operations, some general comments should be made on the subject of investigations.

Clinical neurological examination may be unrewarding in assessing the level or severity of nerve root or cauda equina lesions. Matsuda *et al.* (1977, 1979) have advocated the use of electro-neurophysiological techniques for the identification of compressive lesions of individual nerve roots of the cauda equina or for the study of single nerve root units in degenerative spondylolisthesis, and these may find wider usage in the future.

Radiological examinations which may be essential in helping to establish diagnoses and to plan further surgery in particular cases include:

a) Motion studies of the spine: instability may require spinal fusion.
b) Oblique views of the facet joints and intervertebral foramina: unrecognized foraminal stenosis may require decompression.
c) Antero-posterior and lateral tomograms in any case of failure following spinal fusion or canal exploration: irregular laminal remnants or re-formed bone in scar tissue may require revision of canal decompression.
d) Repeat myelography: to demonstrate space-occupying lesions or arachnoiditis.
e) Discography: to plan the extent of spinal fusion.
f) *Computerized tomography*—especially if reconstructed scans in three planes can be obtained: this offers a wide range of diagnostic information but *does not necessarily supersede the use of (a)–(e).*

The analysis of individual cases of failed spinal operations may be facilitated by using the following classification:

1. Outright Failure

This group comprises patients who show no improvement or who become worse after the first operation.

2. Temporary Relief

These patients may be free of symptoms for months or years after operation.

3. Failures in Spondylolisthesis

These patients are considered separately because of special features of the pathological anatomy in this condition. (See p. 146.)

4. Infection

9.3. Outright Failure

Failure is usually related to wrong diagnosis. Some pain and discomfort are to be expected after any spinal operation. Pain protracted over weeks may follow some operations in which adherent root sleeves have been tediously separated from disc tissue, yet a successful outcome can be predicted. Such special circumstances excluded, patients in this group can usually be identified soon after operation. They complain of pain which is more severe than is normally expected. Those with infections will have elevated temperatures and altered blood counts.

The questions to be determined are simply these:

Is the failure due to an *unrecognized condition?*
Is it due to *wrong diagnosis of the spinal lesion?*
Or finally, has it followed some *technical failure?*

a) Unrecognized Conditions

Investigations should begin as soon as possible, but several months may elapse before the diagnosis can be established. For example, a carcinoma involving the apex of the lung may be the cause of neck pain and brachial neuralgia persisting after anterior cervical fusion. Operation for lumbar spondylolisthesis may fail because the true cause of pain is a secondary prostatic carcinoma of the vertebra.

Rarely, infection after a spinal operation may be caused by tuberculosis or gonorrhoea.

Primary tumours in the spinal canal are relatively rare. They are usually diagnosed before operation by clinical examination and by myelography. However, in cases of failure, the possibility that such lesions may be the cause of continuing symptoms should be considered.

b) Error in Diagnosis of the Spinal Condition

Three questions must be answered:

1. What was the primary diagnosis?
2. What were the operative findings?
3. What was the nature of the operation?

Stenoses of the spinal canal or of a nerve root canal must be excluded as underlying causes of failure. The possibility that the symptoms are those of "claudication" of the cauda equina must be borne in mind. Under such circumstances, myelography is essential to clarify the diagnosis.

c) Technical Errors

i) In Operations for Disc Prolapse

Persistence of severe pain is unusual if the diagnosis of disc prolapse has been confirmed at operation. If a considerable amount of fragmented and dessicated disc material has been removed, it is likely that a further fragment has been displaced beneath the root sleeve after operation, or that a migrating sequestrated fragment has not been removed.

If a pre-operative diagnosis of disc prolapse was made but no disc prolapse was found at the time of operation, it is likely that the intervertebral space at the wrong level has been explored (Fig. 9.1).

Most failures occur when no disc prolapse has been found and perhaps the diagnosis of internal disc disruption should have been established by discography before operation (see pp. 44–56).

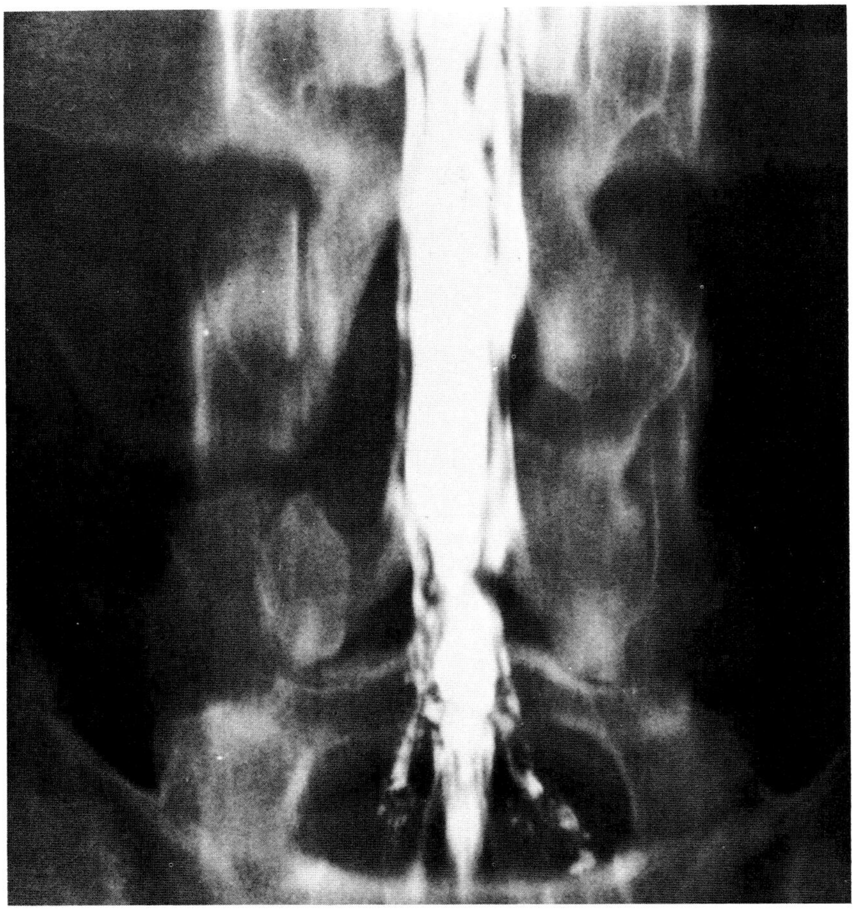

Figure 9.1. An antero-posterior tomograph of the lower lumbar spine in a patient aged 37 years, said to have undergone laminectomy for removal of a left-sided lumbo-sacral disc prolapse. Part of the upper margin of the lamina of the 4th lumbar vertebra has been removed, so that space between the 3rd and 4th vertebrae was probably explored. The outline of the myodil shows that there is bilateral stenosis of root canals at the L4/5 level. This patient's symptoms were relieved by further decompression of the spinal canal, involving removal of the central segment of the arch of the 4th lumbar lamina, combined with bilateral nerve root canal decompression at that level

ii) In Operations for Internal Disc Disruption

If this diagnosis has been established by discography and disc excision and interbody fusion have been done, early failure may indicate that the wrong level has been fused. In the neck particularly, levels should be identified by radiographs taken during operation. The injection of methylene blue at the time of discography is an unreliable method of identifying the level of an affected disc. Even in the lumbar spine, levels may be wrongly identified, especially if there are anomalies such as sacralization.

9.4. Temporary Relief

In this group initial relief of pain after operation may last for weeks or months before the recurrence of disabling pain. The largest number of cases falls into this category.

a) Failure After Operation for Disc Prolapse

Recurrence is usually caused by recurrent prolapse at the level operated on, especially if a large volume of disc material was removed at the original operation, or by a fresh prolapse at another level.

Recurrent but contralateral sciatica occurs after asymmetrical settling of the vertebrae when several grams of disc material have been removed at the initial operation. Radiographs show collapse of one side of the intervertebral space. Recurrence of pain is caused by a fresh prolapse of disc material or by stenosis of the nerve root canal following deformation due to the reduction in height of the intervertebral disc space.

The commonest cause of late recurrence of symptoms after initial successful excision of a disc prolapse is stenosis of the spinal and nerve root canals secondary to degenerative changes (Figs. 9.2a–c). Ectopic ossification or calcification in the remnants of ligamentum flavum may be found at the site of re-exploration in such cases.

Another cause of late recurrence, often associated with secondary canal stenosis but contributing to the overall problem, is the presence of a meningocoele caused by damage to the dural sac at the time of the original operation.

b) Failure After Operation for Internal Disc Disruption

If interbody fusion has been performed for this lesion, early recurrence of severe symptoms within two or three months of operation may be due either to complications of the discography or to trouble arising at the site of grafting.

Chemical discitis may cause severe pain post-operatively if the discography has been followed within a short time by operation. Erosion of the vertebral end-plates and bodies in the area of the nucleus pulposus occurs on either side of the disc, leading to gross narrowing of the intervertebral space at the level of the normal disc above or below the "fused disc". Histological examination of specimens removed at operation shows inflammatory changes with plasma cell infiltration. Cultures are sterile. Injection of steroid into the disc usually controls the pain and promotes healing, though oral Cortisone administered over the course of ten days may also be effective (see Chapter 2, Figs. 2.17, 2.18a–c, 2.19a, b).

Non-union of grafts occurs in a few instances. These problems are discussed in detail on p. 83. The incidence of non-union of interbody grafts has been reduced in recent years following improvements in surgical technique reported by Crock (1976), by Crock (1982) and by Fujimaki, Crock and Bedbrook (1982). Grafts of cancellous bone were shown to have two disadvantages: they are prone to infiltration by disc remnants with subsequent non-union and graft resorption; secondly, even though union occurs, loss of intervertebral height may follow collapse of the cancellous graft and its settling into the vertebral bodies. Stenosis of the nerve

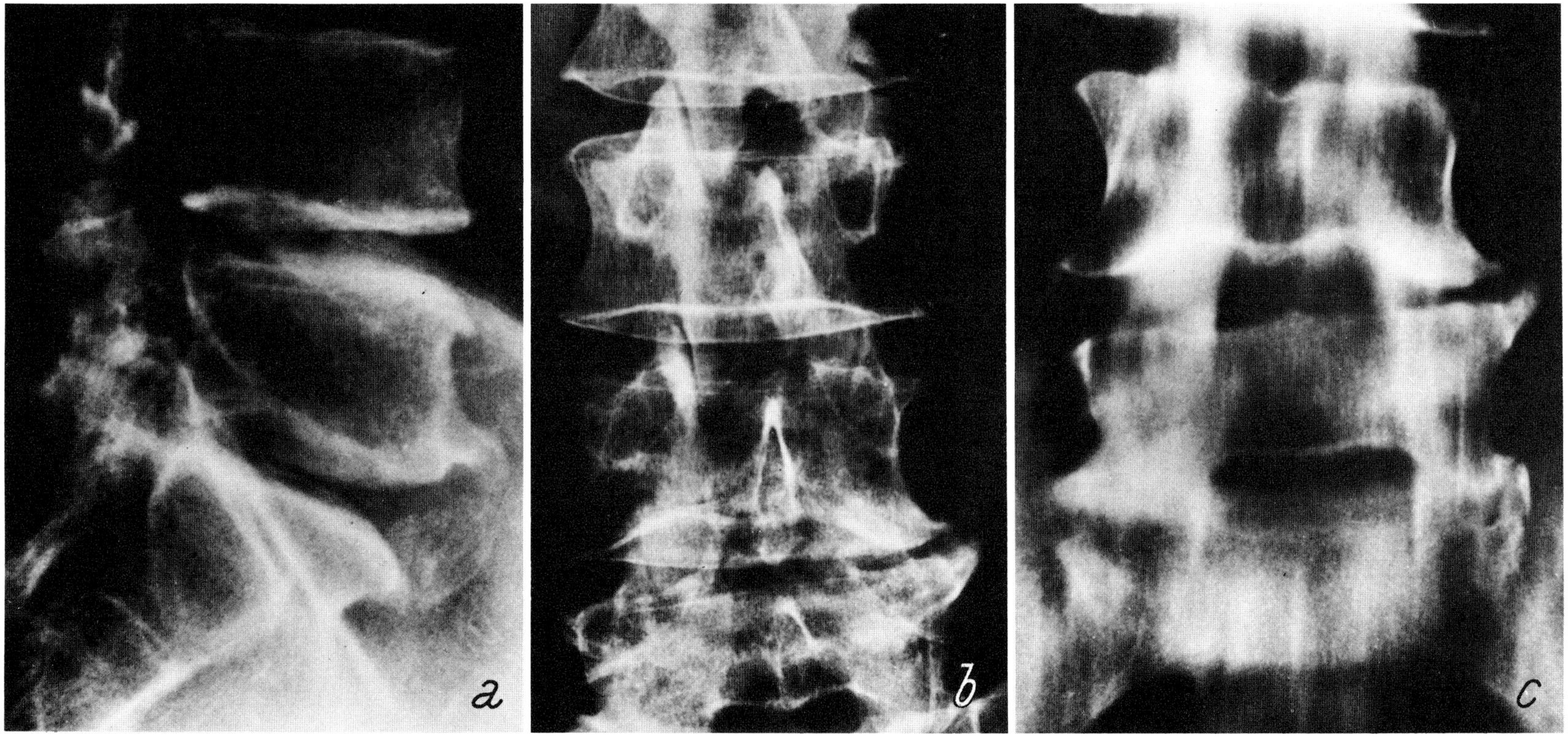

Figures 9.2 a – c. Degenerative changes 30 years after removal of an intervertebral disc prolapse at L 4/5 level in a patient aged 61 years. Note the inter-laminar calcification in the antero-posterior view in Fig. 9.2b. Fig. 9.2c, a tomogram showing the extent of the decompression of the spinal canal and nerve root canals

root canal follows and may cause recurrence of pain in both lower limbs (Figs. 9.3 a, b).

Block or dowel grafts cut from the anterior half of the iliac crest provide grafts which are rapidly revascularized, usually maintain height and always resist infiltration by disc remnants (see Chapter 2, Fig. 2.45).

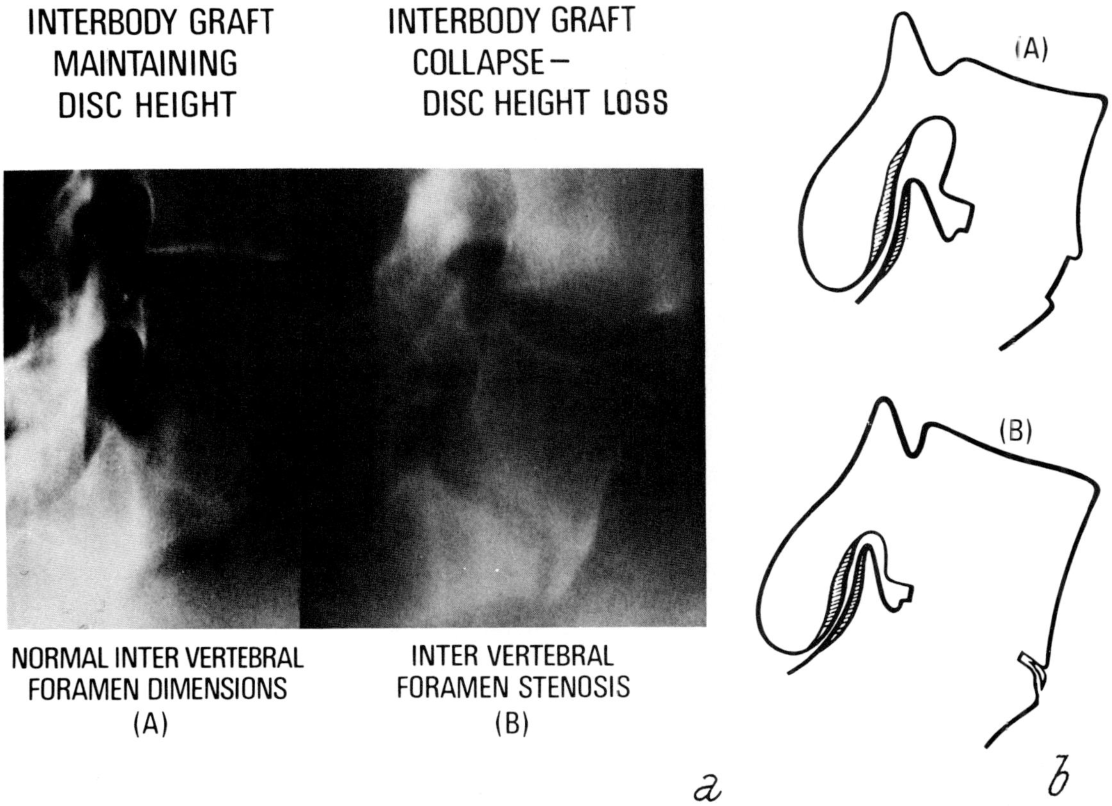

Figures 9.3 a and **b.** Lateral tomographs of the lumbo-sacral junction in man aged 46 years (A) is taken four months after operation, (B) is taken 18 months after operation. The graft has incorporated but secondary disc space collapse has occurred with resultant nerve root canal and intervertebral foraminal stenosis. The diagrams (A) and (B) alongside depict the genesis of the foraminal stenosis

Following successful interbody fusions, the ligamentum flavum related to the fused segment will atrophy, adhering then to the dura and nerve root sleeves. With vertebral column movements above the fused segment, stretching of the dural root sleeves may occur and cause pain. Relief follows total laminectomy and excision of the ligamentum flavum over the area of the fused spinal segment or segments, leaving intact the facet joints between the fused and mobile segments of the column. In the cervical spine, the relevant root canals should also be decompressed, using a very fine forward-angled rongeur.

c) Failure After Operation for Isolated Disc Resorption

This condition has been discussed in detail in Chapter 1. Acquired disc resorption may follow partial disc excision or intradiscal injections of Chymopapain. In such

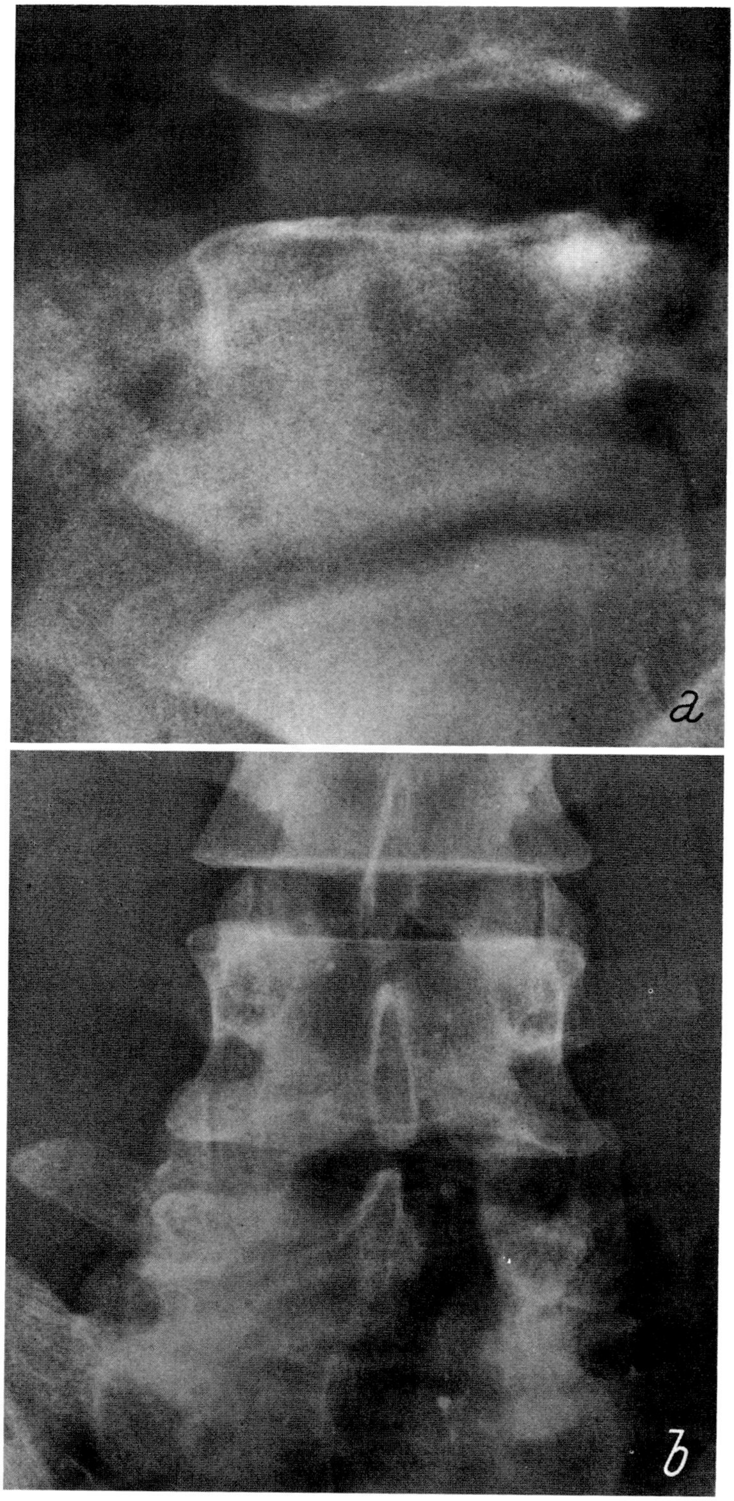

Figures 9.4

cases symptoms usually recur or persist after a second exploration of the disc space with hemi-laminectomy and removal of more disc material (Figs. 9.4a, b). The appropriate surgical treatment of bilateral nerve root canal decompression is discussed in detail on pp. 23–27. If the true significance of the pathology of isolated disc resorption is not appreciated, the patient may be subjected to further major surgery, involving adjacent normal segments of the spine (Figs. 9.5a, b).

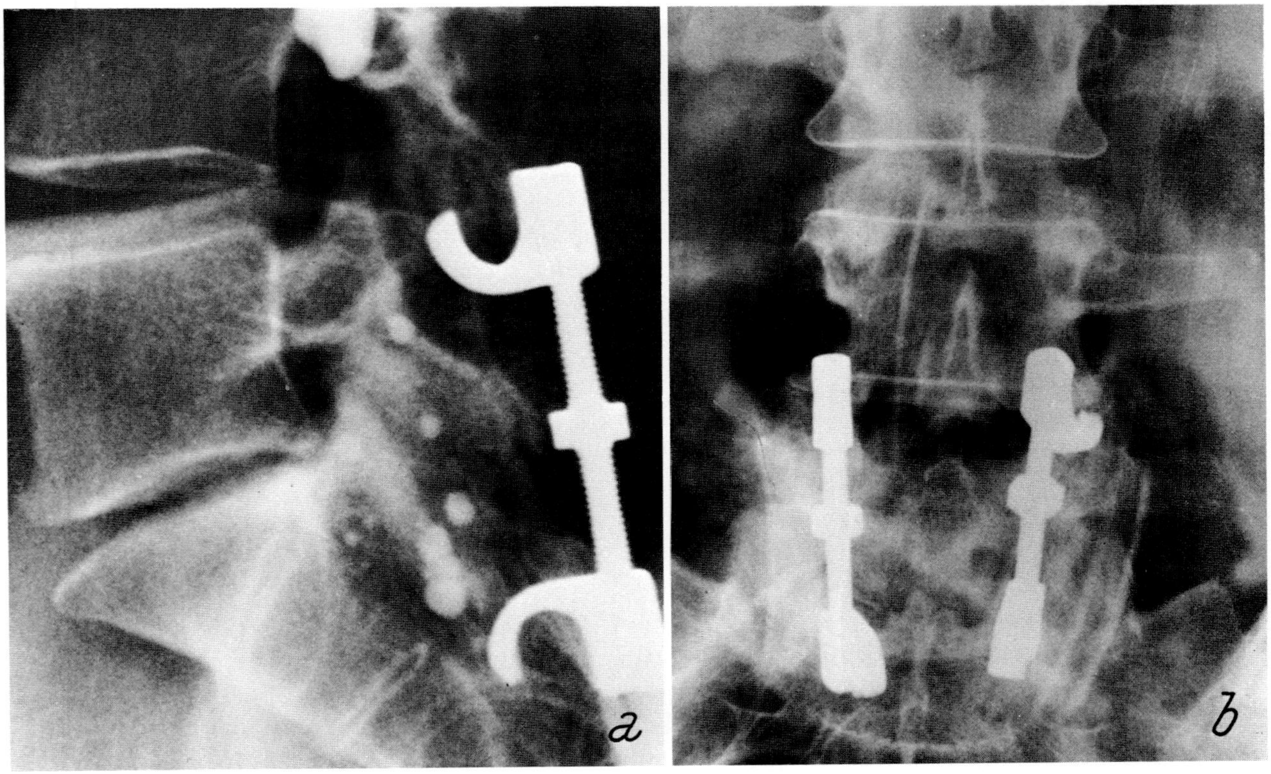

Figures 9.5. **a** A lateral radiograph of the lower lumbar spine. Isolated disc resorption is noted at the lumbo-sacral junction with a degree of retrolisthesis of L5 on S1 and a positive Knuttson sign. The L4/5 disc space is normal. Knodt's rods have been inserted beneath the lamina of L4 above and into the sacrum below. **b** An antero-posterior radiograph of the same spine. Note the bilateral Knodt rods and the segments of graft, some of which extend upwards to lie against the left side of the spinous process of L3. The pathology in this case was present only at the L5/S1 level. *In this patient, two other normal spinal segments have been operated upon unnecessarily.* Supplementary treatment in this case involved removal of the Knodt rods, excision of the unwanted bone at L3/4 and L4/5, and bilateral nerve root canal decompression at L5/S1 level

---

Figures 9.4. **a** A lateral radiograph of the lower lumbar spine of a woman aged 37 years with persistent pain in the back and lower limbs. Note the narrowing of the lumbo-sacral intervertebral disc space, with minimal osteophyte formation and marked sclerosis of the adjacent vertebral body. **b** The antero-posterior radiograph shows the amount of residual laminal bone after two previous operations. This patient's problem was due to acquired disc space narrowing following intervertebral disc surgery, with resultant bilateral nerve root canal stenosis. The second operation has been inadequate, the remnants of the central portion of the 5th lumbar lamina should have been removed, and bilateral nerve root canal decompression performed as described in Chapter 1, pp. 23–27

9.5. Surgical Techniques for Re-Exploring the Spinal Canal

a) Preparation

These procedures are often time-consuming and associated with considerable blood loss. Blood transfusion facilities must be available. Adequate supplies of bone wax, gelfoam or equivalent haemostatic agents should be ready for use.

b) Radiology

Radiographs of the patient's spine should be displayed on a viewing box in the theatre. The most valuable information for the operation of re-exploring the spinal canal is usually provided in antero-posterior views, including tomograms which show the anatomy of the roof of the spinal canal or its remnants most clearly (Fig. 9.6).

c) Positioning

Positioning on the operating table is important and use of the prone position on a suitable frame is recommended.

d) Instruments

Opening of the dural sac may be indicated if arachnoiditis of the cauda equina is recognized during operation. Dural tears may occur accidentally in the course of dissection, especially at the junction of previously operated and non-operated areas. If the dural sac and nerve root sheaths are tethered to the floor of the spinal canal by dense adhesions, it may be necessary to open the dural sac to gain access for removal of prolapsed disc fragments. On rare occasions meningocoeles may be encountered unexpectedly. An adequate array of instruments, including a fine sucker, long handled fine toothed forceps, long handled fine needle holder and long fine "atraumatic sutures" on fine needles (4.0 or 6.0 sizes) should therefore be readily available so that any of these problems may be dealt with promptly during the operation.

e) Exposure

A mid-line incision should be used. Bony landmarks at the extremities of the incision should be palpated with the aim of exposing intact spinous processes and laminae above and below the area to be re-explored.

f) Orientation

The soft tissues relating to the spinous processes should be stripped on one side, then the other. While it may seem too simple to describe these manoeuvres, in fact, this part of the operation assumes great importance. The paraspinal muscles should be

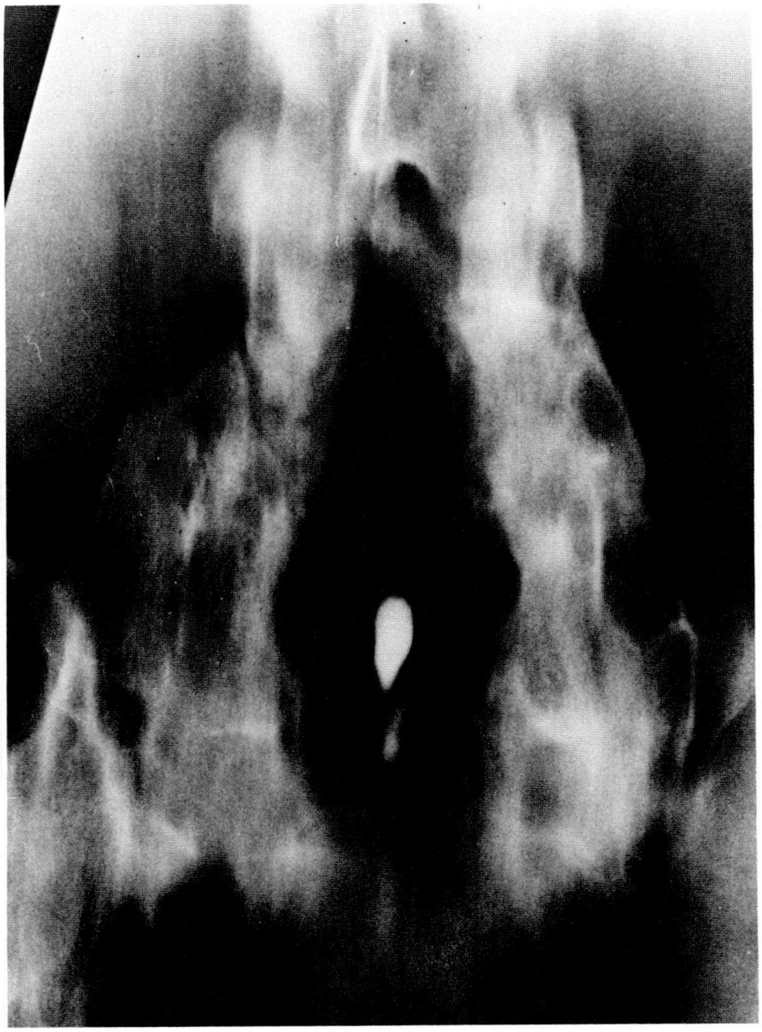

Figure 9.6. An antero-posterior tomogram of the lower lumbar spine of a man aged 52 years who complained of recurrent back and leg pain following two previous spinal operations, including spinal canal decompression and postero-lateral inter-transverse-alar fusion. Note the reformation of the laminal remnant near the top of the picture on the right side at the upper extremity of the previous exploration

separated carefully from the lateral aspects of the spinous processes and the posterior surfaces of the laminae, leaving the periosteum intact and avoiding any disturbance of the capsules of the facet joints. At the upper end of the incision the intact lamina and its inferior facets should be clearly defined, as should the posterior surface of the sacrum below, to the level of its superior laminal edge. Self-retaining retractors should then be inserted before any effort is made to expose the actual area to be re-explored, beyond joining the zones of the sacral exposure and the upper spinous process by a mid-line incision a few centimetres deep into the scar tissue.

The surgeon must re-assess the patient's X-rays at this stage, to be certain of the location of laminal remnants in the dense scar tissue which has usually formed between the paraspinal muscles and the roof of the spinal canal following previous surgery.

Using a sharp scalpel, an oblique incision is made into this scar tissue, starting in the mid-line at the upper extremity of the wound on one side, the direction and depth of the cut being gauged by the orientation of the cleared lamina and its inferior facet joint, laterally and inferiorly to the level of the next joint. The extent of muscle damage resulting from the previous surgical procedure or procedures will be variable. Where it has been slight, there will be a clearly defined fatty layer between the anterior surface of the paraspinal muscles and the bony canal. Through this soft tissue the surgeon can easily palpate the facet joint with the tip of his index finger, thereby determining the plane of dissection. In cases where very dense scar tissue has invaded the paraspinal muscles at the site to be re-explored–a likely finding after multiple explorations–identification of the lateral edge of the pars interarticularis of the lamina and its inferior facet joint is difficult. The site of the pars interarticularis below the normal facet joint at the upper end of the incision can be identified either by removing the extra-synovial fat pad from this facet joint or by locating the main stem of the posterior branch of the lumbar artery which is a constant lateral relation of the pars interarticularis. Using either or both of these guidelines, one can determine the direction of the incision which will lead safely to the exposure of the outer edge of the lamina and its related facet joint. Depending on the findings in particular cases, one may proceed to expose the entire area to be re-explored on one side between the sacrum below and the normal spinous process and lamina above, then repeat the procedure on the opposite side. Where there have been multiple previous operations, it is often wiser to make limited exposures, one level at a time, on the right and left sides alternately, moving the self-retaining retractors progressively as required.

If a meningocoele is present, it will be identified early. Cerebrospinal fluid will fill the wound when the scalpel is used to cut obliquely into the scarred tissue after preliminary exposure of the normal bony segments of the canal, as described above. The inexperienced surgeon will be shaken by the appearance of C.S.F. so early in the operation. The meningocoele should be identified as such and thereafter ignored until the formal exposure of the roof of the spinal canal or its remnants has been completed.

Once the lateral bony margins of the laminae and the facet joints have been exposed on both sides, the self-retaining retractors are positioned definitively.

g) Timing of Retractor Application

The time of their application should be noted because re-exploration operations may last more than two hours. *The retractors should be removed at intervals of 45–60 minutes for 5 minutes,* to restore circulation in the paraspinal muscles. During these rest periods the wound may be irrigated with Ringer's solution.

At this stage of the procedure, a bulky mass of scar tissue of variable depth remains in the mid-line between the lumbar spinous process above and the back of the sacrum below. Its relationship to the underlying dura will vary depending on the amount of laminal bone remaining or reformed after the previous operation or operations. The surgeon should now strip all soft tissues from the outer surface of each lamina or laminal remnant, *referring once again to the patient's X-rays.*

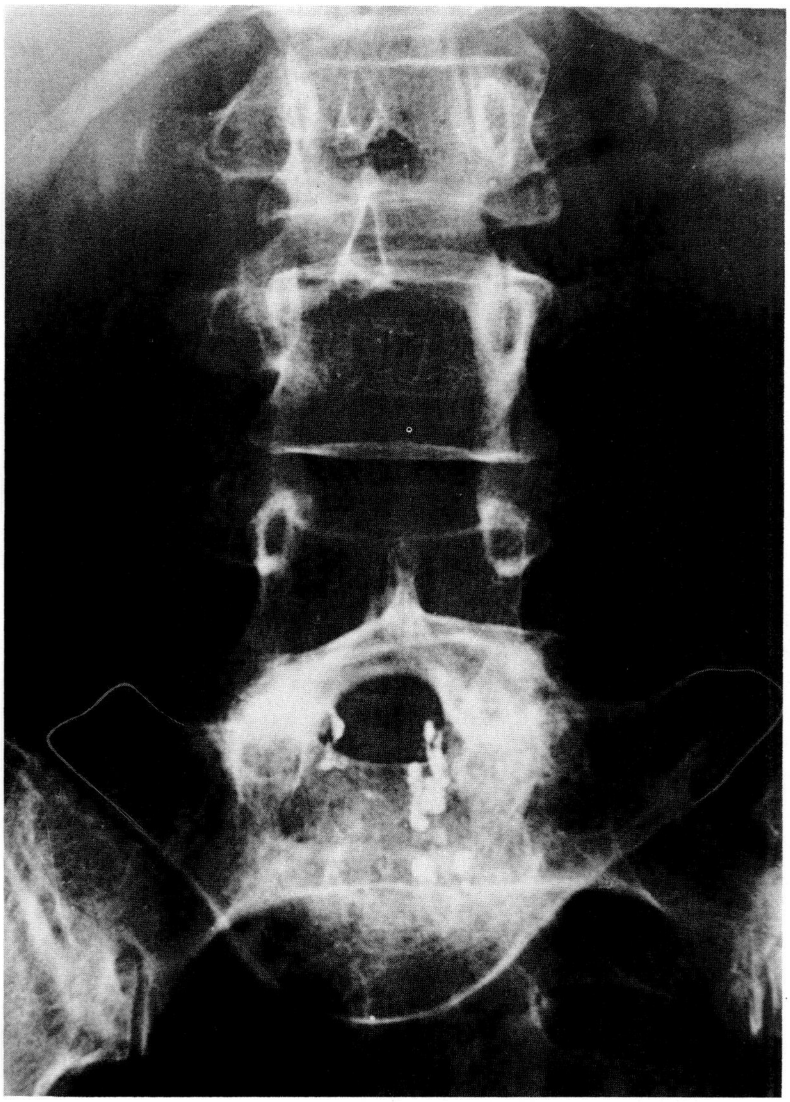

Figure 9.7. An antero-posterior radiograph of the lumbar spine of a woman aged 53, with spondyloptosis of L5. Note the classical radiological sign of "Napoleon's Hat". At operation, identification of vertebral levels can be difficult in such cases. Despite two operations aimed at decompressing the lumbar canal and nerve roots related to the spondyloptosis, the lamina of L5 remains intact. However, the laminae of L2 and L3 have been removed, along with some of their related facets

Identification of laminal levels can be very difficult, particularly in cases with anomalies at the lumbo-sacral junction or in spondylolisthesis with the higher grades of slip of the vertebral body (Fig. 9.7). It may be necessary to take control X-rays in the operating theatre in such cases. This done, at each level between the sacrum and the normal lamina and spinous process above, the bulky mid-line scar tissue can be excised or thinned down to the level of the bony canal, using either a large rongeur with sharp cutting edges or a sharp scalpel.

h) Re-Opening the Spinal Canal

If the upper end of the sacral lamina is in the field of operation, the canal can be re-entered easily in the mid-line, even if the dural sac is covered with densely adherent scar tissue. This can be done by thinning the lamina in the mid-line and then stripping the scar tissue carefully away from its upper edge with a pointed probe (such as the Watson-Cheyne probe). Alternatively, when the bone is very thin, a small gouge directed proximally from a few millimetres distal to the free edge of the lamina can be used. A small plug of laminal bone is turned out, allowing the insertion of a blunt-ended probe into the canal. The dura is pushed away and a 2 or 3 mm sized cup of a 45° forward-angled rongeur then inserted to open the roof of the sacral canal, a few millimetres distal to its upper free edge, from the mid-line outward on both sides to the level of the medial margins of each S1 pedicle. Dural tearing may occur at this stage. It is avoided by careful handling of the fragments of sacral bone created by the use of the angled rongeur. These fragments should not be pulled on forcibly. They are best left attached to the scar tissue, to be dissected free from it by sharp dissection after the canal has been exposed to the level of each S1 pedicle.

Should it be decided to commence the dissection for entry into the spinal canal at the upper end of the operation field, it may be easily done by removing the normal ligamentum flavum from the spinal segment immediately adjacent to the area to be re-explored. The central portion of the lamina on the inferior side of this vertebral interspace is then removed, using the same techniques described in dealing with the removal of the sacral laminal bone at its site of attachment to the scar tissue overlying the dura. Further dissection distally follows, using the landmarks of facet joints, medial pedicular margins and pars interarticularis, obtaining exposure one side at a time, with the careful technique outlined above.

Scar formation between the dura and nerve root sleeves and the paraspinal muscles is prevented by normal ligamentum flavum. This fact should be remembered when re-exploring a spinal interspace, which may have been opened previously on one side only, as it may be put to good use, allowing safe entry into the spinal canal without risk of injuring the dural sac.

Regrettably, notes made at the time of the original surgery are rarely available to a surgeon when he is re-exploring a patient's spine. The identification of a segment of normal ligamentum flavum often assumes great importance. Although the outer surface of this ligamentum may be covered with dense white scar tissue arising from the deep surface of the paraspinal muscles, its presence can be determined most easily by removing the extra-synovial fat pad from the adjacent facet joint, and then defining its characteristic yellow colour, where it attaches to the medial edge of the superior facet at the interspace. Once its presence has been confirmed, the white scar tissue can be cut away, defining its full extent, before incising this ligamentum flavum to gain access to the spinal canal.

In the course of the dissection just described, root canal stenosis or foraminal stenosis can be identified and relieved easily (see pp. 23–27). Once the lateral margins of the dural sac and the regional nerve root sleeves have been exposed on both sides over the whole area being re-explored, the surgeon is then in a position to assess the dural contents by digital palpation. If they are normal, the question of separating all the scar tissue from the dura should be addressed. It is not necessary to remove it entirely, but if scar tissue is left attached, it should be thin and should not contain any remnants of bony spicules. Bone left in scar tissue is likely to grow and it may lead to further canal stenosis after a few years, especially if a hemi-lamina is left nearby (Fig. 9.6).

With the canal thoroughly decompressed and any problems of root canal or foraminal stenosis already resolved, the regional intervertebral discs should be inspected, using digital palpation and probing with the Watson-Cheyne instrument. A nerve root may be bound to a recurrent disc prolapse by dense scar tissue. The use of an operating loop may be necessary to enable the separation of the root sleeve from prolapsed disc tissue, minimizing the risk of nerve injury. If recurrent disc prolapse is found, curettage of the intervertebral disc space may be indicated. The risk of penetration of the abdominal cavity may be high in these circumstances so that realization of this hazard should be uppermost in the surgeon's mind (see Chapter 3, Fig. 3.21).

i) Dural and Epidural Problems

i) Meningocoeles

These lesions are uncommon. They are often only recognized at operation and may be found early in the course of a re-exploration operation. When the spinal canal has been opened as described above, a meningocoele sac may then be dealt with quickly. It will usually have a single ostium which can be closed with a fine atraumatic suture after the bulk of the wall of the cystic cavity surrounding it has been separated from the dural sac and excised.

Dural tears should be avoided with attention to the details of dissecting technique outlined above. They may occur inevitably in some patients in whom the dura is abnormally thin. In such patients multiple tears sometimes occur and closure of the dural defects becomes impracticable. *The closure of the wound at the completion of the operation then becomes critical.* Several layers of sutures should be used in the muscle and fascial layers rendering the wound water-tight. Appropriate chemotherapy should be administered post-operatively until the surgical wound has healed, Penicillins and Sulphonamides being used together when applicable.

Small dural tears should be identified and closed with fine "atraumatic sutures", the area of the tear being kept dry with a fine low-pressure sucker and protective patty. Care should be taken to avoid trapping nerve root filaments in the sutures.

The management of the dura in cases of arachnoiditis of the cauda equina is discussed on p. 175.

The technique of transdural disc fragment excision is found on p. 119.

ii) Unrecognized Epidural Infection

Rarely during re-exploration of the lumbar canal, previously unrecognized epidural or vertebral body infections may be found. The history of a superficial wound infection, followed by *persistent spinal pain out of proportion to what might have been expected post-operatively,* should raise the possibility of this diagnosis. The planned operation of canal decompression should proceed, and intravenous chemotherapy should be commenced during the operation. Special care should be taken to avoid dural injury though the dura in such cases is often thickened. The epidural abscess should be sucked out and its extent defined. If necessary, pus in the intervertebral disc space should be aspirated and sent for immediate bacteriological examination.

The decision for primary or secondary wound closure should be resolved on the assessment of the extent and severity of the infection. It is better to pack the wound open with dry gauze where a large abscess cavity has been discovered, particularly if the vertebral bodies are infected. Secondary closure of the wound may be performed if cultures taken from the granulating surfaces become sterile (Chapter 8, Figs. 8.15a–d). Such wounds, even if they are extensive, will heal by secondary intention in 6–8 weeks. Daily wound care can be managed at home by visiting nurses after the first few post-operative weeks have been spent in hospital.

j) Re-Exploration of the Spine Following Spinal Fusion Operations

The principal indications for these operations are for the treatment of the following complications:

a) Non-union.
b) Graft overgrowth.
c) Development of secondary stenosis.
d) Disc or facet joint lesions above or below fused spinal segments.
e) Fusion at the wrong level.
f) Infection.
g) Spondylosis acquisita.
h) Ligamentum flavum atrophy.

i) Non-Union of Spinal Grafts

The multiplicity of methods of spinal fusion underlines the fact that it is difficult to produce union of the grafts with the vertebral column. The success rate of the lengthy spinal fusions used with Harrington's or Luecke's rods in scoliotics has not been matched when applied to the treatment of degenerative disorders or spondylolisthesis in the lumbar spine.

Non-union of the various spinal grafts used in the lumbar area can be diagnosed usually with plain X-rays, motion X-rays or tomograms. Discography may have a special place in the assessment of persisting pain after posterior spinal fusion with pseudarthrosis, as advocated by MacNab (1977, p. 214). Myelography may also be useful to demonstrate acquired canal stenosis.

Attempts at re-grafting in failed posterior fusions frequently fail. This problem may be managed most effectively in the majority of cases by a supplementary anterior interbody fusion.

Conversely, where an anterior interbody graft has failed, supplementary posterior inter-transverse grafting will often succeed, fusion of the anterior graft occurring pari-passu with the union of the posterior graft.

Particular problems may be encountered when attempting to repeat an anterior lumbar interbody grafting operation when no other method is applicable. The first is the identification of the vertebral interspace which will be obscured by extensive scarring. Facilities must be available for obtaining good quality radiographs in the operating room. The second problem of adherence of the great vessels to the vertebral column is always anticipated–so that a proper range of instruments and sutures should be available to deal with injuries to the great veins or their branches

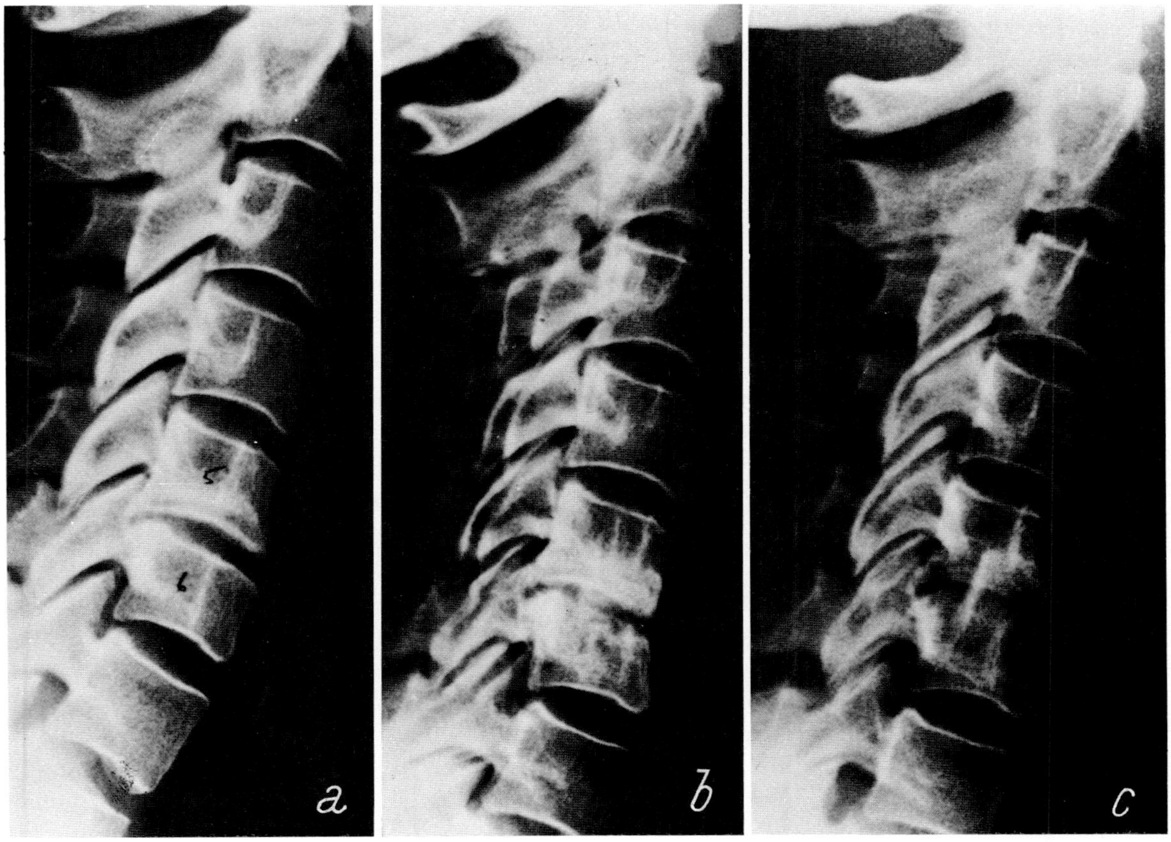

Figures 9.8. Lateral radiographs of the cervical spine of a man aged 39 years. **a** shows an isolated spondylotic degenerative change between the vertebral bodies of C5 and C6, the cause of intractable neck pain, occipital headache and brachial neuralgia. **b** is a lateral radiograph taken nine months after interbody fusion performed by the Cloward method, showing non-union of the graft with some kyphotic deformity. **c** A lateral radiograph taken six months after replacement of the graft using the technique described in Chapter 7, pp. 199–206

which may be inflicted on them inadvertently during dissection. Lumbar interbody fusion operations are usually performed through left-sided abdominal incisions. In the special circumstances of attempting to re-graft in the case of failure, it may be wiser to expose the lower lumbar vertebrae through a right-sided extra-peritoneal approach. *Without doubt, attempted re-fusion of a failed anterior lumbar interbody graft should only be undertaken by a surgeon with special training in the use of these techniques of spinal fusion.* Even equipped with the necessary training and with the help of skilled assistants, it may prove technically impossible to perform a re-fusion by this method. The patient should be informed in advance of the potential problems, including the possibility that the operation may need to be abandoned without completion of the re-grafting.

Non-union of cervical anterior interbody fusions is uncommon. Re-grafting is usually easy, though identification of the site of the pseudarthrosis can be difficult. Special care is needed when inserting the instruments to cut a new graft bed–to ensure proper siting of the dowel cavity between the vertebral bodies, both in the longitudinal and transverse planes. In these cases it is easy to expose the vertebral artery and its venae comitantes if the cutter has been inserted too far laterally. The outlines of the inner margins of the longus colli muscles are usually obscured by the scar tissue formed following the previous surgery–so that the safety factor normally provided by the identification of these landmarks is lost. Damage to the vertebral artery and subsequent efforts to control the ensuing haemorrhage from it may lead to quadriparesis (Figs. 9.8a–c).

ii) Graft Overgrowth After Posterior Spinal Fusion

Attention was drawn to this particular complication by Crock in 1976. It may occur following the use of techniques for posterior spinal fusions involving the use of fragments of cortico-cancellous bone. While every effort should be made to place the bone chips accurately at the time of performing inter-transverse, postero-lateral or Hibb's type posterior fusions, the movement of some of the graft fragments beyond the desired area of fusion may occur and these bony fragments may continue to grow. An extreme example of this problem was seen in an elderly lady who had had multiple spinal operations performed for a lumbo-sacral disc lesion. A dense spicule of bone had extended to the level of the facet joints at L1/2 on one side where the point of this "unwanted graft" impinged upon the facet joint capsule causing chronic pain. Examples of this unwanted overgrowth of graft are shown in Figs. 9.9a–d. Gratifying relief of intractable back pain can be obtained in these cases by simply excising the "unwanted bone", leaving the main body of the graft intact.

iii) Development of Secondary Stenosis Beneath the Graft

Hypertrophy of posterior fusions has been reported and may lead to secondary lumbar canal stenosis after many years. The complication is not common. Currently it is best assessed either by the use of myelography or by C.T. scanning.

Relief of this form of stenosis can be difficult technically because the graft may measure many centimetres in depth. Usually it is possible to relieve the stenosis without interfering with the stability of the graft. This is done by removing the central segment of the graft and exposing the dural sac beneath it, being guided by the principles of re-exploration of the spine which have been outlined above.

iv) Disc or Facet Joint Lesions Above or Below the Fused Spinal Segment

Disc prolapse above a fused spinal segment occurs in a few cases. It usually occurs some years after the fusion and its identification is easy on clinical grounds. Myelography or C.T. scanning are useful investigations when this diagnosis is suspected.

Acute nucleus pulposus calcification may be seen in discs adjacent to a previously fused spinal segment (Chapter 4).

Secondary degenerative arthritic changes may affect the facet joints above and below fused spinal segments, leading to secondary root canal stenosis or even spinal canal stenosis. Limited root canal decompression operations are usually effective in relieving symptoms.

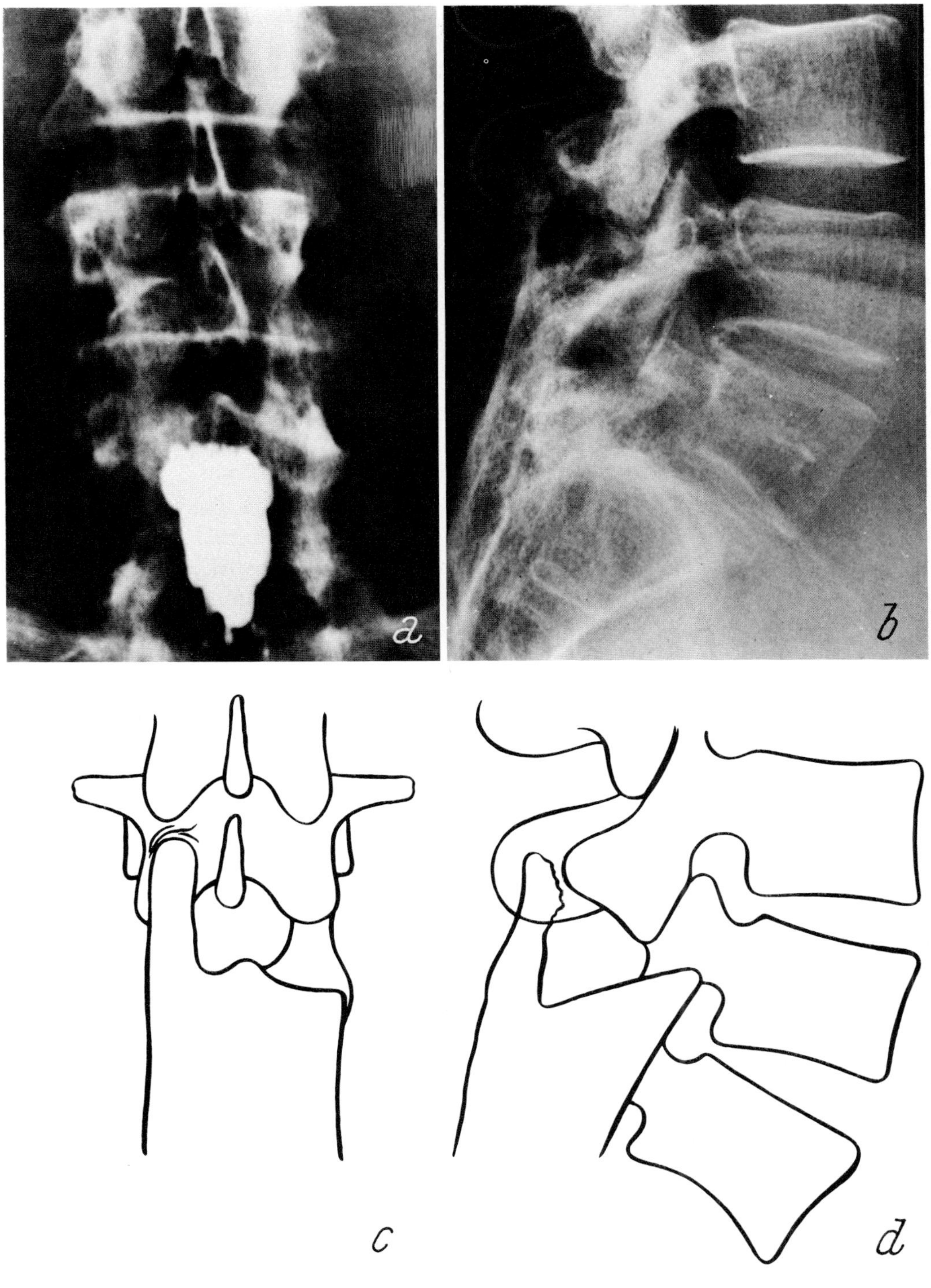

Figures 9.9. **a** and **b** Antero-posterior and lateral radiographs of a posterior spinal fusion for spondylolisthesis in a woman aged 48 years. The prolongation of a bar of grafted bone can be seen on the left side overlying the lamina of L3 with reactive bone formation near the adjacent facet. **c** and **d** Explanatory drawings of the radiographs. **c** shows solid fusion between the posterior elements of L4 and S2, with upward extension of the "unwanted graft"

v) Fusion at the Wrong Level

Surgeons dread this problem which may occur when anterior interbody fusion methods are used at any level in the vertebral column. Readers are referred again to the sections of this book dealing with the operative technique of anterior interbody fusion operations (Chapters 2 and 7).

vi) Infections

Fortunately, infection after spinal fusion is uncommon, though it is usually chronic and often difficult to control.

Early post-operative death from gas gangrene has been reported following inter-transverse-alar fusion.

Chronically infected posterior grafts can be treated successfully by open drainage and the use of long-term chemotherapy; that is, by the same methods which are usually effective in controlling chronic osteomyelitis in long bones.

Infection after anterior interbody grafting operations is rare but serious. Epidural abscess formation is likely and may lead to cervical cord compression or cauda equina compression. Urgent radical drainage is required, with special measures in the neck to prevent the development of secondary kyphotic deformities. Skull traction may be required for some weeks or some form of halo applied, fitted to a thoracic jacket.

If the infection is due to staphylococcal organisms, long-term chemotherapy for at least 6 months is recommended (Fig. 9.10).

vii) Spondylolysis acquisita

This is a well-recognized though uncommon complication of posterior spinal fusion, though as MacNab has pointed out (1977, p. 216) it does not complicate inter-transverse fusions in which the pars interarticularis of the proximal vertebral segment in the spinal fusion is supported by the graft.

Assuming that the disc at the level of the spondylolytic defect is intact, it may be satisfactory to perform a localized foraminal decompression, even on one side only.

viii) Ligamentum flavum Atrophy

Atrophy of the ligamentum flavum occurs following interbody fusion operations, both in the lumbar and cervical regions. In some cases, this may lead to dural root sleeve tethering, so that, with normal movements at the first mobile segment above the fusion, the nerve roots at the level of the fusion may be stretched because the ligamentum flavum adheres to them. In the lumbar region, total laminectomy with excision of the ligamentum flavum over the area of the fused segment of the spine, leaving intact the facet joints at the level of the first mobile segment above the fusion, has been found satisfactory.

Applied to the management of persisting problems of neck and arm pain following successful anterior cervical fusion, this operation of extensive laminectomy and foraminotomy with total excision of the ligamentum flavum has been found less effective probably because of inadequate foraminal decompressions in some cases.

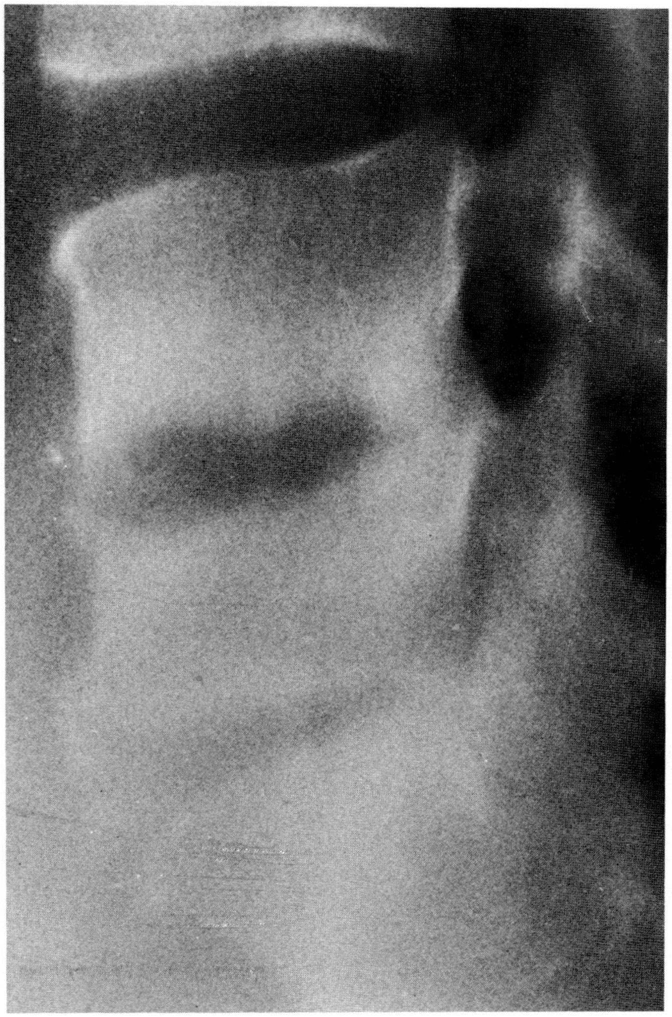

Figure 9.10. A lateral tomogram of the lower lumbar spine of a man aged 45 years. This film was taken more than twelve months after interbody fusions had been performed at L4/5 and L5/S1 levels, following which staphylococcal infection of the spine had occurred, leading to the development of an epidural abscess and to infection of the laminae and spinous processes at both levels. The infection was due to a staphylococcus aureus sensitive to Cloxacillin. The patient was treated by surgical drainage of the paravertebral abscess through the left loin and subsequently by extensive laminectomy for removal of infected laminal bone and for further drainage of an epidural abscess. Long-term chemotherapy was required over the course of 18 months and fibrous union followed

9.6. Summary

The surgical techniques used in re-exploring the lumbar spine have been described in considerable detail in this chapter. In concluding, attention is focussed on a number of important points:

1. Pay particular attention to the muscles of the back which will be further damaged by the re-exploration operation.

Release self-retaining retractors every 45 minutes to allow the muscle blood supply to flow for 5 minutes before proceeding with the surgery.

2. Do not leave jagged remnants of laminal bone in the roof of the spinal canal. Preserve the pars interarticularis, leaving smooth laminal margins adjacent to the dural sac. Coat these bony surfaces with bone wax at the conclusion of the operation.

Do not leave bony spicules in scar tissue covering the dura.

3. Pay particular attention to haemostasis during the operation. Avoid electro-coagulation of vessels in the spinal canal as far as possible, relying rather on the use of haemostatic agents such as gelfoam, packed lightly in the paradural gutters at the end of the operation.

4. Use closed suction drainage post-operatively, except in cases where leakage of cerebrospinal fluid may be anticipated.

5. Before embarking on re-explorations of the spinal canal, *the surgeon must be familiar with techniques for opening and closing the dural sac or nerve root sheaths.* He or she must be aware of the potential danger of cauda equina injury and avoid the use of a strong sucker without the protection of a cotton patty on the sucker tip.

In treating cauda equina arachnoiditis (p. 175) or in circumstances where multiple rents have occurred in abnormally thin dura in the course of the operation, closure of the dura may not be indicated. Special care must then be exercised in closing the wounds and the patient should be given chemotherapy prophylactically.

9.7. Post-Operative Care

Pain control is often particularly difficult in these patients so that special management with continuous intravenous infusions of Pethidine or Omnopon may be required for a few days. Anticoagulant therapy is advised, particularly after lengthy operations.

Mobilization should start soon after operation and in due course a cautious rehabilitation programme should commence. Warm pool therapy is often useful, though if this is not available, then walking progressive distances is to be recommended. Any vigorous muscular exercise is to be avoided.

Light surgical corsets are often helpful for short-term use.

10

Basic Principles in the Management of Spinal Injuries

10.1. Introduction

Descriptions of spinal injuries with neural damage have been found in the earliest of medical writings. Between 1900 and 1935 the incidence of such injuries increased slowly. Since the Second World War further steady increase has led to an incidence of 35 cases per million of population per year in Western countries. Non-traumatic causes of paraplegia account on average for another 15–20 cases per million of population per year.

Motor vehicle trauma accounts for up to 50% of the cases, while injuries resulting from sporting accidents account for about 25% of them.

Spinal injuries are usually classified into three groups:

1. Those without radiological evidence of vertebral fractures.
2. Those with vertebral fractures but without neurological lesions.
3. Those with vertebral fractures and neurological damage including peripheral nerve injuries with or without cord injury.

Life expectancy following spinal injuries has increased until at present, in developed countries, the initial death rate is only 1–2% and life expectancy is normal in the absence of complications.

10.2. Historical

Controversy in the methods of treatment of spinal cord injuries with paraplegia has been a noted feature of their management for more than two hundred years, being first discussed by Gorter in 1742, Sommering in 1793 and Heister in 1750. They were perhaps the first authors to cast doubt on the efficacy of operative procedures in the management of patients with lumbo-dorsal fractures, and particularly those with paraplegia. It was not, however, until 1814 that Henry Klein, a London surgeon, first undertook a laminectomy to reduce a fracture-dislocation of the vertebral column. The controversy concerning the propriety of laminectomy in spinal cord trauma developed into a verbal battle between the giants, Sir Astley Cooper and Sir Charles Bell in 1824. Cooper supported the use of operative procedures while Bell, a leading anatomist and neurologist, wrote a special treatise denouncing Cooper for his support of such ill-timed operative interference.

Even as early as 1845, Bamfield made a number of categorical statements:

1. The operative procedure of laminectomy is difficult.
2. The diagnosis is rarely clear as to whether paralysis has been caused by concussion, extravasation or compression, by puncture, laceration or complete division of the cord, or finally, by general extrusion of osseous tissue from the fractured vertebrae pressing upon the spinal cord.
3. Bamfield further indicated his inability to understand how laminectomy was of assistance when any compression of the cord came from the posterior half of the vertebral body and not from the laminae.
4. He felt that inflammation of the "spinal membranes", as he called the dura and arachnoid, would certainly give rise to further fibrous compression.

Undoubtedly, some of the earliest pathological changes recorded by these authors were due to infection complicating injudicious operative procedures. It was peculiar, however, that in the nineteenth century the surgical method which appeared to be used least was traction with hyperextension as described by Hippocrates, and described again in 1847 by Malgaigne in his treatise on fractures and dislocations. It is noteworthy that he is amongst the first to describe a passive reduction of fracture-dislocation by the use of a postural pillow.

Beckett Howorth, in his treatise on injuries of the spinal column (1964) concluded that the surgical method of traction, extension and de-rotation had great advantages in the overall management of spinal injuries. He showed that attempts to reduce the dislocation by these methods had great effect on the result, both physiologically, posturally and functionally.

It was not until Guttmann started his comprehensive services in 1944, for patients with spinal cord injuries, that the modern care of paraplegia and tetraplegia commenced. Some years earlier, Munro of Boston had shown that management could be materially improved, and thus he sowed the seed for more adequate care of these patients in North America. At about the same time, Botterell in Canada started his service in Toronto, for patients with spinal cord injuries. The service at Stoke-Mandeville was stimulated by the opening of the second front in Europe during the Second World War, and it was shown from there that results in the treatment of these patients could be improved spectacularly.

10.3. Pathogenesis of the Injury

For more than twenty years the present author (G.M.B.) has collected pathological material and examined it in conjunction with Professor Byron Kakulas, so that at the present time, up to 200 cases have been studied and reported in detail (Vinken and Bruyn, Clinical Neurology, Vol. 25, 1976). All spinal fractures and fracture-dislocations are associated with excessive force, usually multi-directional, involving flexion-extension, rotation, compression and stretching. Isolated sharp injuries occurring in association with road trauma are rare. The bone and soft tissues of the vertebral column are usually extensively bruised, crushed and devitalized, with associated spinal cord disruption in many cases. It is unusual to find small discrete areas of damage at post mortem in patients who have died from this type of trauma.

Microscopic damage extends far beyond the macroscopic, accurate delineation of the injury being impossible in the early stages after accident. Avascular necrosis of bone and colliquative necrosis of the cord are concomitant findings. Clinical and pathological estimation of the quantum of damage is impossible until collateral circulation has been established.

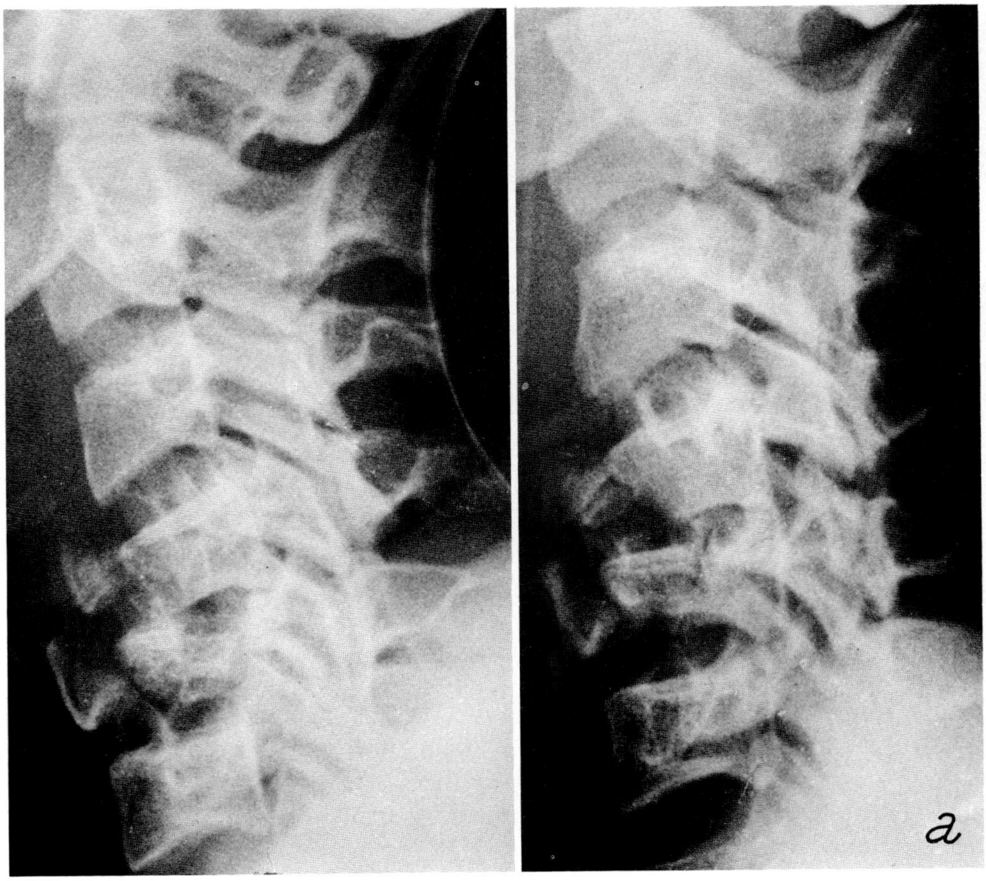

Figure 10.1a. Compression flexion injury of cervical spine associated with haemorrhagic necrosis of spinal cord

The fracture patterns seen on X-ray are either of compressive type or of a flexion type (Figs. 10.1a–c), or a combination of both. The degree of displacement of the fragments varies but there is always some degree of crushing with consequent avascularity of cancellous bone. Replacement and regeneration of this avascular bone is a slow process, and complete reformation of the vertebral body is rare after fracture. In 98% of cases it occurs by paravertebral callus formation. Stability is achieved, with or without reduction of the fracture-dislocation, in the first two or three weeks after injury. Clinical stability of the fracture can be expected when all but one of the ligamentous structures, anterior or posterior to the spinal canal, have

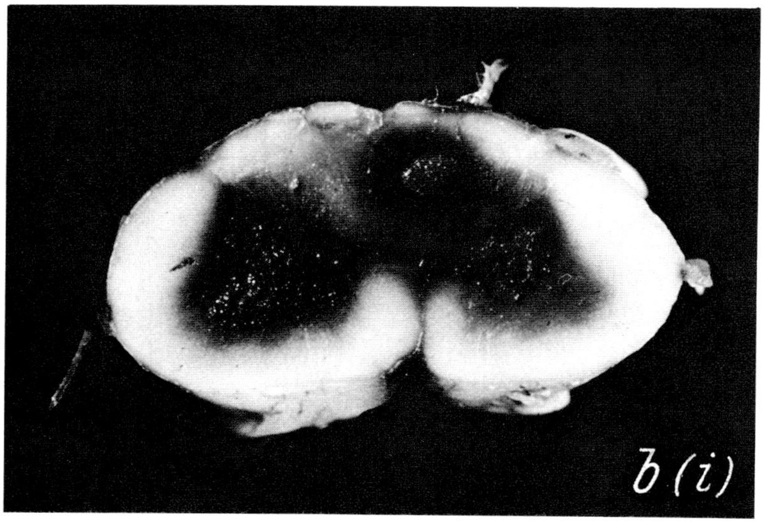

Figure 10.1 b (i). Central haemorrhagic necrosis of spinal cord

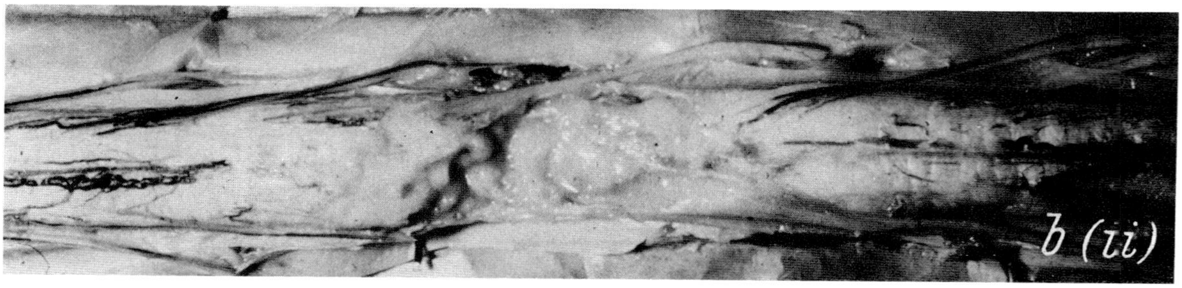

Figure 10.1 b (ii). Necrosis of spinal cord six weeks after injury

been damaged. The terms "stable" and "unstable" should be reserved for the later stages of management rather than in the early stages of assessment. Holdsworth in 1963 indicated the importance of the posterior ligamentous structures in estimating such stability. While he emphasized the importance of the posterior ligamentous complex, it is clear that the anterior ligamentous complex, the disc, and the anterior longitudinal ligament, are also important.

Neural damage may include neuropraxia, axonotmesis, neurontmesis of the spinal rootlets, as well as damage to the spinal cord, varying in degree from patient to patient.

Even in fracture-dislocations which appear to be of comparable severity, neural damage can be quite variable. Various patterns of cord damage emerge, including central necrosis, anterior or posterior necrosis of the cord, complete crushing of the cord, or minor petechial haemorrhages in it.

With the passage of time, the natural history of injury is towards healing, the bony debris being removed and replaced by new bone, while damaged neural tissue is replaced by an intense gliosis in which abortive attempts at nerve regeneration may occur.

The pathology of spinal injuries in the cervico-dorsal spine has features somewhat different from those in the dorsal and lumbo-dorsal column. For example, of the cervico-dorsal injuries with tetraplegia admitted to hospital, over 70% will be incomplete, while root sparing in lumbo-dorsal injuries will be seen in 50%.

Anatomically, the capacity of the neural canal compared with the size of the spinal cord finds its most significant relationship in the lower cervical area where the cervical enlargement usually occupies more than the standard 50% of the canal, and particularly in the older age groups, where with cervical spondylosis the canal may well be almost wholly occupied by the cervical enlargement of the cord. Thus, the

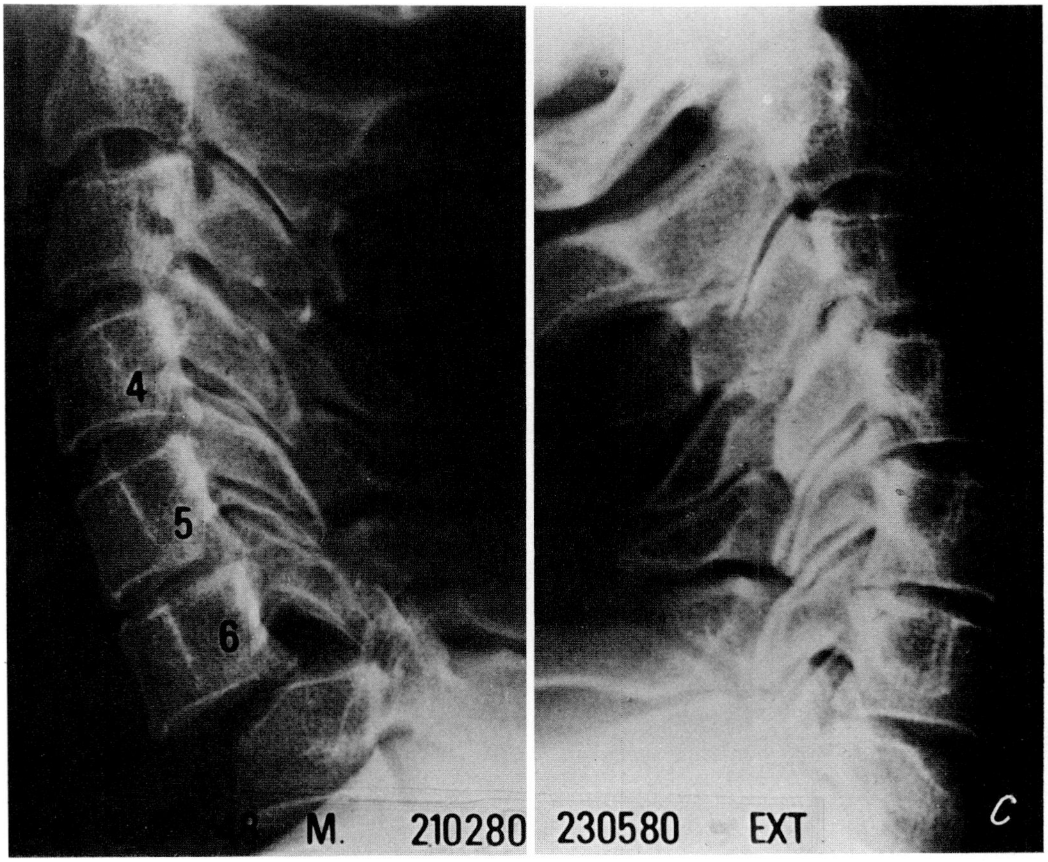

Figure 10.1c. Flexion injury of cervical column with bilateral facet fracture dislocation

anatomical features of the cervical spinal column pre-accident may have a profound effect on the pattern of injury. The spinal cord varies considerably in size from subject to subject. Elliot in 1963, was able to quote variations in the diameter of the cord and the canal, with average measurements showing that the cord occupies only about 50% of the capacity of the canal. In the cervical cord, the cervical enlargement measures, on average, 13.2 mm in width, 7.7 mm in the antero-posterior diameter, while the canal measurements at the same level are 24.5 mm in width and 14.7 mm in the antero-posterior diameter (Figs. 10.2a, b). Caudo-cephalic movements of approximately 1–2 cms occur during flexion and extension of the cervical spine.

Having considered briefly the major anatomical factors which may have a bearing on the outcome of spinal injury, let us examine the common resultant pathological findings.

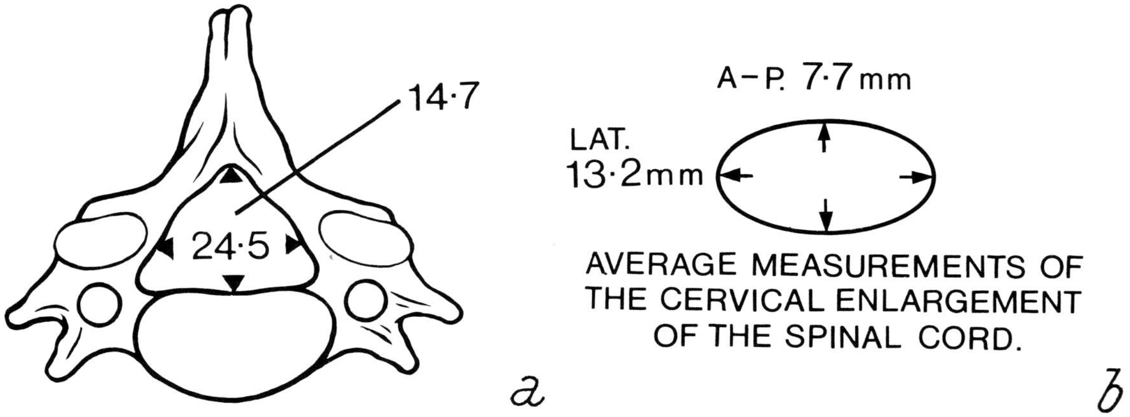

Figures 10.2. A drawing showing average measurements (in millimetres) of the bony cervical canal at the level of the cervical enlargement of the cord

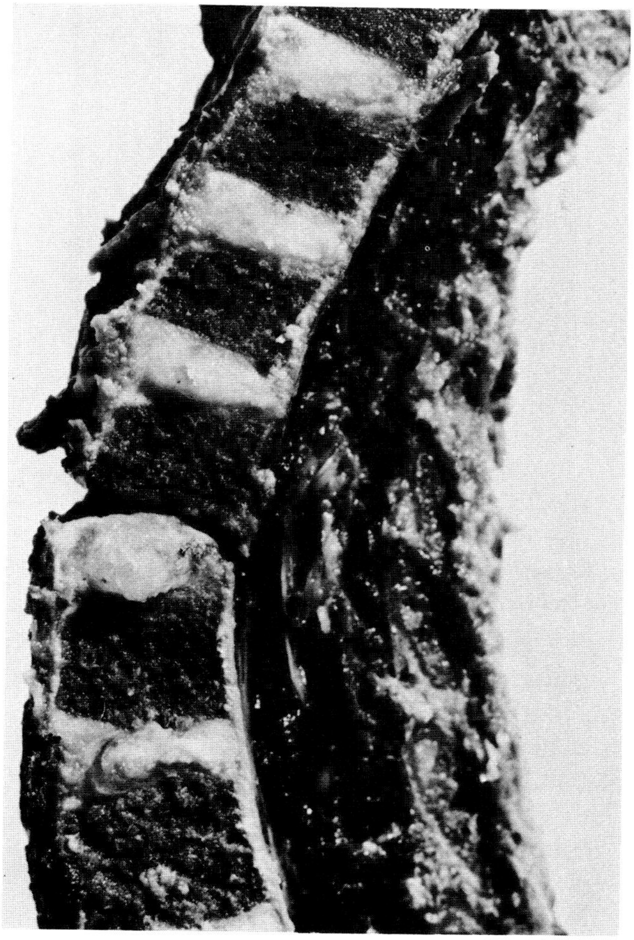

Figure 10.3. Severe extension injury of cervical column. Vertebral end-plate rupture. Gross patchy extra-dural haemorrhage not causing compression

1. Extradural haemorrhage surrounding the spinal cord is seen in all injuries, though it varies in extent from case to case (Fig. 10.3).

In contrast to intracranial extradural haemorrhage, extradural haemorrhage in the spinal column does not give rise to compression of the spinal cord unless the epidural space has been obliterated following previous trauma or operation. Blood which accumulates in the extradural space after spinal injury tends to migrate freely in the canal for several segments above and below the major area of damage. It is unusual to see extradural haemorrhage in the spinal canal as an isolated finding, except in post mortem specimens in patients in whom sudden death has occurred, when there has been insufficient time for the spinal cord to show manifestations of concomitant damage. The clinical significance of extradural-spinal haemorrhage is variable, much of the blood being absorbed, though dural scarring and adherence to the bony canal also occurs. This pathological change in the dura is usually irregular in distribution and may be the cause of discomfort and pain in some patients following spinal injury without associated neurological damage.

2. The completely crushed cord is seen in either flexion or extension injuries, usually in the cervical and rarely in the lumbar enlargement of the cord. Extension injuries in the lumbar column are uncommon (1%) whereas in the cervical column they account for about 26% of the injuries. In 80% of such cervical cases, completely damaged, crushed spinal cords occur where there is no neural continuity (Fig. 10.1b ii).

3. Gross necrosis of the cord may occur following compression injuries or flexion-rotation injuries of the cervical column. Similar injuries of the lumbar column are uncommon and usually occur in association with incomplete cauda equina lesions. However, the conus medullaris may manifest a central necrosis. In all of these cases there is peripherally intact cord tissue with the majority of the damage to central cord tissue usually in the pattern supplied by a central branch from the anterior median longitudinal arterial trunk of the spinal cord, Crock and Yoshizawa, 1977 (Fig. 10.1b i).

4. Anterior necrosis occurs in flexion-rotation injuries usually of the unilateral type and usually in the cervical column. Such necrosis does not follow the pattern of the arterial supply and it commonly involves, in this instance, both grey matter and white matter, leaving the posterior columns intact. The aetiology of such a pattern of cord injury may be due both to anterior compression momentarily and to venous haemorrhage in the cord due to rupture of the ligamentum denticulatum. These injuries are usually associated with gross extradural haemorrhage.

5. Cauda equina injuries occur in the lumbar column and in the lumbo-dorsal column where the conus medullaris finishes at a variable level–from T11 to L2. It must be remembered that the rootlets of the cauda equina can be avulsed from the conus medullaris or severely stretched with flexion-rotation strains. At the same time, a vertical rent can occur in the dura, through which nerve roots may prolapse. Thus at a later stage of examination, the nerve roots appear to have lost their usual vertical alignment and appear to be knotted. Typical Wallerian degeneration occurs at a later stage still; plaques of calcified material can be observed among the rapidly forming gliotic scar tissues.

To summarize, injuries of the spinal cord may occur after severe trauma, where various combinations of flexion, extension, rotation, compression and longitudinal stresses are exerted on a tissue which has a very low coefficient of elasticity and does not tolerate injury well. The spinal cord normally acts as a very soft spring and while it has some resilience during the normal processes of spinal movement and even occasionally in situations of abnormal stress such as may occur during an extension injury of the cervical column without neural damage, nevertheless spinal cord tissue will not stand severe trauma.

Pathologically, the following fractures will usually be stable (Figs. 10.1, 10.2):

1. The crush fracture or dispersion fracture, both of the lumbar and the cervical column; because the ligamentous complexes remain intact.
2. Extension injuries of both the lumbar and cervical column are usually stable because the posterior ligamentous complex is intact along with the posterior longitudinal ligament.

On the other hand, the clinically and pathologically unstable fractures are those in the following groups:

1. Fractures manifested mainly by the flexion-rotation injury where all of the posterior ligaments are ruptured or damaged, including the interspinous, the capsular ligaments and the ligamentum flavum, while one of the anterior group, e.g. the anterior longitudinal ligament, usually remains intact and thus will, on reduction, maintain spinal stability. However, pathologically this injury must be considered to be unstable.

2. Vertebral body fractures, with one vertebral body displaced in front of another, are associated with gross disruption of spinal ligaments. Pathologically, when all of the displaced fractures and fracture-dislocations have been adequately reduced, there will be rapid healing in the ligamentous structures and slow but sure healing in the osseous tissues, so that stability will occur either:

i) by ligamentous healing over a period of six to eight weeks, or
ii) by paravertebral callus in the ruptured ligamentous structures where some osteogenic tissue is found.

In a survey of spinal injuries, over 90% were shown to heal by local means, often with fusion of only two segments, or three at the most, leaving the rest of the vertebral column mobile. However, even when the maximum injury occurs at one mobile spinal segment, e.g. between T12 and L1, it is important to remember that the mobile segment between T11 and T12, and L1 and L2, may have sustained soft tissue damage (i.e. to disc and longitudinal ligaments), which will not be manifested for some years and which can explain the late onset of pain in a paraplegic who otherwise has remained well since accident. *Late pathological manifestations are common and must not be forgotten.*

Finally, it must be remembered that injuries may be multiple in the spinal column so that segments may be "jumped". Only by recalling that such patterns of injury may occur can diagnosis be complete.

In the cervical column the common bony injuries include:

1. Extension injuries with rupture of the anterior longitudinal ligament and/or disc.
2. Compression fractures with intact ligamentous structures.
3. Flexion-rotation injuries, either a unilateral fracture-dislocation or a bilateral fracture-dislocation.

In the lumbar column, the following patterns of injury may occur:

1. Severe flexion-rotation injuries, either unilateral or bilateral facetal fracture-dislocations giving greater than one-half vertebral body displacement in the sagittal plane.
2. Compression injuries or dispersion injuries of the vertebral column.
3. Rarely, extension injuries.

The pattern of vertebral injury will depend on which segment of the column absorbs the damage. The physical stresses are absorbed either by a single vertebra, by a two-vertebrale complex, or even occasionally by a three-vertebrale complex. Experimentally, different patterns will emerge when force is directed to either one, two or three segments of the vertebral column and whether the force is dissipated in either the static bony structure or the more mobile discal segment between two vertebral bodies.

10.4. Recognition of the Injury

Despite technical advances in studying neural impulses which may help to monitor neural disruption, *techniques of diagnosis of all spinal injuries, including spinal cord dysfunction, remain predominantly clinical.* Physical examination continues to require great acumen on the part of clinicians, both in the elucidation of signs and in the interpretation of their significance. In acute spinal fractures with or without spinal cord interruption, physical examination either by a doctor or by a person trained in first-aid, should give, in the conscious patient, an immediate basic diagnosis of the level and extent of neural damage–both sensory and motor. With the arrival of more skilled personnel at the scene of the accident, accurate physical diagnosis in three-dimensional terms of the spinal column and cord can be made. In the case of spinal cord injury, early admission to a comprehensive spinal unit is mandatory to reduce secondary problems as well as to obtain maximal recovery from neural sparing.

It is relevant to state dogmatically that all cases of paraplegia or tetraplegia must be treated as acute emergencies. Following spinal cord injury there are some specific signs which are of great diagnostic significance:

1. A definite "sensory level".
2. Bradycardia and low blood pressure–indicating neurogenic shock.
3. The presence or absence of perineal "neurological sparing".
4. Early intense priapism in the male indicates severe cord damage.
5. Complete areflexia in the lower limbs or upper limbs, significant in the unconscious patient.
6. Associated injuries are common so that a thorough general examination of the patient is essential.

Tenderness over a spinal segment always indicates a spinal fracture until proven otherwise, while restriction of movement is also to be carefully observed and is always a significant factor. The neurological state at the end of six to eight hours after the episode of trauma will help to elucidate prognosis in the paraplegic and enable the examiner to continue to build up a three-dimensional picture of the injuries. Early special examinations such as X-rays and blood investigations should be deferred until a clinical diagnosis has been made.

a) Clinical Examination

No other investigation is as important in those patients suspected of having a spinal injury. Too often the surgeon comes to rely heavily on special examinations and not enough on his clinical acumen. The first medical examiner has a great responsibility to conduct a thorough and complete examination; accurate diagnosis is usually possible and is vital before definitive treatment is carried out. Features that need to be stressed in establishing a diagnosis in these patients are:

i) History

1. The police, ambulance officers and original medical examiners can all be helpful in getting accurate historical information.

ii) General Assessment

2. Resuscitation does not mean just intravenous therapy and oxygen, but should include airway control and lower limb support by bandaging or abdominal compression. Occasionally, laparoscopy, if intra-abdominal blood loss is suspected.

3. The surgeon needs to have patience. Time spent in examination should be of no consequence once life has been preserved by the use of urgent resuscitative methods.

4. No special examinations should be ordered until a thorough physical assessment of the patient has been made, allowing a clear cut diagnosis in nearly all cases. A review of our acute cases has confirmed the accuracy of diagnosis which can be established purely on careful clinical assessment.

5. Many patients are alcoholic and fractious. Firm handling is essential to get the maximum amount of information. *All patients must be turned and all clothing removed.* The lessons of leprosy apply: *All* surface areas must be examined meticulously by the time-honoured methods of inspection, palpation, auscultation, including inspection of the oropharyngeal and rectal cavities.

6. Cranial trauma is a common accompaniment, so that the conscious state needs adequate assessment and if necessary immediate attention. Respiratory distress needs early assessment, particularly if associated with chest injuries. Abdominal diagnosis in the flaccid paraplegic can depend simply on the early detection of peristalsis which is rarely affected in the early stages unless there is an associated abdominal injury.

7. Less than 1% of acute cases will need urgent surgery within a few hours of admission. Drama must give way to meticulous examination before definitive treatment can commence.

iii) Examination of the Spine

Too often the examination of the spine is left to the examination of an X-ray. Careful, clinical examination by palpation of all vertebral segments and movement of the mobile segments within the limits of pain will give information as to the level and extent of damage. Palpation of the interspinous ligaments will determine the level of severe dislocation, for there is usually a gap admitting more than one horizontally applied digit. Even a subluxation is palpable.

iv) C.N.S. Examination

A paraplegic, or tetraplegic, complete on examination after five to six hours will probably remain so. In tetraplegia, however, all authorities agree that care should be exercised in predicting prognosis until six to eight weeks have elapsed, for up to 15% of so-called complete tetraplegics may be incomplete. At post mortem, complete disruption of the cord and meninges in the cervical area is uncommon.

The important points in neural examination include

1. Develop a routine of examination, for example:

a) Examination of all reflexes including evidence of spinal reflexes seen in disruption. These will depend on time after accident, early flaccidity and absence of any complications. Special reflexes such as the bulbocavernosus, or the anal reflex, may be absent, while priapism and the dartos response must be searched for. Early return of such reflexes usually means the loss of spinal shock and spinal cord isolation. The bulbocavernosus response may be slow to return in the presence of urinary infection. Its absence in the otherwise complete paraplegic must be treated with caution and provided there are no complications, it may be evidence of an intact cord.

b) Motor examination of all muscle groups, using Medical Research Council standards, including observations of spasm and pain is vital. In some cases individual muscles may be flaccid, while others may be spastic. There may be an associated irregular loss of reflexes and thus a three-dimensional clinico-pathological picture of the cord damage will be built up.

c) Detailed sensory charting and marking of the sensory chart on the patient's body is essential. *Every dermatome must be examined.* A finite level of sensory loss is an indication of complete transection of the spinal cord. Absence of a finite sensory level with a variable amount of hyperaesthesia indicates that cord injury is incomplete. *Sacral sparing is a vital clinical finding:*

i) it may mean that excellent recovery overall is likely to occur;
ii) it will mean that excellent visceral function can be expected;
iii) it may be the only evidence of incomplete spinal cord injury to be found during the original clinical examination.

d) A detailed examination of the cranial nerves is always necessary.

2. Remember always that sensory neurones, axons and sensory nerves withstand trauma better than the motor elements and that motor sparing frequently takes a long time to be finite.

3. Clinical examination, both in patients with spinal cord injury and in those with spinal column injury alone, needs to be repeated after six to eight hours, to provide confirmation of observations and record changes, either of regression or resolution. Accurate recording is the only way to follow up the continuing changes of pathology now well documented in many centres.

4. Recording each examination on a chart is essential, also the regular recording of skin sensory loss.

5. The surgeon can only really help continuing signs of compression. He cannot as yet regularly help acute incomplete cases whose chances of recovery can easily be made worse by meddlesome surgery. What, therefore, are the probable signs of compression? In the acute stages of spinal trauma they include:

a) Massive dislocation with incomplete lesions.
b) No bony displacement with acute neural changes.
c) Those cases seen with an upper motor neurone onset.

In later stages it includes:

a) A plateauing of improvement of the central nervous system changes, in the absence of complications such as urinary tract infection.
b) Deterioration, usually seen in compression of slow onset which includes spasm and paresis.

It is important for the surgeon at this stage to know the common pathological changes seen in both acute osseous trauma and acute spinal cord trauma. The latter includes complete disruption, central cord necrosis, varying degrees of necrosis, neural disruption of varying degrees, and lastly, gross extradural haemorrhage seen in all cases but rarely of clinical significance (see pp. 272, 273).

Correlation of the clinico-pathological features leads to more accurate diagnosis and so to better care. All lesions in the vertebral column are three-dimensional, either major or minor, and bear no relationship to the X-ray appearances as seen for the elucidation of the bony fracture types. Head injuries are commonly associated with spinal column injuries. All patients admitted to hospital with head injuries should be X-rayed to exclude cervical injury and vice versa.

Unconscious patients should be carefully examined peripherally, the following signs being suspicious:

a) absence of all reflexes;
b) total flaccidity in the lightly unconscious state;
c) urinary retention in similar states;
d) a decerebrate state with uneven development of spasm.

Spinal injury should always be suspected in unconscious patients following head injury. There is *no* substitute for repeated physical examination in such cases.

Having completed a full physical examination including both a spinal examination and neurological examination, the examiner, before any other diagnostic measures are applied, should be able to say that this is a fracture or fracture-dislocation at the level "x" or "y" with complete, incomplete, or no spinal paralysis below the appropriate level. This neurological segment has been designated as the last intact one as defined by Michaelis and Guttmann.

Asymmetry of spinal cord injuries is usual. Longitudinal signs, sensory changes with variations in type and intensity will help in determining the three-dimensional character.

Spinal shock, consisting of total areflexia, flaccidity, total sensory loss and bladder atonia frequently delays final assembling of the pathological evidence for a few days.

Confirmatory diagnostic methods will include X-rays, lumbar puncture, the use of contrast methods, and occasionally others, e.g. peritoneal lavage.

b) Radiological

Radiological evidence is essential to confirm the clinical diagnosis. It must be remembered that injuries so demonstrated have no quantitative relationship to the neural lesion present. Requests must be precise as to the level or levels of examination required in multiple level injuries and the types of special views needed should be clearly designated. When routine antero-posterior, lateral and oblique films have been studied, the surgeon may require special views and special methods. Sagittal and coronal tomography in 1–2 mm cuts are invaluable; I believe they have helped considerably in our diagnostic facility. However, computer assisted tomography, although investigated and used for research purposes, has not so far been proven to be useful routinely, except in some upper cervical spine injuries.

c) Special Problems

Each area of the spinal column has its own diagnostic problems (see Fig. 10.4).

In the cervical spine poor radiology of C6 to T1 and C1/2 is the best known, and can be easily overcome by using the special swimmer's and open mouth views. Preservation of sensation infra-clavicularly does not mean that the upper limbs are preserved as the presence of the intact infra-clavicular nerve comes from C3 and C4. Asymmetry of upper limb signs in tetraplegics is to be expected. Some lack of motor and sensory correlation can be explained on the basis of pre- and post-fixation of the brachial plexus.

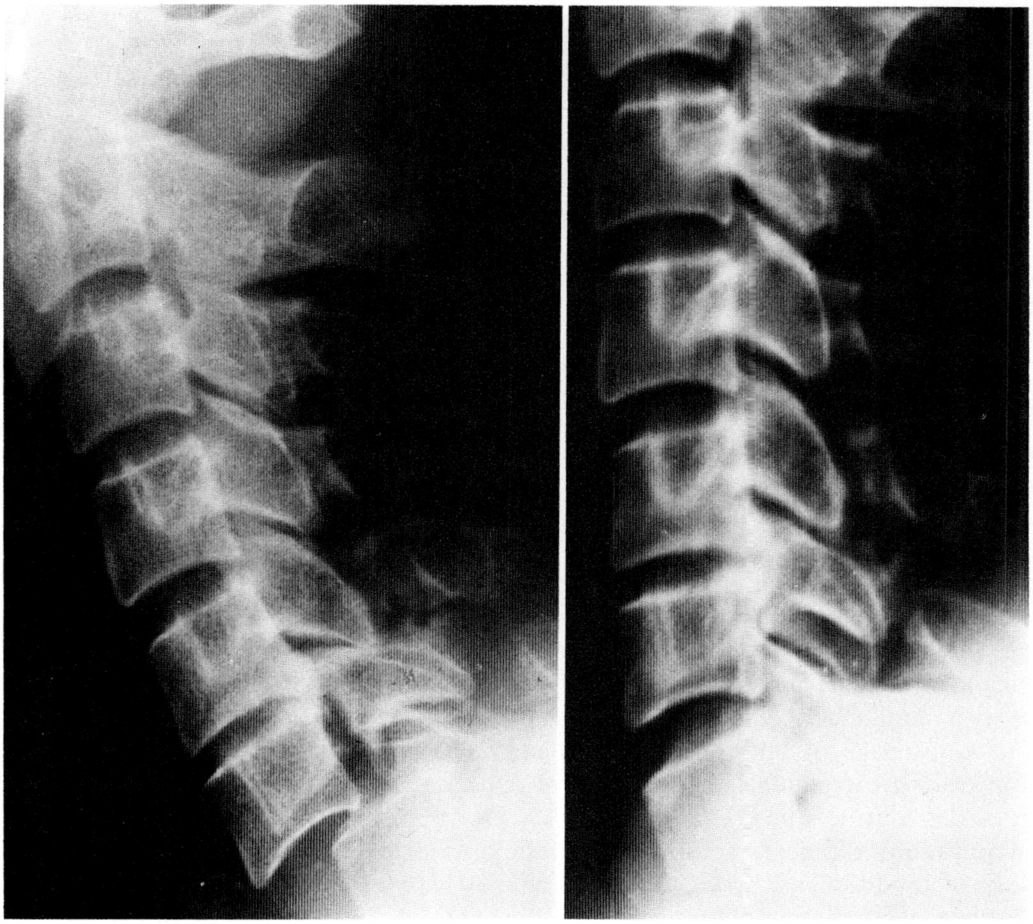

Figure 10.4. Fracture-dislocation of C6 on C7. Poor radiography failed to demonstrate the fracture-dislocation in the film on the right

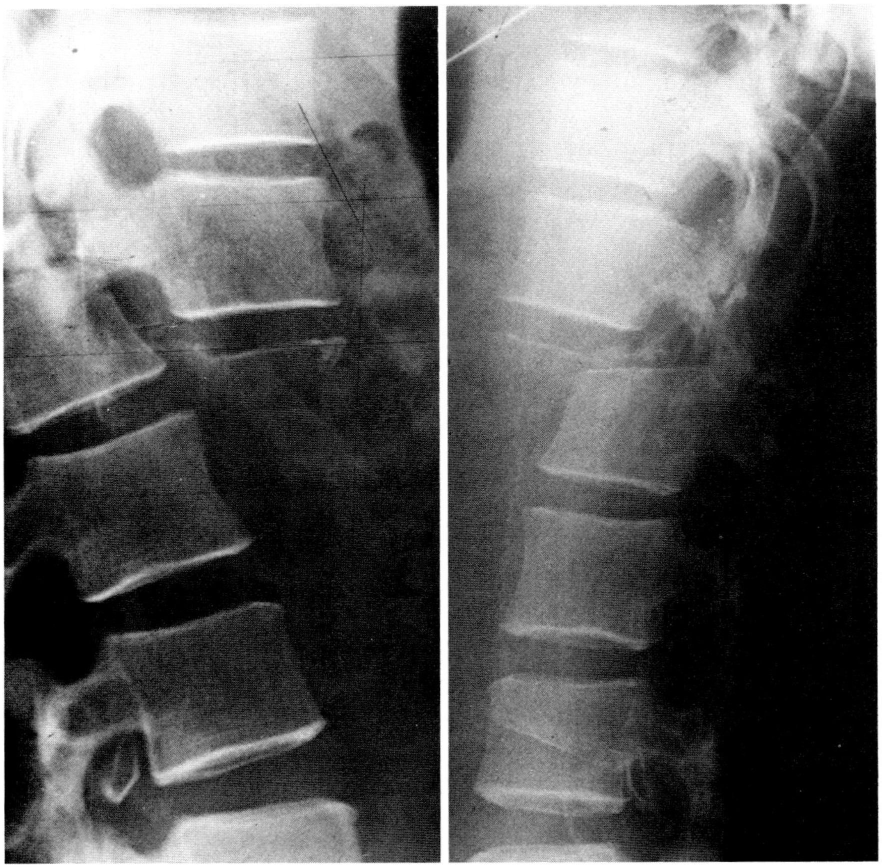

Figure 10.5. Fracture-dislocation of T12/L1. Posturing has assisted in obtaining better radiographs

In the thoracic column, poor examination by palpation and failure to examine the dorsal surface of the trunk is usually the cause of difficulty, while failing to remember that fractures of the sternum are often associated with thoracic fractures is another area of concern. Radiology needs to be exact. Tomography is useful.

In the lumbo-dorsal column (Fig. 10.5), errors result from failure to examine the dorsal area of the spine and failure to realize that if two fingers can be placed between adjacent spinous processes at the painful area, fracture-dislocation is certain. Good radiology depends on accurate pre-clinical diagnosis and then extra oblique and tomographic views can be ordered, if necessary. Mixed upper motor neurone, lower motor neurone lesions with sensory sparing, and a variety of neural lesions with similar bony injury create a challenging area that can be resolved by an accurate knowledge of both the anatomy and the pathology of injury to this area. Sacral injuries are frequently missed, largely because of failure to examine this area as part of the routine spinal examination. This is an area of the spine where accurate clinical and radiographical examination will help to reduce the iatrogenic problems of disorders of bladder and bowel function.

The use of lumbar puncture and myelography has been debated for years. The use of lumbar puncture with pressure studies has not been useful as a diagnostic aid, in our hands, because of the variability of the pathology, extradural haemorrhage, and intraneural necrosis which becomes defined in the first days. Likewise, myelography as an acute diagnostic tool has not usually been valuable. The introduction of irritant contrast material into the spinal theca carries certain risks. Scher in Cape Town sums up well when he states, "Myelography in acute spinal cord injury is technically difficult and has not regularly led to positive help as well as being hazardous for the patient". Opinions differ, but until more positive evidence is available, this is the generally held opinion. Air contrast techniques, with C.T. scanning, can assist in the definition of the pathology, but has not given much more information than is obtainable by using standard X-ray techniques. Again, the surgeon is regularly seeking evidence of continuing compression by "space-occupying lesions" or bony masses. These are very rare; even discs may be space-occupying, but rarely, if ever, cause compression when cases are first seen after severe injury.

No surgical procedure has yet been proven to be useful in spinal cord lesions, either anterior decompression or posterior release. The very pathology itself, being three-dimensional over three to four segments, does not lead to such surgery being useful. Myelography must, however, be used in some cases where neural findings are deteriorating (despite their poor prognosis) and in some cases where paraplegia is of late onset. Cord lesions amenable to relief by surgical means are uncommon.

Other procedures, such as discography, have little place, particularly if the clinical examination is well done by an examiner who understands the pathology of spinal injuries.

d) Associated Injuries

The diagnosis of associated injuries is important and must always be sought. Neural, vascular, bony and soft tissue injuries are common. Only by careful repeated examination can these injuries be discovered. Ruptures of the diaphragm at the lumbo-dorsal area must always be excluded, while fractures of the pelvis may account in large measure for profound shock. Peritoneal lavage has ben advised as a subsidiary diagnostic measure.

The methods found to be of greatest use in the diagnosis of peripheral injuries associated with spinal column lesions are:

1. Careful palpation of all limb bones.
2. Careful passive movements of joints.
3. Detection of severe bruising.
4. Auscultation of the abdomen and chest and major blood vessels. Abdominal palpation and testing for shifting dullness.
5. Good sensory charts in incomplete lesions to determine peripheral nerve injuries.
6. Careful radiography of suspicious areas always including the chest and frequently the abdomen in various positions.

The effects of first-aid and time in diagnosis have not been sufficiently emphasized and need to be. Once again, stress must be placed on the importance of re-examination a short time after admission and early careful recording by the first clinical examiner. Good first-aid will reduce shock. Any suspicion of greater shock than is usual should be an indication for another search for associated injuries. The consequences of poor diagnosis are immense in terms of complications, treatment and final disability. Nothing is of greater importance in reducing final disability in medicine generally than early adequate diagnosis.

Finally, having made a diagnosis, the examiner must carefully consider a differential diagnosis. Diagnoses which have been confused with spinal injury and paralysis include:

1. Hysteria.
2. Secondary malignancy.
3. Old fractures of the spine.
4. Previous spinal cord injury with a new non-paralytic episode.
5. Very occasionally, minor accidents of spinal dysfunction with purpura and/or vascular catastrophies.

Hysteria is the most serious. Signs which assist are:

a) Normal reflexes immediately, which remain unaltered.
b) Changing patterns of non-anatomical sensory disturbances.
c) Normal visceral function.
d) Abnormal behaviour.

However, it should be remembered that hysteria can exist in genuine cases of cord damage.

Secondary malignancy can become manifested by injury, but usually the patient's antecedent history will help to clear up misunderstandings.

Old fractures and previous spinal cord injury will be excluded if a careful history is obtained in *all* cases as well as adequate X-rays. They do constitute a group to be remembered, particularly if the patient is unconscious.

Diagnosis and differential diagnosis of spinal fractures with and without cord transection are, I believe, clinically solvable matters. In summary, the most useful methods of diagnosis are based on:

a) Knowledge of the pathological changes which may follow spinal cord injury.
b) Careful, repeated examination by all clinical methods.
c) Proper recording of results by standard methods.
d) Adequate radiological examination of the vertebral column, including computerized tomography if available.

11

The Management of Spinal Injuries With and Without Neural Damage

11.1. Introduction

Management of spinal fractures and fracture-dislocations starts immediately after the accident; at the roadside, in the mine or on the farm. Good first-aid will result in a decrease in morbidity and disability and a decrease in the number of complete paraplegics being admitted to paraplegic units.

First-aid measures for the management of spinal injuries have been clearly set out in manuals by the St. John Ambulance Association and other bodies. The guiding principle must be gentleness with adequate lifting and turning of the patient in one piece. Life-saving procedures such as overcoming airway obstruction and reducing blood loss are first priorities, followed by the establishment of an adequate diagnosis of the nature of the injuries.

In many parts of the world flying squads are now available for emergency calls and these coordinated teams have improved the standard and efficiency of first-aid care, especially for victims of spinal injury.

In any unconscious patient the airway must be maintained so that anoxia is prevented, while a diagnosis of spinal injury should always be suspected. Serious associated injuries will occur in about 40% of paraplegics, e.g. lower limb fractures. Splinting of limb injuries at the site of the accident is essential.

With the arrival of a flying squad, additional care can be given, such as:

a) The use of prepared splints and cervical collars.
b) The use of intravenous therapy.
c) The use of airways or endotracheal tubes.

Overall, however, the aim of first-aid management in these cases is to secure satisfactory posture for the patient in a comfortable, normal supine or lateral position, preventing further potentially damaging spinal movement during transport to hospital. Patients with suspected cervical spinal injuries should be treated with traction, while those with suspected injuries to the lumbar vertebral column should be transported with adequate lateral splinting.

11.2. Transport

During the early stages of the first-aid management of the patient with spinal injuries, arrangements should be made to transport them to the nearest major emergency centre, or preferably, to a comprehensive spinal unit. If the patient is to be transported by air, then facilities for the use of some form of rotor stretcher are usually available. The standard stretchers available in most ambulances are satisfactory, providing firm support can be assured for the lumbar and cervical spinal curves.

It is dangerous to transport patients with severe respiratory insufficiency, with severe head injuries and anoxia, or with associated major injuries and profound shock in unpressurized aircraft.

On admission to hospital, the following routines should be established as soon as possible:

1. Disciplined nursing with a turning technique to maintain all normal curves of the spine and to maintain extension postures in the lower limbs.
2. Strict monitoring of blood pressure, pulse and respiratory rates. Recording of urinary output is essential, following intermittent catheterization or the use of a temporary indwelling catheter.
3. Management of the associated injuries with the use of temporary plasters or splints.
4. Occasionally, skeletal traction may need to be applied urgently.

During the early stages of the patient's management in the original medical centre, diagnosis of the spinal injury should be confirmed on an emergency basis, following careful physical examination and the use of appropriate radiographic examinations as discussed in Chapter 10.

11.3. Prevention of Secondary and Tertiary Complications

In all cases with spinal injuries, complications can be prevented by strict attention to simple details in the early stages of management. Complications include:

1. Deterioration of the spinal fracture.
2. Early introduction of urinary tract infection.
3. Pressure sores.
4. Limb oedema, contractures and muscle spasm, aggravated by poor posture.

The appearance of these complications may create tertiary states which can aggravate the patient's condition throughout his or her life. Central to the management of these patients is the maintenance of cleanliness and the prevention of infection, especially in relation to the care of the bladder.

11.4. Early Care in the Resuscitation Unit and/or Spinal Cord Injury Centre

Advance notice of the patient's admission to a spinal injuries centre should be given so that a consultant can be available for consultation at the time of admission. Further care may be required as follows:

1. Replacing blood loss.
2. The use of intercostal tubes for the treatment of haemopneumothorax.
3. Positive pressure ventilation or occasionally tracheostomy.
4. Continuation of the postural care of the spinal fractures.
5. *All* minor injuries, at this stage, should be carefully diagnosed and managed.
6. All associated injuries should be checked.

The basic plans for the management of the patient in the six or eight weeks following his admission to the spinal injuries centre are laid down in the acute emergency area. Careful thought is needed before a programme of balanced care can be planned. Clinically, all systems need to be fully investigated, with particular reference to changes that have occurred in the time between the original examination at the site of accident and the findings on admission to the spinal injuries centre. Radiological examination must now be precise and accurate, and requests to the radiographer should be precisely set down, detailing the levels of the vertebral column to be examined and the special views required. Particular attention is to be paid to the difficult areas in the upper and lower cervical vertebral column so that the risks of missing lesions at C1/2 or at the C6 to T1 levels are minimized. *Flexion and extension films should only be carried out by consultants or medical officers with experience and should only be used as an extension of diagnosis in those cases where it is felt necessary,* for example, where the original X-rays failed to reveal a fracture-dislocation which is suspected to be present. Special examinations may be used on occasions. They include:

1. Computerized tomography. This is especially useful following injuries in the upper cervical spine. However, it has not yet replaced standard radiological techniques in the general investigation of spinal injuries.

2. Routine tomography is of great value in defining the pathological anatomy of any fracture. This should be performed in both coronal and sagittal planes.

3. Myelography. This investigation has little use in the early management of patients with spinal fractures and neural damage. It is useful in the rare cases of spinal stenosis which may occur late after injury.

11.5. General Considerations

Once again, emphasis should be placed on the general care of patients under treatment in a spinal cord injury unit. The basic principles of management have been laid down: adequate posture, adequate visceral care, adequate cleanliness, careful procedural activity and early attention to the reduction of fracture-dislocations of the spine. Spinal surgery can be safely delayed until the admission of the patient to a major neurosurgical-orthopaedic service, or particularly to a comprehensive spinal injuries unit. There are well documented reasons for this advice:

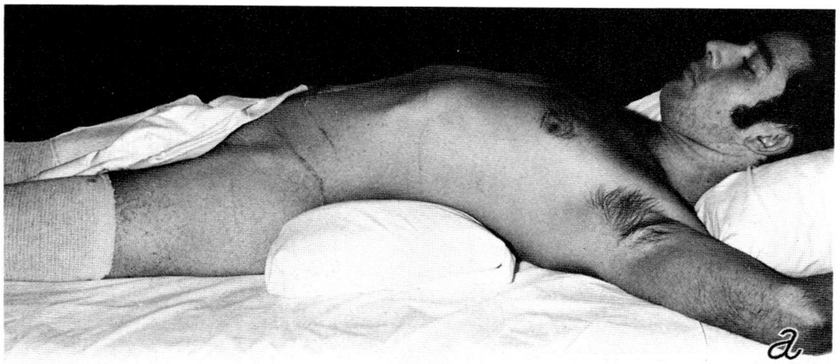

Figure 11.1 a. Postural reduction of lumbo-dorsal fracture-dislocation, the supine position

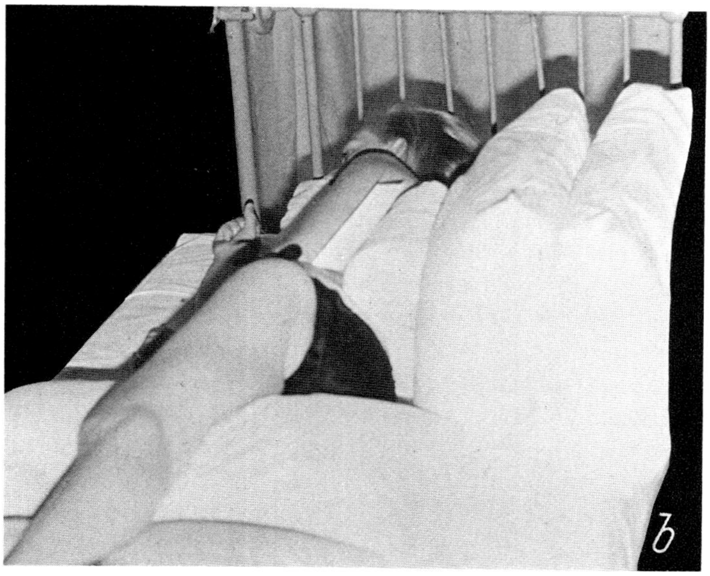

Figure 11.1 b. Postural reduction of lumbo-dorsal fracture-dislocation, the lateral position, showing placement of the pillows

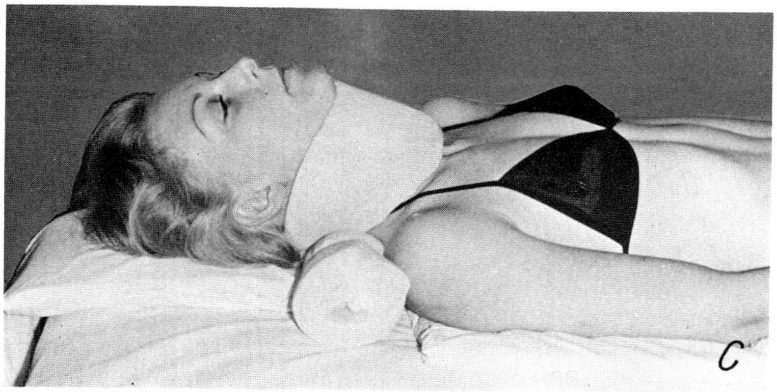

Figure 11.1 c. Postural maintenance after reduction of cervical fracture-dislocation, the supine cervical position

1. Poor surgery is likely to increase the neurological damage; the "occasional surgeon" should avoid becoming involved in the care of such problems.

2. There is no proof that early surgery is of value in aiding neurological recovery.

3. Urgent surgery is rarely required. Distinctions between indications and contra-indications can be more clearly drawn 48 hours after admission.

It should be remembered that early social care of the patient and relatives is important.

11.6. The Role of Special Procedures in Specific Areas of Spinal Injury

a) Postural Reduction of the Fracture (Figs. 11.1a–c)

Watson-Jones, Nicoll and others agree that most fractures and fracture-dislocations can be reduced by postural methods using either a pillow technique as described by Guttmann, or by using a two-table technique for plastering as described by Watson-Jones during the Second World War. In cases with severe fracture-dislocations treated by postural reduction and nursed in hyperextension, a dead space is left in the vertebral bodies. This fills with haematoma and secondary deformity follows inevitably. It is doubtful whether one should persist with the use of plaster casts as a general technique in such cases. Nicoll has advocated early muscle activity in the erector spinae and abdominal muscle groups to encourage a better functional recovery of vertebral column movements.

b) Traction, Including Flexion and Extension, Effecting Reduction of the Fracture-Dislocation (Fig. 11.2)

This method has proven of great value both historically and in contemporary use. Ambrose Paré in 1575 described the method of pelvic-thoracic traction which is well illustrated in Howorth's book "Injuries of the Spine" (1964). Most surgeons attempt to reduce severe lumbo-dorsal and cervico-dorsal fractures and fracture-dislocations with bilateral facet dislocations by postural methods without general anaesthesia. After admission, skeletal traction in cervical injuries with careful traction first in flexion and then in extension over a 24-hour period will result in reduction (Bedbrook, 1981). In lumbo-dorsal injuries, good postural methods can be supplemented by traction. These methods are safe and effective and should always be used initially in the management of these patients.

c) Manipulative Reduction (Figs. 11.3a, b)

Manipulative reduction of cervico-dorsal injuries and lumbo-dorsal injuries may be tried slowly, usually without anaesthesia, or rapidly under anaesthesia. In the case of the cervico-dorsal injuries, some type of skeletal traction should be applied. Without anaesthesia, the head should be shaved and prepared, noting the sagittal line and the

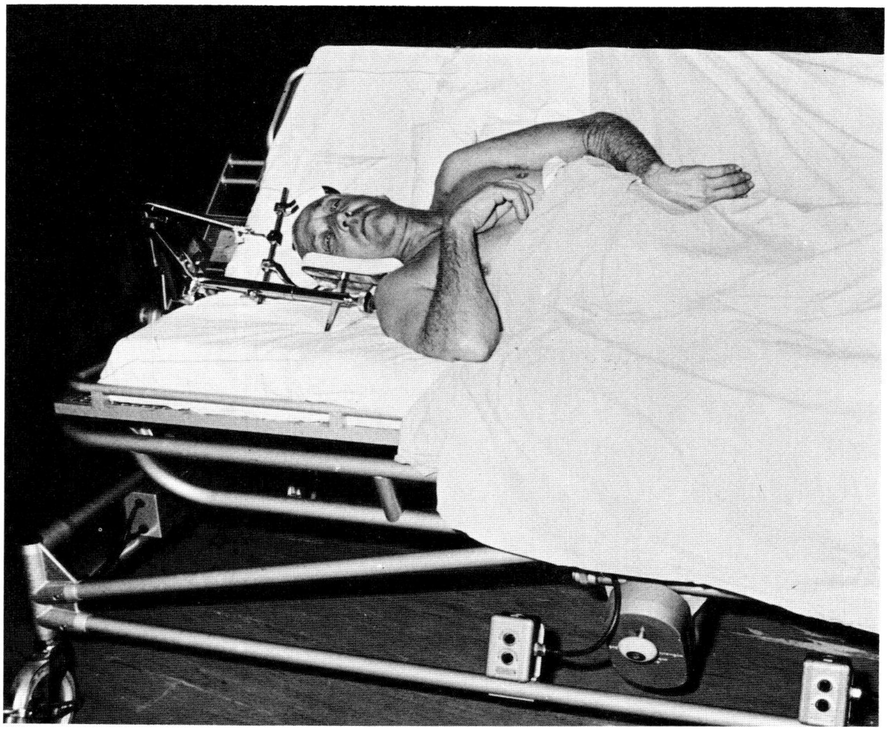

Figure 11.2. The Stoke Mandeville Edgerton bed used in this instance with traction for a cervical injury

inter-aural line, both of which are marked on the scalp with Bonney's Blue. The points at which the calipers will enter the skull are then marked carefully, holding the open calipers over the skull. Flexion of the cervical spine can be obtained by placing the calipers behind the transverse plane, while extension can be produced if they are set anterior to this plane. Local anaesthetic is then infiltrated into the selected points and the skull exposed with half inch incisions, the underlying pericranium being reflected. A 7/16th inch drill is then used to drill the outer table of the skull on both sides; this is fitted with a protective device to prevent penetration of the inner table. When both sides have been carefully drilled, the calipers are then inserted firmly. Weights of up to 80 kg can be applied if necessary.

In cervico-dorsal fractures, traction should be applied first in flexion of 35° to unlock the fracture. If the fracture-dislocation is unilateral, the traction should be applied more to one side than to the other to unlock the dislocation. After the dislocation has been unlocked then the head can be brought slowly into extension, thus reducing the fracture-dislocation. In using a manipulative measure, Walton's manoeuvres for the reduction of unilateral fracture-dislocations of the cervical spine can be performed under general anaesthesia, as illustrated in the diagrams in Fig. 11.3a.

Occasionally, cervical dislocations will reduce spontaneously after induction of anaesthesia, during intubation, when a soft click is heard in the spine.

In the lumbo-dorsal column a similar technique can be used for the reduction of locked facets or locked fracture-dislocations. With the patient adequately anaesthetized and relaxed, pelvic traction and thoracic counter-traction in some

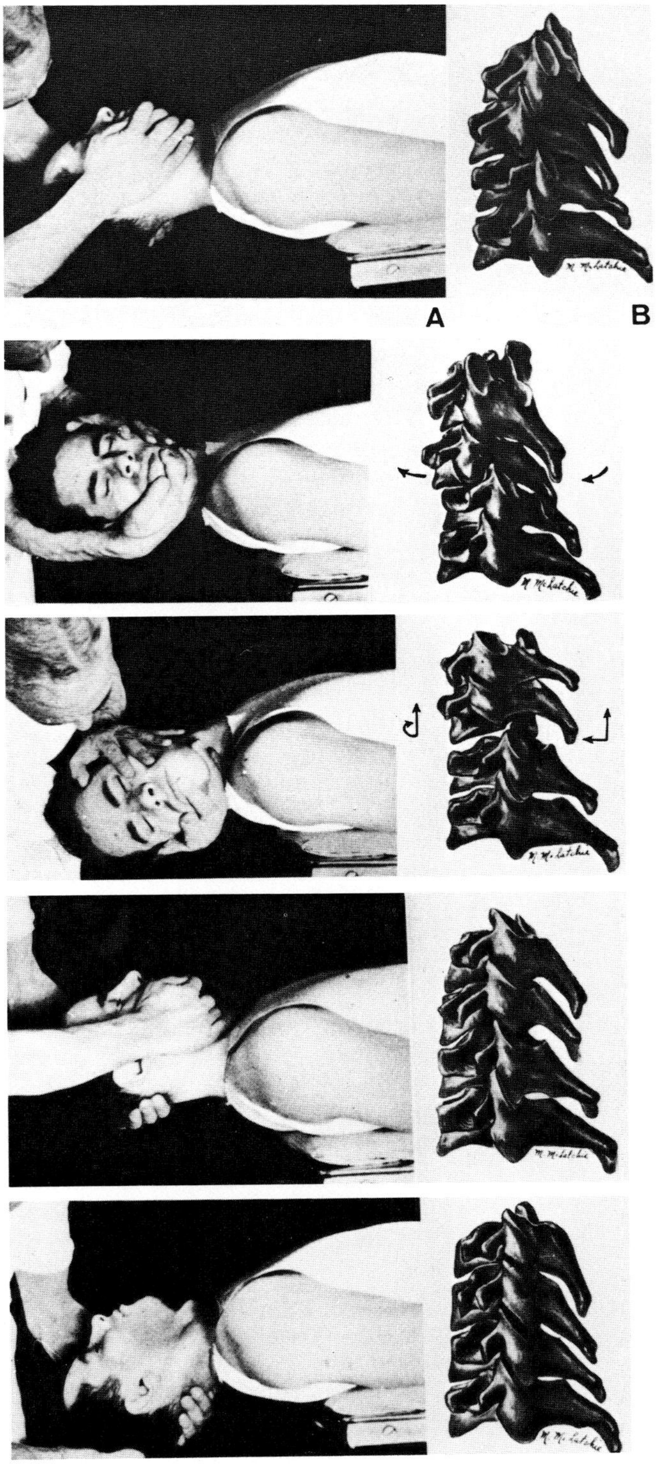

Stage I

A Position for reduction at the start. Walton manipulative reduction

B Rotary dislocation of the cervical spine

Stage II

Walton reduction. Rotation away from the side of the lesion

Stage III

Walton reduction. Retrolateral flexion

Stage IV

Walton reduction. Rotation back to neutral. Lateral flexion maintained

Stage V

Walton reduction. Extension in neutral. Complete reduction

a

Figure 11.3 a. The procedure used for manual manipulation of displaced fracture-dislocations of unilateral type

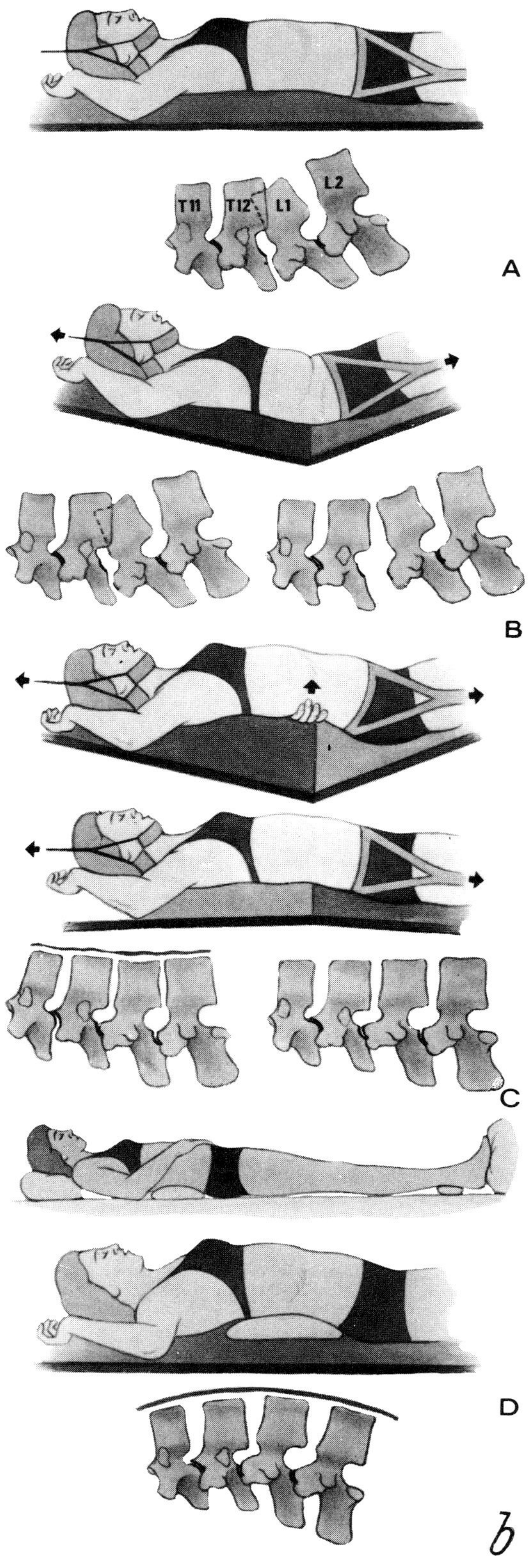

Indications

1. When postural reduction fails.
2. When open reduction is contra-indicated by:
   a) infection;
   b) multiple injuries;
   c) other complications such as pulmonary; or
   d) psychological or religious reasons.
3. Before open reduction.

Method

Reduction under general anaesthesia.

A The patient is placed supine with relaxation, ensuring that the fracture site is at the break in the table so that the spine can be flexed or extended.

B Traction is applied manually or via harness to the head or thorax and pelvis to distract the fracture in the flexed position by "breaking" table.

C With traction continuously applied the operator exerts a forward thrust to the prominent spinous process, thus lifting (patient supine) the lumbo-dorsal spine lordosis. The lumbar column below the fracture-dislocation can usually be felt to move forward and be locked by the anterior longitudinal ligament.

D Traction and extension are maintained. The table is reversed and a gall-bladder rest is raised under a pillow to give hyperextension, thus "fixing" the intact anterior longitudinal ligament. Traction is released but postural reduction is maintained.

The X-ray is checked. The above process is repeated if necessary, then the patient is allowed to recover from relaxant anaesthesia so that the muscle tone assists.

The patient is taken off the operating table by the sliding method onto a rigid surface to hold reduction. The rigid surface is removed in the ward when the patient is fully conscious.

Postural reduction is maintained.

b

Figure 11.3b. Closed reduction of fracture-dislocation of lumbo-dorsal spine with locked facets, with and without paraplegia [from: Bedbrook, G. M.: Spinal Injuries, pp. 222–241; in: Operative Surgery, Orthopaedics (Bentley, G., ed.). Butterworths. 1979] flexion will serve to unlock the fracture-dislocation which can then be hyperextended, reducing the dislocation by local manipulation. All of these procedures should be regarded as gentle techniques having a regular application in treatment, leading frequently to complete reduction of fracture-dislocations.

In the cervico-dorsal column such methods have almost superseded open techniques, while in the lumbo-dorsal column the results are not quite as good, though often satisfactory.

d) Open Reduction and Internal Fixation

The usual indications for such procedures are said to be – to ensure stability, for ease of nursing, to control pain, for failure to reduce by other methods, or for reduction of the kyphos.

Operative procedures have been used in all areas of the vertebral column, but particularly in the lumbo-dorsal area. Early operative reduction is indicated, in the author's opinion, only in the following circumstances:

a) Following failure to reduce by postural or manipulative measures gross fracture-dislocations which have resulted from flexion and rotation forces.

b) In cases where, after reduction, difficulties in nursing management may produce recurrent deformity at the fracture site.

However, such procedures are rarely indicated. There are, in fact, no absolute indications for open reduction and fixation in either the cervico-dorsal or the lumbo-dorsal area, particularly within the first 48 hours after injury. Gross disruption of the vertebral column and early scoliosis may eventually need fixation. Patients should have operations only after the indications and the contra-indications, e.g. urinary infection, pressure sores etc., have been adequately assessed and where the surgeon can review carefully all aspects of care before deciding that surgery can be of assistance.

e) Laminectomy

This operation has been generally abandoned, except in occasional cases. Post-operative instability following laminectomy may require anterior spinal fusion, and there is mounting concern for its role in the production of arachnoiditis (Comarr, 1968). The history of this operation in the management of patients with spinal cord injury is black. Schneider (1951), Morgan and Wharton (1970) have reported series of patients with cervical injuries treated by laminectomy, in which cases with incomplete spinal cord damage ended with complete paralysis following operation. Comarr and Kaufman in their classical review of 850 cases in 1956 showed that results of neurological recovery were significantly better in patients who had not been subjected to exploratory laminectomy.

f) Use of Exoskeletons

Exoskeletons are used regularly in the management of patients with cervico-dorsal and lumbo-dorsal fractures. Many patients whose spinal injuries have been managed conservatively need an exoskeleton when allowed to get up, particularly if they complain of pain. Exoskeletons are regularly used in most patients at the end of six weeks. Many varieties of these devices are now available.

a) Plaster of Paris jackets are still widely used, applied by a number of methods including the two-table technique, traction on a scoliosis frame or simply by applying anterior and posterior shells which can be subsequently connected.
b) The use of polythene supports which are constructed around plaster moulds of the patient's trunk.
c) The use of functional splints such as cervical collars. Many varieties are now available commercially.
d) Special functional splints such as the SOMI Brace providing neck support based on four pillars attached to a thoracic jacket.
   Most of these exoskeletons will be much more comfortable with the patient in the erect position and should not be considered to be perfectly satisfactory in the supine position. They are made for functional activity. Careful fitting to maintain adequate posture with the use of such exoskeletons is essential.
e) Halo cast. Over the last decade since Halo pelvic apparatus has been described in the management of scoliosis there have been various ways of applying such exoskeletal appliances to fractures of the spine. Pelvic fixation is now rarely used; most have become variations of halo cast techniques whereby a skull halo is applied and fixed to a custom built body cast. These appliances have been used from any time between one and six weeks after injury for periods up to three months after accident. For tetraplegics this method has limited application as it runs all the risks of skin stress and sores. A trial made by this author (G. M. B.) led to an initial abandonment of the method as not adequate and not improving rehabilitation. For non-tetraplegics the method has advantages of early mobility, allowing early discharge from hospital, but there are disadvantages:
   (i) Considerable maintenance is required.
   (ii) Scalp infection along the pin tracks is likely to occur.
   (iii) Unstable fractures treated in this device may displace quietly and unobtrusively.
   (iv) Halo casts may be comfortable with the patient in the erect posture but uncomfortable in the supine position. Casts tend to ride upwards. These appliances require adjustment often two or three times daily.

These are the procedures which are available to the surgeon caring for patients with spinal injuries. The majority of cases are treated best by the use of posture, postural reduction, regular isometric exercise and occasionally non-operative manipulative reduction. Rarely indeed is early open surgery required. Physical rehabilitation using isometric and graded resisted muscle exercises is essential.

11.7. Management in Specific Areas

a) Cervico-Dorsal Fractures and Fracture-Dislocations in Early Stages

i) Acceleration/Deceleration Injury

This so-called "whiplash" injury of the neck usually results from motor vehicle accidents when the driver and passenger are seated in a stationary vehicle which is hit from behind. These injuries occur in considerable numbers in all major cities. This mechanism of neck injury may be associated with lower motor neurone paralysis in the upper cervical trunk, particularly if there has been a sudden lateral flexion injury of the spine. Plain X-rays of the spine taken at the time of the accident usually show no abnormality, though occasionally minor fractures may be noted. In many of these cases the maximal effects of injury are exerted on the cervical intervertebral discs (see Chapter 7) and on the anterior ligamentous structures of the neck. Associated peridural and epineural extradural haematomas may occur.

The majority of patients who have sustained this injury respond to careful conservative treatment for pain, including the use of a collar and the early introduction of isometric muscle activity. Many develop major psychological problems, and quite a few may require surgical treatment in the long term for disc excision and interbody fusion at the affected level (see Chapter 7).

ii) Fractures and Fracture-Dislocations from C3 to T1

(i) Hyper-Extension Injury: Incidence of 23% (Fig. 10.3, Chapter 10)

In these cases there is usually a history of a blow on the head and clinical examination may show abrasions on the forehead. On palpation of the spine there may be tenderness anteriorly along the anterior longitudinal ligament. Neurological examination may be normal, while in others there may be complete or incomplete tetraparesis.

Lateral X-rays in flexion and extension may reveal wide opening of the disc space at the affected level. With this mechanism of injury, damage to multiple discs occurs frequently.

The majority of these patients can be immobilized simply in bed with the neck in flexion (Fig. 11.1c); the length of bed rest will depend entirely on the severity of the injury and its association with spinal cord damage.

(ii) Axial Compression Injuries – Sometimes Associated With Flexion Injuries (Fig. 10.1a, Chapter 10)

Following this mechanism of injury, vertebral body fragments may be displaced anteriorly, posteriorly and laterally. Vertebral body fragments displaced posteriorly into the canal may damage the spinal cord. Injuries of this type may occur with little or no final displacement as seen on X-ray, though major neurological damage may have occurred.

Having determined that these injuries are stable by careful X-ray study, the majority need no further treatment other than collar support and isometric neck muscle exercises until the fracture subluxation has healed. In this group, flexion and extension X-rays are required at the time of the initial management to determine whether or not the spine is stable.

(iii) Flexion Rotation Injuries With Unilateral Facet Fracture-Dislocation: Incidence 25% of Injuries (Fig. 11.4)

Fracture-dislocation of the cervical spine with associated subluxation of a single facet, with or without cord injury is known as a Beatson Type I injury. Reduction of this type of injury is necessary. Some of the fractures will reduce spontaneously when the neck is postured in extension to restore the cervical

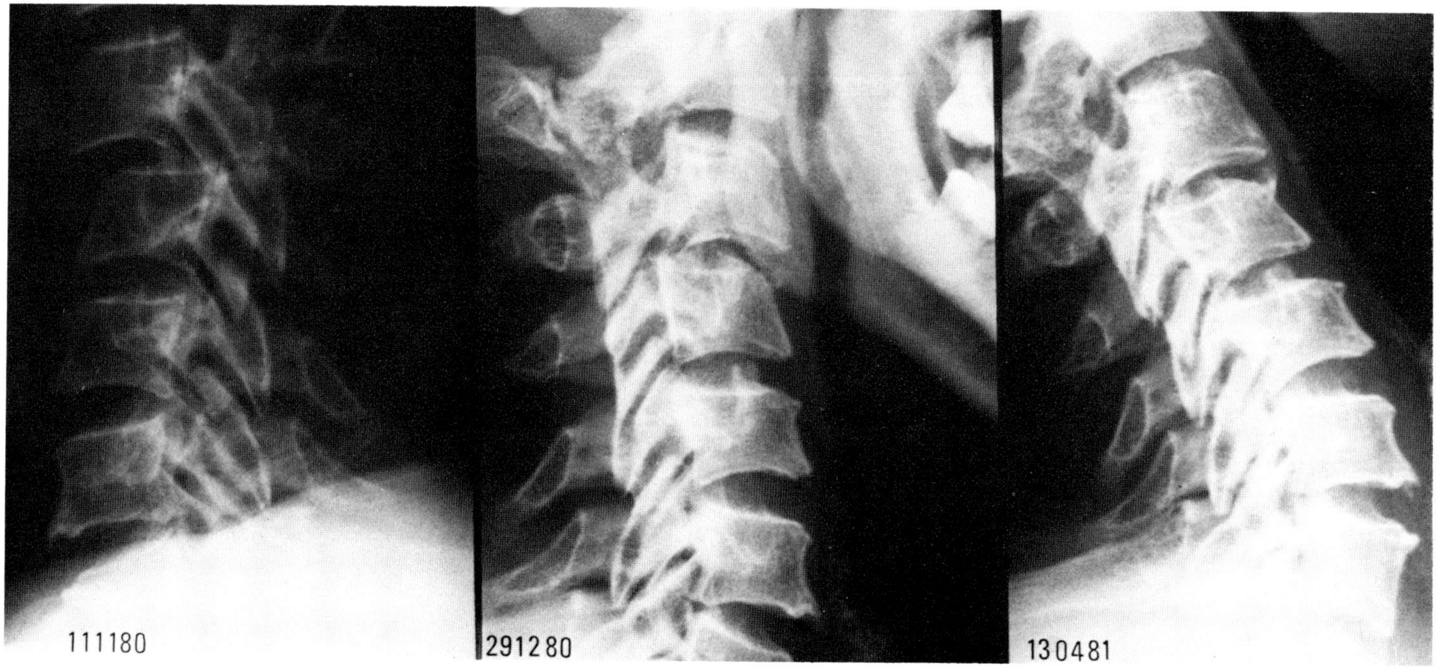

Figure 11.4. Unilateral C3/C4 fracture-dislocation associated with fracture of lamina of C2, emphasizing the multiplicity of injuries in the same cervical spine

lordotic curve. In cases with unilateral facet dislocation, reduction is usually necessary. However, if there is an associated fracture-dislocation then spontaneous reduction may occur, Key (1976).
In the acute management of these injuries, simple posturing, occasionally with cervical traction, may only be required to effect reduction. Occasionally, manipulative reduction with the use of the Walton method is required (Fig. 11.3a). Surgical treatment is rarely indicated but may be necessary if spinal instability persists after six or eight weeks of treatment. In addition, open reduction may be required where conservative reduction has failed and the patient refuses prolonged conservative treatment. However, failure to reduce this type of injury is not necessarily an indication for surgery, as the majority of cases of unilateral fracture-dislocations heal well in the unreduced position. The spinal cord is not really in jeopardy, this fact being well demonstrated in computerized tomography studies.

(iv) Gross Vertebral Fractures and Fracture-Dislocations of the Beatson Type II: Constituting 25% of Injuries With Tetraplegia (Fig 10.1c, Chapter 10)

These fractures and fracture-dislocations always need reduction. Those associated with gross fractures of the apophyseal joints can usually be reduced without anaesthesia after skeletal traction has been applied. With careful increase in traction, first in flexion to unlock the facets, and then with extension, the fracture-dislocation will usually reduce within 24 hours. Dislocations not associated with gross fractures are rare. (Fractures were found in every case of 65 specimens examined at post mortem.) These gross dislocations and fracture-dislocations are best reduced by the manipulative measures which have already been discussed. Maintenance of the reduction can be achieved by the application of adequate skeletal traction using 4–6 kgs for a period of six to eight weeks. In the post-operative management, one should stress again the importance of adequate attention to the maintenance of cervical lordosis by posturing the head and neck. In these cases surgical treatment is rarely indicated in the early stages. Bony union will occur in 85% of cases; 10% will stabilize with fibrous unions and only 5–6% will be found unstable in the long term, requiring stabilization.

b) *Lumbo-Dorsal Injuries* (Fig. 11.5)

In lumbo-dorsal injuries 95–98% of cases will result from flexion-rotation strains, while compression forces will account for 2–3% of the injuries and extension forces for only 1%. In dealing with these cases, it is important that the surgeon should understand the mechanism of injury in each case. Injuries resulting from hyperextension forces can be nursed in flexion and therefore need to be nursed carefully in bed without a pillow under the lumbar spine. Stability results from adequate healing of the perivertebral soft tissues and ligaments. Crushing injuries of the vertebral column in this region may also be treated conservatively providing they are not associated with flexion-rotation injuries. Even in paraplegics, providing the sensory level is in the groin at L1 or L2, plaster fixation may be satisfactory with either of these types of injuries.

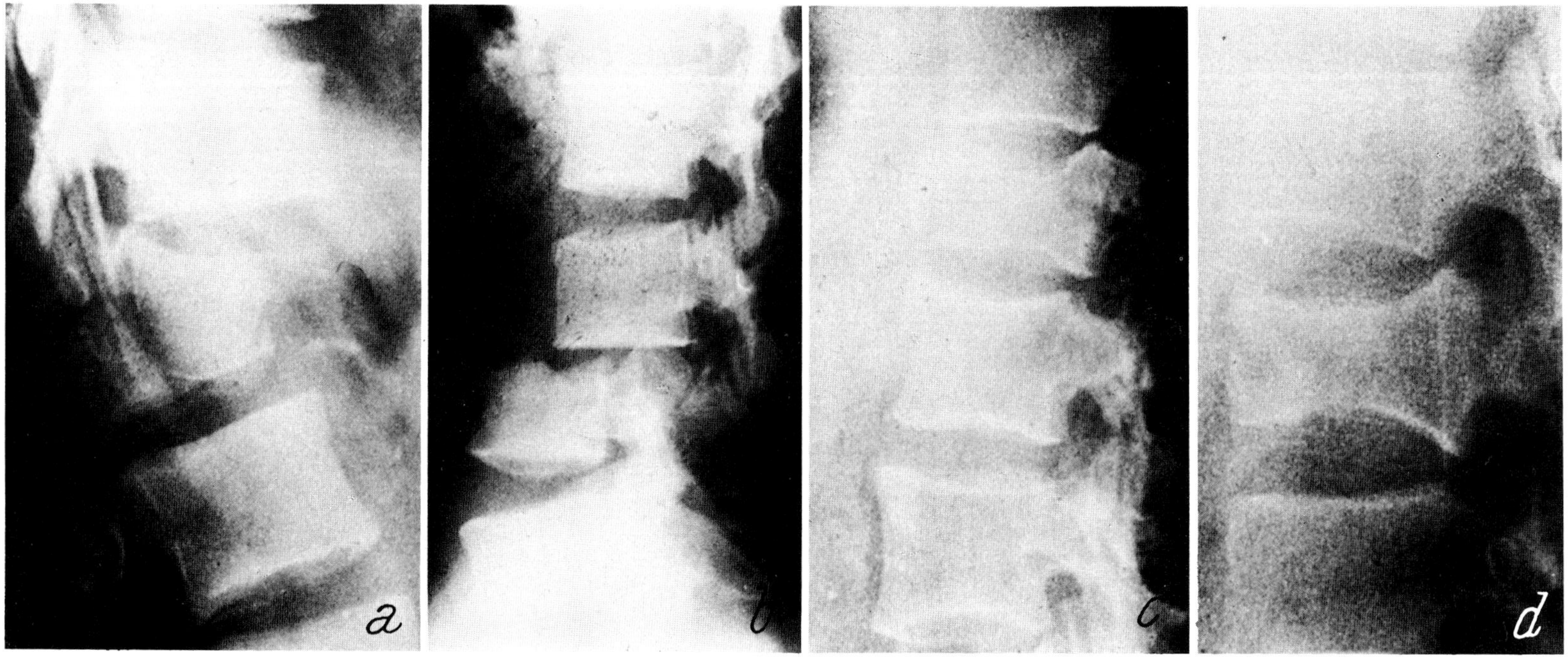

Figure 11.5. The lumbo-dorsal fractures and fracture dislocations. **a** Flexion-rotation. **b** Hyperextension. **c** and **d** Axial compression

The most difficult problems in management are seen in cases with flexion-rotation injury. Even in these cases, the majority can be managed adequately by postural methods. Postural reduction should always be attempted as soon as possible after the patient's admission to hospital. It is important to remember that 95% of these fractures and fracture-dislocations will heal by conservative measures, resulting in fusion of only two vertebral segments. By contrast, if surgical procedures are undertaken, at least four or five vertebral segments may fuse. This will inevitably give rise to a stiffer spine, the patient being left without full mobility. One of the reasons put forward by proponents of internal fixation is that earlier mobility of the patient is allowed. This, in fact, is not regularly so in units which institute early mobility in bed and still provide postural reduction. Most patients using a postural reduction technique can be fitted with an exoskeleton, usually of a polythene type, at the end of five to six weeks, with mobilization out of bed at that stage. Prior to that particular stage, most patients will be mobile in bed, undertaking many activities in physical therapy, exercising their erector spinae and abdominal muscles in the lumbo-dorsal area. If surgery is undertaken, it should be remembered that some surgical procedures inevitably denervate areas of the erector spinae muscles, unnecessarily causing further paralysis for the patient. After most lumbo-dorsal fractures and fracture-dislocations with paraplegia, the nerve supply to the erector spinae muscles remains intact at least two to three segments below the level of the injury (Bedbrook and Donovan, 1979). Thus the erector spinae and the latissimus dorsi muscles particularly may be damaged further during surgical exploration. There will, however, be a small group of patients where early–as opposed to emergency–surgery must be considered. The indications for surgical treatment are as follows:

a) For complete disruptive lesions of the vertebral column with scoliosis.
b) For those patients in whom adequate reduction of the fracture-dislocation cannot be achieved by conservative means.
c) For those who have locked facets. Even in this group the present author finds no absolute indication for open reduction.

Definite contra-indications to surgery exist if there are any infected areas on the skin, if early urinary tract infection occurs and if there are other injuries which need preferential surgical treatment. The surgeon should recognize the fact that an early surgical procedure on the spine could prove too much for his or her patient. When surgical procedures on the spine are undertaken, they should be performed by those who are best qualified and who regularly use surgical techniques for other indications in the spine, e.g. for scoliosis corrections. Internal fixation using plates has been generally abandoned. Currently, the Harrington distraction rod system is the one most widely used.

The application of plates through screws fixed to the pedicles has been described by Roy-Camille, though the method carries potential hazards if the screws are wrongly positioned in the pedicles.

11.8. Surgical Technique

Patients are placed in the prone position, avoiding too much flexion. The fracture-dislocation is exposed through a mid-line incision and the paravertebral muscles separated. Frequently the muscles will have been torn from their mid-line attachments so that further surgical separation should be limited. Reduction of the fracture may not occur until facetectomy has been performed in some cases. The question of fixation must be decided in each case, depending on the local findings after reduction.

Harrington distraction rods are placed two segments above and two segments below the lesion on both sides. Occasionally the distraction rods will produce distraction of the fracture-dislocation; however, as the anterior longitudinal ligament is intact in most cases, this is not a common problem. Over-distraction should be avoided as it may lead to non-union at the fracture site.

Some surgeons advise bone grafting, while others claim it is unnecessary. The present author feels that grafting of the area of the fracture-dislocation is essential. The laminae should be preserved, but if there is a fractured fragment found indenting the posterior surface of the dura it should be carefully removed.

11.9. Indications and Contra-Indications for Specific Surgical Procedures

a) Anterior Decompression of Acute Fractures of the Cervical Spine

There is really no absolute indication for anterior decompression of acute cervical fractures. Comparisons between groups of patients treated by surgery or by conservative methods indicate that the results achieved by conservative methods are as good and probably better than those achieved surgically.

There are a number of contra-indications to surgery:

a) Incomplete tetraplegia–operative intervention can aggravate the tetraplegia, rendering it complete (Morgan and Wharton, 1971, Sussman, 1978). A malpractice suit in this context was settled recently in the United States of America for 3.5 million dollars.
b) Urinary infection.
c) Any other associated major injury.

b) Open Reduction and Internal Fixation of Lumbo-Dorsal Fractures

Indications for surgery are:

a) Gross disruptive fracture-dislocations that cannot be maintained and reduced by postural methods.
b) Locked facets, rarely.

Contra-indications to the use of Harrington internal fixation procedure are:

a) Infection arising either from bed sores or from the urinary tract.
b) A patient with incomplete paralysis showing signs of improvement clinically, with adequate reduction achieved conservatively.
c) Associated minor injuries.

c) *Antero-Lateral Decompression*

This operation may have some place in the management of secondary canal stenosis occurring late after injury.

d) *Spinal Fusion*

Spontaneous union of spinal fractures can be expected in approximately 95% of lumbo-dorsal fractures and in 85% of cervico-dorsal injuries. Accordingly, there should be no indication for spinal fusion in the early stages of management.

In later stages, fusion is indicated for non-union or for pain proven to arise from a disc space higher or lower than the fracture or fracture-dislocation. The operation finds a valuable place in the management of progressive kyphoses following vertebral injuries in children or adolescents.

In a group of 750 cases with spinal injuries, 50 patients required spinal fusion for the following reasons:

a) Following failure of conservative management where traction had been removed too early.

b) Following extensive spinal injuries in young children between the ages of 12 and 13 years where vertebral epiphyseal growth had been disturbed.

c) For non-union following unsatisfactory reduction of fracture-dislocations.

d) For progressive spinal deformity following fractures of multiple vertebral bodies.

11.10. Management of Problem Cases

Cases presenting to the orthopaedic surgeon with a fracture or fracture-dislocation unreduced at the end of seven to ten days should be managed initially in exactly the same way as acute cases. In many of these, reduction can be achieved using postural methods or manipulative techniques combined with slow traction.

Most surgeons avoid the use of acute manipulative reduction of fractures or fracture-dislocations presenting 48 hours after injury.

Patients who present even later, up to two to three weeks from the initial injury, can usually be managed with adequate traction, and if reduction is not achieved in cases with fractures of the fracture-dislocation type, then a decision about the use of surgical methods must be taken. At this later stage the operative procedure does not carry the risks which may lead to disastrous results with its use in the acute phase of management, because the blood supply of the cord, by then, has been re-established. Facetectomy can be undertaken without fear of further damaging the blood supply of the spinal cord. However, facetectomy does not always result in reduction of the fracture and fracture-dislocation and then fusion in situ may be required.

In cases in which reduction has not been achieved at the three to six weeks period it is wiser to allow fusion to occur spontaneously in situ. Should symptoms arise from spinal stenosis in such cases, a supplementary decompression of the area can be undertaken, either through the spinal canal or by an anterior approach to the vertebral column. If there is obvious evidence of instability four to five weeks after injury then spinal fusion is required.

11.11. Summary

The risks following the use of surgical procedures early after spinal injury are summarized below:

1. The anterior longitudinal ligament–which is usually intact after fracture-dislocation of the spine–may be damaged, rendering the spinal segment unstable.
2. After anterior interbody fusion, the graft may slip forwards into the retro-oesophageal position because of poor fixation. [This problem may not occur if a dowel graft is inserted transversely across the disc space (Cornish, 1968).]
3. Posterior operations in the early stages can interfere with the blood supply of an already damaged spinal cord, as reported by Schneider (1951), Cheshire (1964) and Morgan (1971).
4. Operative interference in the early and even in the late stages following injury may be difficult, with the risk of further damage to an already damaged cord.
5. Early operative procedures aimed at producing spinal fusion are contra-indicated when it is known that spontaneous fusion can be expected in a high percentage of cases.
6. *Operative procedures in the early stages following spinal cord injury have a definite mortality rate.*

Surgical procedures should be restricted to the following general indications:

a) For gross dislocation with or without fractures, where conservative methods have failed.
b) For spinal injuries resulting from gunshot wounds in the acute stage.
c) For non-union of fractures.
d) For the stabilization of fracture-dislocations with proven instability six to eight weeks after the initial injury.
e) Following the failure of conservative management in any case.
f) *For neurological deterioration after incomplete paraplegia.* Regrettably even in this situation good results cannot always be guaranteed.

11.12. Conclusions

The surgeon's attitudes to his or her role in the overall management of spinal trauma should be strongly influenced by knowledge of the surgical pathology of spinal injuries.

There is no indication to operate on a patient with spinal injuries merely because the surgeon is "concerned" or because the patient deserves to be given the "benefit of the doubt".

After careful consideration of the mechanisms of injury and following evaluation of the resultant spinal lesions, doubts about indications for surgical treatment should not exist.

In most patients in whom paralysis does not complicate the spinal injury, the use of postural methods of reduction or reduction with manipulative procedures followed by physical rehabilitation in the manner described by Watson-Jones in 1952 will be found effective. In paraplegic patients the clinical methods discussed must be followed carefully, and only a few patients will need to be submitted to surgical treatment of the spine (less than 5%). The indications for surgery need to be precisely defined.

References

Adkins, E. W. O.: Lumbo-sacral arthrodesis after laminectomy. J. Bone Joint Surg. *37B,* 208–223 (1955).

Albee, F. H.: Transplantation of a portion of tibia into the spine for Pott's disease. JAMA *57,* 885–886 (1911).

American Academy of Orthopaedic Surgeons Symposium on the Spine, p. 289. St. Louis: C. V. Mosby. 1969.

Armstrong, J. R.: Lumbar disc lesions. Edinburgh: E. & S. Livingstone. 1965.

Aronson, H. A., Dunmore, R. H.: Herniated upper lumbar disc. J. Bone Joint Surg. *45A,* 311–317 (1963).

Arseni, C., Nash, F.: Protrusion of thoracic intervertebral discs. Acta Neurochir. (Wien) *11,* 3–33 (1963).

Bailey, R. W., Badgley, C. E.: Stabilization of the cervical spine by anterior fusion. J. Bone Joint Surg. *42A,* 565–594 (1960).

Bampfield, R. W.: An essay on curvature and diseases of the spine. Philadelphia: 1845.

Beadle, O. A.: The intervertebral disc (Medical Research Council, Special Report series 161), p. 79. London: His Majesty's Stationery Office. 1931.

Beals, R. K., Hickman, N. W.: Industrial injuries of the back and extremities. J. Bone Joint Surg. *54A,* 1593–1611 (1972).

Bedbrook, G. M.: Spinal injuries. In: Operative surgery, fundamental international techniques (Bentley, G., ed.) (Orthopaedics, Part I, 3rd ed.), pp. 222–241. London: Butterworths. 1979.

Bedbrook, G.: The care and management of spinal cord injuries. Berlin-Heidelberg-New York: Springer. 1981.

Bedbrook, G. M., Donovan, W. D.: Denervation of erector spinae of H rods. Personal communication, 1979.

Bell, C.: A system of operative surgery, pp. 132–139. London: Longmans. 1807.

Bell, C.: Observations on injuries of the spine and thigh bone, pp. 3–31. London: Thomas Tegg. 1824.

Bickerstaff, E. R.: Neurological examination in clinical practice, 3rd ed. Oxford-London-Edinburgh-Melbourne: Blackwell. 1973.

Blikra, G.: Intradural herniated lumbar disc. J. Neurosurg. *31,* 676–679 (1969).

Bobechko, W. P., Hirsch, C.: Autoimmune response to nucleus pulposus in the rabbit. J. Bone Joint Surg. *47B,* 574–580 (1965).

Epstein, B.: The spine. New York-London: Lea & Febiger. 1969.
Epstein, J. A., Epstein, B. S., Lavine, L.: Nerve root compression associated with narrowing of the lumbar spinal canal. J. Neurol. Neurosurg. Psychiat. *25,* 165–176 (1962).

Farfan, H. F., Cossette, J. W., Robertson, G. H., Wells, R. V., Krause, H.: The effects of torsion on the lumbar intervertebral joints: the role of torsion in the production of disc degeneration. J. Bone Joint Surg. *52A,* 468–497 (1970).
Farfan, H. F., Huberdeau, R. M., Dubow, H. I.: Lumbar intervertebral disc degeneration. J. Bone Joint Surg. *54A,* 492–510 (1972).
Ferguson, A. B.: Roentgendiagnostic. Extremities and spine. New York: Hoeber. 1949.
Fineschi, C.: Anatomical anomalies of the lumbar spinal roots. Arch. Putti *2,* 222–236 (1952).
Finneson, B. E.: Low back pain. Philadelphia: J. B. Lippincott. 1973.
Flynn, J. C., Hoque, M. A.: Anterior fusion of the lumbar spine. J. Bone Joint Surg. *61A,* 1143–1150 (1979).
Frankel, H. L., Hancock, D. O., Hyslop, G., Michaelis, L. S., Ungar, G. H., Vernon, J. D. S., Walsh, J. J.: The value of postural reduction in the initial management of closed injuries of the spine with paraplegia and tetraplegia, Part I. Paraplegia *7,* 179–192 (1969).
Fraser, R. D.: A wide muscle-splitting approach to the lumbosacral spine. J. Bone Joint Surg. *64B,* 44–46 (1982).
Freebody, D., Bendall, R., Taylor, R. D.: Anterior transperitoneal lumbar fusion. J. Bone Joint Surg. *53B,* 617–627 (1971).
Frykholm, R.: Deformities of dural pouches and strictures of dural sheaths in the cervical region producing nerve root compression. A contribution to the aetiology and operative treatment of brachial neuralgia. J. Neurosurg. *4,* 403–413 (1947).
Fujimaki, A., Crock, H. V., Bedbrook, G. M.: The results of 150 anterior lumbar interbody fusion operations performed by two surgeons in Australia. Clin. Orthop. and Related Res. *165,* 164–167 (1982).

Gill, G. G., Manning, J. C., White, H. L.: Surgical treatment of spondylolisthesis without spine fusion. J. Bone Joint Surg. *37A,* 493–518 (1955).
Gimeno, A.: Arachnoid, neurenteric and other cysts. In: Handbook of clinical neurology: congenital malformations of the spine and spinal cord (Vinken, P. J., Bruyn, G. W., eds.), pp. 393–448. Amsterdam: North-Holland. 1978.
Gonsette, R.: An experimental and clinical assessment of water-soluble contrast medium in neuro-radiology. A new Medium-Dimer–X. Clin. Radiol. *22,* 44–56 (1971).
Gorter, O.: Chirurgia repurgata. Ludgum Batavorum *8,* 377 (1742).
Graham, C. E.: Backache and sciatica. Med. J. Aust. *1,* 5–8 (1974).
Grollmus, J., Perkins, R. K., Russel, W.: Erythrocyte sedimentation rate as a possible indicator of early disc space infection. Neurochirurgia (Stuttg.) *17,* 30–35 (1974).
Gross, D.: Treatment of prolapsed lumbar intervertebral disk. Folia Rheumatologica (Basel) *2,* 1–16 (1965).
Gurdjian, E. S., Webster, J. E., Ostrowski, A. Z., Hardy, W. G., Lindner, D. W., Thomas, L. M.: Herniated lumbar intervertebral discs–an analysis of 1,176 operated cases. J. Trauma *1,* 158–176 (1961).
Guttmann, L.: The conservative management of closed injuries of the vertebral column resulting in damage to the spinal cord in spinal roots. In: Handbook of clinical neurology (Vinken, P. J., Bruyn, G. W., eds.), pp. 285–306. Amsterdam: North-Holland. 1976.
Guttmann, L.: The treatment and rehabilitation of patients with injuries of the spinal cord. In: Medical history of the second world war: surgery (Cope, Sir Zachary, ed.), p. 44. London: His Majesty's Stationery Office. 1953.

Hakelius, A., Nilsonne, U., Pernow, B., Zetterquist, S.: The cold sciatic leg. Acta Orthop. Scand. *40,* 614–623 (1969).

Happey, F., Johnson, A. G., Naylor, A., Turner, R. L.: Preliminary observations concerning the fine structure of the intervertebral disc. J. Bone Joint Surg. *46B,* 563–567 (1964).

Harrington, P. R.: Treatment of scoliosis: correction and internal fixation by spine instrumentation. J. Bone Joint Surg. *44A,* 591–610 (1962).

Hartman, J. T. (Dean, Faculty of Medicine, Texas Tech. University, Lubbock, Texas): Personal Communication, unpublished.

Hasue, M., Ito, R.: Sacral nerve root cyst as a cause of low back pain and sciatica. J. Jap. Orthop. Ass. *46,* 65–72 (1972).

Heister, L.: Institutiones Chirurgiae, Part I, Book II, Chapter IX, p. 200. Amelstod: 1750.

Helfet, A. J., Gruebel Lee, D. M.: Disorders of the lumbar spine. Philadelphia: J. B. Lippincott. 1978.

Hirsch, C., Bobechko, W. P.: Auto-immune response to nucleus pulposus in the rabbit. J. Bone Joint Surg. *47B,* 574–580 (1965).

Hirsch, C., Zotterman, Y.: Cervical pain. Proc. Intern. Symp. Wenner-Gren Center, Stockholm, 1971. Oxford: Pergamon Press. 1972.

Hodgson, A. R., Stock, F. E.: Anterior spinal fusion: A preliminary communication of the radical treatment of Pott's disease and Pott's paraplegia. Brit. J. Surg. *44,* 266–275 (1956).

Holdsworth, F. W.: Fractures, dislocation and fracture dislocations of the spine. J. Bone Joint Surg. *45B,* 6–20 (1963).

Holdsworth, F. W., Hardy, A. G.: Early treatment of paraplegia from fractures of the thoraco-lumbar spine. J. Bone Joint Surg. *35B,* 540–550 (1953).

Hooper, J.: Low back pain and manipulation. Med. J. Aust. *1,* 549–551 (1973).

Houdart, R., Djindjian, R., Hurth, M.: Chirurgie des angiomes de la moelle. Neuro-Chirurgie *15,* Suppl. 1 (1969).

Howarth, B. M., Petrie, J. G.: Injuries of the spine. Baltimore: Williams & Wilkins. 1964.

Hudgins, W. R.: The predictive value of myelography in the diagnosis of ruptured lumbar discs. J. Neurosurg. *32,* 152–162 (1970).

Hult, L.: The Munk Fors investigation. Acta Orthop. Scand. Suppl. *16,* 1–76 (1954).

Inman, V. T., Saunders, J. B. DeCM: Anatomico-physiological aspects of injuries to the intervertebral disc. J. Bone Joint Surg. *29,* 461–475 (1947).

Jackson, R. K.: The long-term effects of wide laminectomy for lumbar disc excision. J. Bone Joint Surg. *53B,* 609–616 (1971).

Jayson, M.: The lumbar spine and back pain. London: Sector Publishing. 1976.

Jenkins, D. H. R., Weeks, R. D., Yau, A. C. M. C., Du, R. R.: Manual of spinal surgery. London: Butterworths. 1981.

Johnson, R. H.: Cerebro-spinal fluid. In: Scientific foundations of neurology, pp. 281–288. London: W. Heinemann. 1972.

Jones, R. A. C., Thomson, J. L. G.: The narrow lumbar canal. J. Bone Joint Surg. *50B,* 595–605 (1968).

Kakulas, B. A., Bedbrook, G. M.: Pathology of injuries of the vertrebral column, with emphasis on the macroscopical aspects. In: Handbook of clinical neurology (Vinken, P. J., Bruyn, G. W., eds.), Vol. 25, pp. 27–42. Amsterdam: North-Holland. 1976.

Kellgren, J. H.: Sciatica. Lancet *1,* 561–564 (1941).

Key, A.: Cervical spine dislocations with unilateral facet interlocking. In: Proc. Ann. Sci. Meeting I.M.S.P., Stoke Mandeville Hospital, Aylesbury, England, July 1975. Paraplegia *13,* 208–215 (1976).

Keyes, D. C., Compere, E. L.: The normal and pathological physiology of the nucleus pulposus of the intervertebral disc: an anatomical, clinical and experimental study. J. Bone Joint Surg. *14,* 897–938 (1932).
Kirkaldy-Willis, W., Hill, R. J.: A more precise diagnosis for low back pain. Spine *4,* 102–109 (1979).
Kirkaldy-Willis, W. H., Paine, K. W. E., Cauchoix, J., McIvor, G.: Lumbar spinal stenosis. Clin. Orthop. and Related Res. *99,* 30–50 (1974).
Knutsson, F.: The vacuum phenomenon in intervertebral discs. Acta Radiol. (Stockh.) *23,* 173–179 (1942).
Köhler, A., Zimmer, E. A.: Borderlands of the normal and early pathologic in skeletal roentgenology. New York-London: Grune & Stratton. 1968.
Kramer, J.: Intervertebral disk diseases: causes, diagnosis, treatment and prophylaxis. Stuttgart: G. Thieme. 1981.
Kudelka, P.: Laminectomy in lumbar disc syndrome. Med. J. Aust. *1,* 1120–1122 (1968).
Kulak, R. F., Schultz, A. B., Belytschko, T., Galante, J.: Biomechanical characteristics of vertebral motion segments and intervertebral disc. Orthop. Clin. North Am. *6,* 121–133 (1975).

Lancourt, J. E., Glenn, W. V., jr., Wiltse, L. L.: Multiplanar computerized tomography in the normal spine and in the diagnosis of spinal stenosis: a gross anatomic-computerized tomographic correlation. Spine *4,* 379–390 (1979).
Le Vay, D.: A survey of surgical management of lumbar disc prolapse in the United Kingdom and Eire. Lancet *1,* 1211–1213 (1967).
Lindblom, K.: Diagnostic puncture of intervertebral discs in sciatica. Acta Orthop. Scand. *17,* 231–239 (1948).
Lowther, D. A. (Monash University, Melbourne): Personal communication, 1972.
Lowther, D. A., Baxter, E.: Isolation of a chondroitin sulphate protein complex from bovine intervertebral discs. Nature (Lond.) *211,* 595–597 (1966).

MacCartee, C. C., Griffin, P. P., Byrd, B. E.: Ruptured calcified thoracic disc in a child. J. Bone Joint Surg. *54A,* 1272–1274 (1972).
McCulloch, J. A.: Chemonucleolysis. J. Bone Joint Surg. *59B,* 45–52 (1977).
McKenzie, J. A., Williams, J. F.: The dynamic behaviour of the head and cervical spine during "whiplash". J. Biomech. *4,* 477–490 (1971).
Macnab, I.: Acceleration-extension injuries of the cervical spine. In: American Academy of Orthopaedic Surgeons Symposium on the Spine, p. 16. St. Louis: C. V. Mosby. 1969.
Macnab, I.: Chemonucleolysis. Clin. Neurosurg. *20,* 183–192 (1973).
Macnab, I.: Backache. Baltimore: Williams & Wilkins. 1977.
Macnab, I., McCulloch, J. A., Weiner, D. S., Hugo, E. P., Galway, R. D., Dall, D.: Chemonucleolysis. Can. J. Surg. *14,* 280–289 (1971).
Malgaigne, J.: Traité des fractures et des luxations, Vol. I, pp. 410–426; Vol. II, pp. 318–391. Paris: 1847.
Maroudras, A., Nachemson, A., Stockwell, R. A.: Factors involved in the nutrition of the adult human intervertebral disc. J. Bone Joint Surg. *55A,* 658–659 (1973).
Mathews, J. A.: Epidurography. In: Modern trends in orthopaedics, pp. 148–166. London: Butterworths. 1972.
Matsubara, T., Karube, F., Terashima, I.: Atypical course observed following discography–cases of discitis and disappearing backache. J. Orthop. Surg. (Tokyo) *17,* 124–130 (1966).
Matsuda, H. M., Hirose, T., Shimazu, A., Yoshimura, M., Yamano, Y., Nakajima, K.: Electro-neurophysiological diagnosis by the approach from single nerve root unit in the degenerative spondylolisthesis. Osaka City Med. J. *23,* 155–165 (1977).

Matsuda, H., Hirose, T., Hashimoto, T., Shimazu, A., Yamano, Y., Nakajima, K.: Electrodiagnosis of compression of individual nerve roots of the cauda equina. Intern. Orthop. *2,* 121–131 (1979).

Med. J. Aust. (Editorial): Comments on: Backache and sciatica: a new breakthrough or a new controversy? Med. J. Aust. *1,* 3 (1974).

Mercer, R., Duthie, R. B.: Orthopaedic surgery, 6th ed. London: Edward Arnold. 1964.

Michaelis, L. S.: Prognosis of spinal cord injury. In: Handbook of clinical neurology (Vinken, P. J., Bruyn, G. W., eds.), Vol. 26, pp. 307–312. Amsterdam: North-Holland. 1976.

Miller, H.: Accident neurosis. Brit. Med. J. *1,* 919–925 (1961).

Mitchell, P. E. G., Hendry, N. G. C., Billewicz, W. Z.: The chemical background of intervertebral disc prolapse. J. Bone Joint Surg. *43B,* 141–151 (1961).

Mixter, W. J., Barr, J. S.: Rupture of the intervertebral disc with involvement of the spinal canal. New Engl. J. Med. *211,* 210–215 (1934).

Moll, J., Wright, T. V.: Measurement of spinal movement. In The lumbar spine and back pain (Jayson, M., ed.), pp. 93–112. London: Sector Publishing. 1976.

Morgan, F. P., King, T.: Primary vertebral instability as a cause of low back pain. J. Bone Joint Surg. *39B,* 6–22 (1957).

Morgan, T. H., Wharton, G. W., Austin, G. N.: The results of laminectomy in patients with incomplete spinal cord injuries. Paraplegia *9,* 14–23 (1971).

Munro, D.: Thoracic and lumbo-sacral cord injuries, study of 40 cases. JAMA *122,* 1055 (1943).

Murphey, F., Simmons, J. H. C., Brunson, B.: Surgical treatment of laterally ruptured cervical disc. Review of 648 cases, 1939–1972. J. Neurosurg. *38,* 679–683 (1973).

Murphey, M. G., Gado, M.: Anterior cervical discectomy without interbody bone graft. J. Neurosurg. *37,* 71–74 (1972).

Nachemson, A.: Mechanical stresses on lumbar disks. In: Current practice in orthopaedic surgery, pp. 208–224. St. Louis: C. V. Mosby. 1966.

Nachemson, A.: Intradiscal measurements of pH in patients with lumbar rhizopathies. Acta Orthop. Scand. *40,* 23–42 (1969).

Nachemson, A. L.: The lumbar spine an orthopaedic challenge. Spine *1,* 59–71 (1976).

Nachemson, A., Morris, J. M.: In vivo measurements of intradiscal pressure. J. Bone Joint Surg. *46A,* 1077–1092 (1964).

Nashbold, B. S., Hrubec, Z.: Lumbar disc disease: a twenty year follow-up study. St. Louis: C. V. Mosby. 1971.

Naylor, A.: The biophysiological and biochemical aspects of intervertebral disc hernation and degeneration. Ann. Roy. Coll. Surg. Engl. *31,* 91–114 (1962).

Naylor, A.: The late results of laminectomy for lumbar disc prolapse. J. Bone Joint Surg. *56B,* 17–29 (1974).

Naylor, A., Happey, F., Turner, R. L., Shentall, R. D., West, D. C., Richardson, C.: Enzymic and immunological activity in the intervertebral disc. Orthop. Clin. North Am. *6,* 51–58 (1976).

Newman, P. H.: Surgical treatment for derangement of the lumbar spine. J. Bone Joint Surg. *55B,* 7–19 (1973).

Nicoll, E. A.: Fractures of the dorsal lumbar spine. J. Bone Joint Surg. *31B,* 376–394 (1949).

Northfield, D. W. C., Osmond-Clarke, H.: Surgical treatment. In: Cervical spondylosis (Brain, R., Wilkinson, M., eds.), p. 215. London: W. Heinemann. 1967.

O'Connell, J. E. A.: Maternal obstetrical paralysis. Surg. Gynec. Obstet. *79,* 374–382 (1944).

O'Connell, J. E. A.: Protrusions of the lumbar intervertebral discs. A clinical review based on five hundred cases treated by excision of the protrusion. J. Bone Joint Surg. *33B,* 8–30 (1951).

Ohki, K.: Biochemical studies on lumbar disc lesions, changes in the protein-polysaccharide complex. J. Jap. Orthop. Ass. *48,* 567–579 (1974).

Paine, K. W. E., Haung, P. W. H.: Lumbar disc syndrome. J. Neurosurg. *37,* 75–82 (1972).
Palmer, J. J.: Spinal arachnoid cysts. J. Neurosurg. *41,* 728–735 (1974).
Pankovich, A. M., Korngold, L.: A comparison of the antigenic properties of the nucleus pulposus and cartilage protein polysaccharide complexes. J. Immunol. *99,* 431–437 (1967).
Parker, N.: Malingering. Med. J. Aust. *2,* 1308–1311 (1972).
Paulson, S., Sylven, B., Hirsch, C., Snellman, O.: Biophysical and physiological investigations on cartilage and other mesenchymal tissues. The diffusion rate of various substances in normal bovine nucleus pulposus. Biochim. Biophys. Acta (Amst.) *7,* 207–213 (1951).
Peacock, A.: Observations on the post-natal structure of the intervertebral disc in man. J. Anat. (Lond.) *86,* 162–179 (1952).
Peck, F. C., Jr.: A calcified thoracic intervertebral disk with herniation and spinal cord compression in a child. Case report. J. Neurosurg. *14,* 105–109 (1957).
Penning, L.: Functional pathology of the cervical spine. Amsterdam: Excerpta Medica. 1968.
Pennybacker, J. (Oxford University): Personal communication, 1959.
Perot, P. L., Munro, D. D.: Transthoracic removal of mid-line thoracic disc protrusions causing spinal cord compression. J. Neurosurg. *31,* 452–458 (1969).
Putti, V.: New conceptions in the pathogenesis of sciatic pain. Lancet *2,* 53–60 (1927).

Ransford, A. O., Harries, B. J.: Localized arachnoiditis complicating lumbar disc lesions. J. Bone Joint Surg. *54B,* 656–665 (1972).
Rathke, F. H., Schlegel, K. F.: Surgery of the spine. In: Atlas of orthopaedic operations (Hackenbroch, M., Witt, A. N., eds.), Vol. 1. Stuttgart: G. Thieme. 1979.
Reynolds, F. C., Katz, S. F.: Herniated lumbar intervertebral disc. In: American Academy of Orthopaedic Surgeons Symposium on the Spine, pp. 84–96. St. Louis: C. V. Mosby. 1969.
Riley, L. H., Robinson, R. A., Johnson, K. A., Walker, A. E.: The results of anterior interbody fusion of the cervical spine. Review of 93 consecutive cases. J. Neurosurg. *30,* 127–133 (1969).
Robinson, R. A., Smith, G. W.: Anterolateral cervical disc removal and interbody fusion for cervical disc syndrome. Bull. Johns Hopkins Hospital *96,* 223–224 (1955).
Robinson, R. A., Walker, A. E., Ferlic, D. C., Wiecking, D. K.: The results of anterior interbody fusion of the cervical spine. J. Bone Joint Surg. *44A,* 1569–1587 (1962).
Rothman, R. H., Simeone, F. A.: The spine, Vol. II. Philadelphia: W. B. Saunders. 1975.
Roy-Camille, R., Saillant, G., Berteaux, D.: Osteosynthesis of thoraco-lumbar spine fractures with metal plates screwed through vertebral pedictes. Reconstruct. Surg. and Traumatol. *15,* 2–6 (1976).

Sacks, S.: Anterior interbody fusion of the lumbar spine. J. Bone Joint Surg. *47B,* 211–233 (1965).
Sarpyener, M. A.: Congenital stricture of the spinal canal. J. Bone Joint Surg. *27,* 70–79 (1945).
Schatzker, J., Pennal, G. F.: Spinal stenosis, a cause of cauda equina compression. J. Bone Joint Surg. *50B,* 606–618 (1968).
Scher, A. T.: The high rugby tackle–an avoidable cause of cervical spinal injury. S. African Med. J. *53,* 1015–1018 (1978).
Schmorl, G.: Die pathologische Anatomie der Wirbelsäule. Verh. Dtsch. Orthop. Ges. *21,* 3–41 (1926).
Schmorl, G., Junghanns, H.: The human spine in health and disease (translated by Wilk, S. P., Groin, L. S.), p. 38. New York: Grune & Stratton. 1959.

Schneider, R. C.: A syndrome in acute cervical spine injuries for which early operation is indicated. J. Neurosurg. *1,* 360–367 (1951).

Simeone, F. A.: The modern treatment of thoracic disc disease. Orthop. Clin. North Am. *2,* 453–462 (1971).

Simpson, J. A.: Electromyography. In: Scientific Foundations of Neurology, pp. 341–356. London: W. Heinemann. 1972.

Smith, B. H.: Clinical spondylosis and its neurological complications. Springfield, Ill.: Ch. C Thomas. 1968.

Smith, J. W., Serafini-Fracassini, A.: The distribution of the protein polysaccharide complex in the nucleus pulposus matrix in young rabbits. J. Cell. Sci. *3,* 33–40 (1968).

Smith, L., Brown, J. E.: Treatment of lumbar intervertebral disc lesions by direct injection of chymopapain. J. Bone Joint Surg. *49B,* 502–519 (1967).

Sommering, J.: Bemerkungen über Verrenkung und Bruch des Rückgraths, pp. 3–40. Berlin: 1793.

Sonnabend, D. H., Taylor, T. K. F., Chapman, G. K.: Intervertebral disc calcification syndromes in children. J. Bone Joint Surg. *64B,* 25–31 (1982).

Spangfort, E. V.: The lumbar disc herniation. Acta Orthop. Scand., Suppl. *142,* 1–95 (1972).

Spurling, R. G., Grantham, E. G.: The end results of surgery for ruptured lumbar intervertebral discs. A follow-up study of 327 cases. J. Neurosurg. *6,* 57–64 (1949).

Stauffer, R. N., Coventry, M. B.: Anterior interbody lumbar spine fusion. Analysis of Mayo Clinic series. J. Bone Joint Surg. *54A,* 756–768 (1972).

Stauffer, R. N., Coventry, M. B.: Posterolateral lumbar spine fusion: analysis of Mayo Clinic series. J. Bone Joint Surg. *54A,* 1195–1204 (1972).

Stevenson, H. G.: Back injury and depression–a medico-legal problem. Med. J. Aust. *1,* 1300–1302 (1970).

Stewart, D. Y.: Current concepts of the "Barré syndrome" or the "posterior cervical sympathetic syndrome". Clin. Orthop. *24,* 40–48 (1962).

Sussman, B. J.: Fracture dislocation of the cervical spine. A critique of current management in the United States. Paraplegia *16,* 15–38 (1978).

Taylor, T. K. F., Akeson, W. H.: Intervertebral disc prolapse: a review of morphologic and biochemic knowledge concerning the nature of prolapse. Clin. Orthop. *76,* 54–79 (1971).

Torgerson, W. R., Dotter, W. E.: Comparative roentgenographic study of the asymptomatic and symptomatic lumbar spine. J. Bone Joint Surg. *58A,* 850–853 (1976).

Venner, R. M., Crock, H. V.: Clinical studies of isolated disc resorption in the lumbar spine. J. Bone Joint Surg. *63B,* 491–494 (1981).

Verbiest, H.: A radicular syndrome from developmental narrowing of the lumbar vertebral canal. J. Bone Joint Surg. *36B,* 230–237 (1954).

Verbiest, H.: Further experience of the pathological influence of a developmental narrowness of the bony lumbar vertebral canal. J. Bone Joint Surg. *37B,* 576–583 (1955).

Verbiest, H.: The lateral approach to the cervical spine. Clin. Neurosurg. *20,* 295–305 (1973).

Verbiest, H.: Neurogenic intermittent claudication. Amsterdam: North-Holland. 1976.

Vogelsang, H.: Intraosseous spinal venography. Amsterdam: Excerpta Medica. 1970.

von Torklus, D., Gehle, W.: The upper cervical spine. London: Butterworths. 1972.

Waddell, G., Kummel, E. G., Lotto, W. N., Graham, J. D., Hall, H., McCulloch, J. A.: Failed lumbar disc surgery and repeat surgery following industrial injuries. J. Bone Joint Surg. *61A,* 201–206 (1979).

Waddell, G., McCulloch, J. A., Kummel, E., Venner, R. M.: Nonorganic physical signs in low-back pain. Spine *5,* 117–125 (1980).

Watkins, M. B.: Postero-lateral bone grafting for fusion of the lumbar and lumbo-sacral spine. J. Bone Joint Surg. *41A,* 388–396 (1959).

Watson-Jones, R.: Fractures and joint injuries, 8th ed. Edinburgh: E. & S. Livingstone. 1952.

Weinstein, P. R., Ehni, G., Wilson, C. B.: Lumbar spondylosis: diagnosis, management and surgical treatment. Chicago: Year Book Medical Publishers. 1977.

White, A. A., Southwick, W. O., Deponte, R. J., Gainor, J. W., Hardy, R.: Relief of pain by anterior cervical spine fusion for spondylosis: Report of 65 patients. J. Bone Joint Surg. *55A,* 525–534 (1973).

Williams, P. C.: Reduced lumbosacral joint space: its relation to sciatic irritation. JAMA *99,* 1677–1682 (1932).

Wilson, P. H., MacCarty, W. C.: Discography: its role in the diagnosis of lumbar disc protrusion. J. Neurosurg. *31,* 520–523 (1969).

Wiltberger, B. R.: The dowel intervertebral body fusion as used in lumbar disc surgery. J. Bone Joint Surg. *39A,* 284–292 (1957).

Wiltberger, B. R., Abbott, K. H.: Dowel intervertebral body fusion as used in lumbar disc therapy. J. Int. Coll. Surg. *29,* 204–213 (1958).

Wiltse, L. L.: Spondylolisthesis in children. Clin. Orthop. *21,* 156–163 (1961).

Wiltse, L. L.: The etiology of spondylolisthesis. J. Bone Joint Surg. *44A,* 539–560 (1962).

Wiltse, L. L.: Common problems of the lumbar spine: spondylolisthesis and its treatment. JCE Orthop. *7,* 13–31 (1979).

Wiltse, L. L., Bateman, J. G., Hutchinson, R. H., Nelson, W. E.: The paraspinal sacrospinalis-splitting approach to the lumbar spine. J. Bone Joint Surg. *50A,* 919–926 (1968).

Wiltse, L. L., Hutchinson, R. H.: Surgical treatment of spondylolisthesis. Clin. Orthop. *35,* 116–135 (1964).

Wiltse, L. L., Rocchio, P. D.: Preoperative psychological tests as predictors of success of chemonucleolysis in the treatment of the low-back syndrome. J. Bone Joint Surg. *57A,* 478–483 (1975).

Wiltse, L. L., Widell, E. H., Jr., Jackson, D. W.: Fatigue fracture: the basic lesion in isthmic spondylolisthesis. J. Bone Joint Surg. *57A,* 17–22 (1975).

Wullenweber, R., Brock, M., Hamer, J., Klinger, M., Spoerri, O.: Lumbar disc. Adult hydrocephalus. (Advances in Neurosurgery, Vol. 4.) Berlin-Heidelberg-New York: Springer. 1977.

Yoshizawa, H., O'Brien, J. P., Smith, W. T., Trumper, M.: The neuropathology of intervertebral discs removed for low-back pain. J. Path. *132,* 95–104 (1980).

Subject Index